MEDICINE-BY-POST

THE CHANGING VOICE OF ILLNESS IN EIGHTEENTH-CENTURY BRITISH CONSULTATION LETTERS AND LITERATURE

THE WELLCOME SERIES
IN THE HISTORY OF MEDICINE

Forthcoming:

Healing Bodies, Saving Souls:
Medical Missions in Asia and Africa

Edited by David Hardiman

The Wellcome Series in the History of Medicine series editors are
V. Nutton, M. Neve and R. Cooter.
Please send all queries regarding the series to Michael Laycock,
The Wellcome Trust Centre for the History of Medicine at UCL,
210 Euston Road, London NW1 2BE, UK.

MEDICINE-BY-POST

THE CHANGING VOICE OF ILLNESS IN EIGHTEENTH-CENTURY BRITISH CONSULTATION LETTERS AND LITERATURE

Wayne Wild

Amsterdam – New York, NY 2006

First published in 2006
by Editions Rodopi B. V., Amsterdam – New York, NY 2006.

Editions Rodopi B.V. © 2006

Design and Typesetting by Michael Laycock,
The Wellcome Trust Centre for the History of Medicine at UCL.
Printed and bound in The Netherlands by Editions Rodopi B.V.,
Amsterdam – New York, NY 2006.

Index by Indexing Specialists (UK) Ltd.

British Library Cataloguing in Publication Data
A catalogue record for this book is available from the British Library

ISBN-10: 90-420-1868-2
ISBN-13: 978-90-420-1868-6
'Medicine-by-Post:
The Changing Voice of Illness in Eighteenth-Century
British Consultation Letters and Literature' –
Amsterdam – New York, NY:
Rodopi. – ill.
(Clio Medica 79 / ISSN 0045-7183;
The Wellcome Series in the History of Medicine)

Front cover:
Three affluent doctors congratulating themselves on their profession, coloured
mezzotint 1793 after R. Dighton. Courtesy: Wellcome Library, London.

© Editions Rodopi B. V., Amsterdam – New York, NY 2006
Printed in The Netherlands

All titles in the Clio Medica series (from 1999 onwards) are available to
download from the IngentaConnect website: http://www.ingentaconnect.com

Contents

List of Illustrations   3

Acknowledgements   5

Introduction   7

1   Patients and their Doctors in Eighteenth-Century Britain: Etiquette, Eclecticism, and Ethics   17

2   New Science Rhetoric in Medicine-by-Post: The Private Practice Correspondence of Dr James Jurin   61

3   George Cheyne: A Very Public Private Doctor   113

4   The Correspondence of Dr William Cullen: Scottish Enlightenment and New Directions in Medicine-by-Post   175

5   Literary Applications of Medicine-by-Post   243

Bibliography   263

Index   275

For my very special grown-up son and daughter,
Nicholas and Zoe,
with immense love and pride.

And thank you both, so much, for the years of support and
enthusiasm for my career change, and the work on this book.

List of Illustrations

1.1   Two doctors quarrelling whilst their patient deteriorates.
Coloured engraving by I. Cruikshank, 1794.   22

2.1   Portrait of James Jurin (1684–1750) by James Worsdale;
signature of James Jurin.   63

2.2   Example of corrections on the letter dated 28 July 1733,
from Mordecai Cary to James Jurin.   88

2.3   Letter dated 1 August 1733,
from Mordecai Cary to James Jurin.   90

3.1   George Cheyne (1671–1743). Line engraving by J. Tookey,
1787, after J. van Diest; signature of George Cheyne.   115

4.1   William Cullen (1710–90), portrait by William Cochrane;
signature of William Cullen.   177

Acknowledgements

Very special thanks are owed to several people who have guided and inspired the writing of this volume, who have made the experience of scholarship always challenging and fulfilling. Most particularly, I am grateful to Professor Susan Staves at Brandeis University. Her faith in her students and dedication to their work, along with her immense knowledge of the eighteenth-century world, made her the genius behind our endeavours. She, along with Professor Tom King, taught me how to allow my primary sources to speak in their own voices while helping me to find my own voice to narrate what I was discovering in those eighteenth-century texts. Both Susan and Tom were always ready to stimulate new research through questions that were critical to the final form of this work.

I am also greatly indebted to the late Roy Porter of the Wellcome Trust Centre for the History of Medicine at UCL. Every medical historian is familiar with his staggering output of articles and books on all facets of eighteenth-century medicine and the social world in which that medicine was practiced. However, for those of us who were fortunate enough to have spent a little time under Roy's tutelage, and to have experienced his great personal charm and energy, he proved that his generosity towards budding scholars was as immense as his own contributions to medical historiography.

Also, I owe much thanks to Iain Milne, Librarian for the Royal College of Physicians of Edinburgh. He not only helped to guide me through the huge collection of William Cullen's correspondence, but he also introduced me to the basics of Scottish medicine, including correct Scottish pronunciation! Both David Shuttleton, University of Wales, Aberystwth, and Andrea Rusnock, University of Rhode Island, have been especially generous in sharing letters with me that they had found and transcribed previous to my own research, letters from George Cheyne and James Jurin, respectively. Towards the final stages of this book, Guenter Risse and Christopher Lawrence have been most kind and encouraging in reading the manuscript and making suggestions.

The Burroughs–Wellcome Fund provided me with an especially generous grant that sponsored my research at the Royal College of Physicians of Edinburgh; and a Sachar Grant from Brandeis University facilitated my research at the then Wellcome Institute in London (now The Wellcome

Trust Centre for the History of Medicine at UCL). I am most grateful for both.

Finally, throughout the trying period of making revisions, it has been good to know that Michael Laycock was there at the Wellcome Trust Centre to help me keep the faith and get the text up to par for publication. It was forever reassuring to know that Michael was only an email away.

Introduction

Medicine-by-post, the subject of this book, refers to the eighteenth-century practice of medical consultation through an exchange of letters between patient and physician. It was an extension of the doctor's private practice, a service provided to middle and upper class patients. As such, the doctor–patient correspondence of Drs James Jurin, George Cheyne, and William Cullen, all highly esteemed physicians in their time, offers a unique window into the doctor–patient relationship in England and Scotland, and most particularly the rhetoric of that relationship.

In the case of James Jurin and William Cullen, the majority of the private-practice letters presented here have never been published previously, and certainly there has been no equivalent thorough rhetorical analysis attempting to discover what this correspondence tells us about the eighteenth-century doctor–patient relationship (including ethics), the patient experience of illness, and the interrelationship of medical theory and societal self-image as reflected in the microcosm of private practice medicine. The collection of William Cullen's correspondence is particularly unusual in that it contains both sides of the doctor–patient correspondence. George Cheyne's medical practice, including his medical consultation letters, have been of interest to many authors before this study, but his letters are revisited here in a new light, placing them in the context of an evolving eighteenth-century medical rhetoric, and focusing on his role in creating and popularising that rhetoric. In this context, Cheyne's correspondence provides an important, transitional, link between the iatromechanical rhetoric of Jurin and the Scottish Enlightenment rhetoric of Cullen. Still more, the correspondence of all three doctors, I believe, offers new insights into the metaphor of illness and the meaning of the doctor–patient encounter in the eighteenth-century novel.

In a recent edition of the Swiss journal *Gesnerus*, concerned with medical correspondence in early modern Europe, Piloud, Hächler, and Barras, help us appreciate the wide spectrum of doctor–patient correspondence in the eighteenth century.[1] The authors urge scholars to recognise that this rich and complex source of medical history, which has been used primarily as background material to support studies on medical theory and practice, is a genre that deserves full attention in its own right. Not only must scholars examine the professional correspondence network of the

7

physician–correspondent at any given moment in his career, but also scholars need to consider the often-conflicting perspective of healer and patient, and the great variety in personal character of physicians in terms of sympathy with their clients. Furthermore, writes Piloud, scholars should also recognise that medical theory had little to do, in practice, with the prescription patterns of doctors – a finding generally (if not entirely) corroborated in my own work in *Medicine-by-Post*. Basic and familiar remedies (recipes) were prescribed by established physicians of all theoretical schools and speculative bent and were remarkably similar throughout the seventeenth and eighteenth centuries. Nonetheless, the strongly theoretical 'dietetical' advice of Dr George Cheney certainly strained against the common treatments of his time, and against his patients' well-established food preferences, yet Cheyne achieved enormous popularity because of his theoretical ideas and the manner in which he presented his case to the public in his published medical treatises and, equally, in his private consultation letters (see Chapter 3).

This raises an important point not addressed by Piloud and his co-writers – that while medical theory may have had little influence on a patient's reason to consult a doctor, or the physician's standard prescription practices, yet the rhetoric of doctor and patient, as I show in this study, is affected dramatically by current medical theory and popular medical culture. *Medicine-by-Post* places a microscope on the particular rhetorical contents of the doctor–patient correspondence and the influences on that rhetoric. The influence of medical theory and popular medical culture on rhetoric is so pervasive that, as demonstrated in my final chapter, it spills over into the novel and other literary genres in distinctly recognisable patterns, colouring all aspects of the representation of illness and trauma in the literature of various decades of the eighteenth century.

In crucial ways, the experience of being sick is a social construct shaped by rhetoric. Popular conceptions about illness conjoin with prevailing medical discourse to generate a common language – a rhetoric that shapes the patient's experience as much as it describes it. Furthermore, the patient's endorsement of an established medical rhetoric is a precondition to acquiescence in therapeutic intervention and can profoundly influence the outcome of such intervention.

David Harley, in 'Rhetoric and the Social Construction of Sickness and Healing', has argued cogently for the key role of rhetoric in medical historiography. He emphasises that in science of any kind, '[w]henever a new style of enquiry is developed, a rhetorical campaign is required to legitimate it and differentiate it from earlier styles.'[2] But in medicine, 'the objects of enquiry' are 'alert to the rhetoric' and, indeed, 'most patients can answer back or walk away, so persuasion is crucial, not only as a market strategy but for the very process of healing.'[3] Harley concludes, 'it is the rhetorical engagement, based on trust in the system and the practitioners, that is at the heart of the healing process.'[4]

While in Harley's construction rhetoric retains its classical meaning as an art of persuasion, it is equally a process of negotiation. The propagation of a particular medical rhetoric – whether originating with an elite of 'established' physicians or popularised by a fringe of 'unorthodox' healers – is only half the story. Eighteenth-century patients of the upper classes and upper-middle class were well-informed clients who, as patients today, challenged their physicians with alternative and often antagonistic medical rhetorics; they probed the knowledge and competence of their doctors by engaging them in current medical jargon, thereby declaring their determination to play a role in therapeutic decisions. Any study of rhetoric in doctor–patient letters must be sensitive to the tensions and the vying for authority that describe this complex relationship.

A common doctor–patient rhetoric also establishes the parameters of acceptable behaviour in the medical dialogue, the operating ethics of private practice: what may be said, what should be said, the implied obligations of both parties to one another. Until the first attempts at codification of a modern medical ethics in the late-eighteenth and early-nineteenth century in the works of John Gregory and Thomas Percival, it was almost entirely the gentleman's code of behaviour and its associated rhetoric that defined the moral character of the physician. Carey McIntosh, in *The Evolution of English Prose, 1700–1800: Style, Politeness, and Print Culture*, underscores the important ties between, on the one hand, standards of rhetoric and politeness and, on the other hand, societal and individual moral virtues.[5] Indeed, a doctor's good character, as revealed in manner and language, was the cornerstone of the established physician's credibility and authority. A kind of private practice aesthetic served to support patient confidence in the healer even through the trials of therapeutic disappointment. Only in the latter part of the century, when the public grew more sceptical about the gentleman's code of conduct, did doctors begin to develop an independent and more formal code of medical ethics.

A proper medical rhetoric not only served to instil patient trust in the doctor but, equally, lent credibility to patients' version of their medical history. Doctor–patient negotiation depended on the trustworthiness of the patient's account of clinical detail, including response to medications; and in this regard, the patient's character mattered greatly. So in the context of this study of doctor–patient correspondence, I use the term rhetoric to signify what McIntosh defines as those language 'skills' that 'produce belief' for a particular culture within a particular historical period.[6] Eighteenth-century doctor–patient rhetoric must be viewed as intimately concerned with matters of trust and with the social and moral obligations that comprised the roots of an emerging modern medical ethics. Contained within the decorum of this epistolary relationship, absent the physical body, are the seeds of modern medical ethics.

Eighteenth-century medicine-by-post reveals several paradigm shifts in doctor–patient rhetorical modes; in particular, it reveals that eighteenth-century medicine was not dominated by a single rhetoric of sensibility. Nevertheless, it is true that the language of sensibility, most brilliantly ushered into medical private practice parlance by George Cheyne, signalled a major alteration in the way patients and doctors described disease and the experience of being sick. In the first decades of the eighteenth century, the rhetoric of doctor–patient correspondence had been hugely influenced by the impersonal and objective language adopted from the 'new science' rhetoric of Royal Society, which viewed the human body as a hydraulic mechanism, applying Newtonian principles to human physiology. But in the years approaching mid-century, 'new science' rhetoric was supplanted by a rhetoric of sensibility, based on a physiology that gave pre-eminence to the role of the nervous system in control of overall body functions. The rhetoric of sensibility encouraged patients' narration of their case histories as experiential, not merely as a compendium of exact physical symptoms. The vocabulary and expression of medicine-by-post letters was in keeping with the cultural vogue that held ultra-refined feeling to be the mark of civilised society, but it also complemented a growing eighteenth-century acceptance of the idea of personal identity as experiential, distinct from identity based primarily on one's societal role, social rank or religious affiliation.[7] This new paradigm encouraged the idea of feeling, and of self-expression, subjectivity, and a metaphorical view of illness by the patient – of illness as a sign of moral habits. But even the new medical rhetoric of sensibility, though extroverted and dramatic (and frequently characterised by irritability and melancholy) was itself as predictable, even formulaic, as 'new science' rhetoric had been. And it was not until the final decades of the eighteenth century that the rhetoric of sensibility was joined to utilitarian purpose, derived largely from the Scottish Enlightenment, to produce a more varied, less self-conscious and individual patient voice. Thus, in the rhetoric of doctor–patient correspondence there is an ongoing dialectic between medical speculation and cultural beliefs.

At a period in medical history in which therapeutic success was highly unpredictable, and in which patients were indifferent to the institutional affiliations of the physician, a doctor's professional stature with patients finally depended on his professional demeanour and skill in matching his rhetoric to prevailing social expectations – expectations derived, in turn, from prevailing medical theories. However, physician authority also was greatly served through attention to whatever was the prevailing medical rhetoric. In the early decades of the eighteenth century, medicine's emulation of the so-called 'plain' rhetorical style authorised by Bacon, Boyle, and the Royal Society, and the application of Newtonian principles to medical physiology, announced to the public that the medical profession was following in the footsteps of natural philosophy and was a branch of an unassailable empirical tradition. With the advent of a culture of sensibility, physician authority rested even more on the demonstration of exemplary moral character as manifested by a rhetoric which proclaimed the doctor to be a man able to combine a rigorous rational judgment with the utmost in compassion. In the eighteenth century, medical science and cultural refinements crisscross regularly.

The rhetorical paradigm shifts I describe in medicine-by-post letters are equally recognisable in the eighteenth-century novel (and other literary genres, even poetry) and contribute to our understanding of the role of illness as a measure of character in these texts (both physician and patient character), and of the precise metaphorical intention of the eighteenth-century authors in introducing medical matter into their work. Illness, doctors, doctor–patient encounters, and the patient's response to injury and illness reflect both a personal and a societal self-image.

It is the changing metaphorical meaning of medicine and medical encounters in eighteenth-century literature (as discovered in the rhetoric of medicine-by-post) that I believe has been under-appreciated in literary criticism of the period. What Defoe and Fielding conceived of as the sick body differed vastly from Richardson's conception of illness. And even though the literature of the latter half of the eighteenth century was dominated by the idea of sensibility, still the manifestations of disease experienced by persons of sensibility changed over time. Sensibility was represented quite differently in the works of Richardson, Sterne, or Smollett if one pays attention to medical details. In common for all these authors, however, the human body and the doctor–patient relationship presented ready microcosms of larger social ideals, and the tensions between the patient's personal needs and the doctor's professional will were played off regularly against the backdrop of those social ideals.

One area of literature that is, in particular, influenced by a more complete view of medical rhetoric in the eighteenth century is the way in which women's bodies were represented. Jessie Van Sant has described the creation of the 'idealised, *feminised* body' in the culture of sensibility, a composition of ultra-fine microscopic nerves joined to literary metaphor to produce a being that verged on the immaterial.[8] But the letters of women patients to their doctors, and the written responses of those doctors, reveal a view of women as having substantive bodies that experience physiological

11

distress in ways not so different from the experience of male patients. While the mid-to-late eighteenth-century woman was regarded by her society (in both medical and non-medical writings) as a being of heightened sensibility, and therefore more delicate and subject to certain ills such as hysteria, women patients wrote explicitly to their physicians about physical disorders (even of the most private kind) relatively unfettered by ideals of sensibility. Rather, the rhetoric of sensibility seems to have served an increasingly liberating role by encouraging the female patient to convey to the doctor the full drama of being sick. Persons of great sensibility were 'entitled' to intense feelings, that became inextricably linked to the narrative of being sick. Equally important, doctor consultation letters show that physicians did not dismiss the drama of illness but regarded the complaints of women patients seriously, without shying away from necessary regimens that were often inconvenient or even painful. The many letters from Dr George Cheyne to the Countess of Huntingdon, or between Dr William Cullen and his female patients, confirm that women were frank about their bodies and only conformed to the rhetoric of sensibility as it served their purpose: to express the urgency of their situation, or to describe specific medical conditions associated with nervous disorders that might be alleviated by specific remedies. The study of medicine-by-post, thus, enlarges our panorama in respect to the representation of women's physicality in the eighteenth century.

Indeed, the larger representation of both male and female bodies in eighteenth-century fiction is given an extra vividness through the experience of medicine-by-post letters. Samuel Richardson's understanding of 'nervous sensibility', formed by his friendship with Dr Cheyne, went hand in hand with a concept of illness as an opportunity for revealing individual moral integrity, for turning physical distress into metaphor, whereas men's and women's bodies in Defoe and Fielding – writers more influenced by the iatromechanical school of medicine – suffer very real bumps and bruises and physical decline as a function of daily life and serving, incidentally, as a commentary on societal ills. In the latter part of the century, influenced by the character of Scottish Enlightenment medicine, with its combination of refined sensibility and utilitarian philosophy, authors as different as Frances Burney and Tobias Smollett are similar in being able to conjoin the stark descriptions of pain and discomfort with the rhetoric of sensibility. As I describe in my conclusion, Frances Burney's epistolary account of her mastectomy is a particularly rich example of vivid physical detail enveloped within a novel-like portrait of the fine sensibility of her doctors, friends, and family. Smollett celebrates his own incessant physical discomfort as the natural consequence of irritable nerves, enwrapping his very real physical miseries in a blanket of irascibility woven out of the fabric of 'hypersensibility', like Matthew Bramble, the fictional protagonist in Smollett's *The Expedition of Homphrey Clinker* (1771).

Medicine-by-Post, therefore, is an interdisciplinary study intended both for readers whose main interest is the social history of medicine and readers of eighteenth-century literary criticism. The aim of this work is threefold: first, to contribute to a new and growing body of eighteenth-century medical historiography, that of medical correspondence, and to enlarge on that corner of medical history by the addition off an important corpus of doctor–patient letters and a close look at the rhetoric of that genre of letter writing;[9] second, through rhetorical analysis, to discover the strategies of self representation by eighteenth-century healers; and third, to reinterpret the meaning of illness and the doctor–patient encounter in eighteenth-century literature in the light of actual medical experience as reflected in medical correspondence of the period. All of these purposes serve to enlarge and clarify our sense of the interplay between culture, medicine, and literature.

The structure of this study remains largely chronological. I chose this organisation for two reasons: first, such an approach is appropriate for an argument that describes changes in the doctor–patient relationship over time; second, from the medical–historical point of view, it is most useful to have the letters of a specific doctor grouped together to form a picture of that individual physician and his practice over specific decades of the eighteenth century. Chapter 1 describes some of those common themes of medicine-by-post that remained constant over the century and against which the changes in rhetoric can be measured. For this purpose I take examples from letters and the epistolary fiction of various canonical authors, but especially the correspondence of Samuel Johnson. The foundations of eighteenth-century medical ethics are also described in the first chapter; understanding the pre-eminence of physician character in any discussion of Enlightenment medical ethics explains the important role of medicine-by-post as a means for doctors to reveal their moral integrity and, at the same time, to define their expectations of patient behaviour in the doctor–patient collaboration. The subsequent three chapters focus on the correspondence of three physician practices from different decades of the century, each representing the predominant medical theory and rhetorical strategies of their time. Chapter 2 considers the influence of New Science rhetoric in doctor–patient correspondence in the early part of the century as evidenced in the private practice correspondence of James Jurin (1684–1750), physician, and secretary to the Royal Society from 1721–27. Jurin was a Newtonian and follower of iatromechanical medical theory. Chapter 3 re-examines, but in a new light, the previously published correspondence of Dr George Cheyne (1671–1743) to the Countess of Huntingdon over the period 1730–39, and to Samuel Richardson from 1733–43. Cheyne brilliantly popularised the notion of a national illness – the 'English malady' – a 'fashionable' nervous disorder which primarily affected upper-class Britons whose nerves were debilitated, literally, by rich diet and lack of exercise and from living the sweet life made possible by national prosperity. In James Jurin's later private practice correspondence and Cheyne's developing consultation rhetoric in the 1730s, one discovers a transitional period in patient correspondence with their doctor, a move from mostly objective discussions of physical illness to more subjective accounts of the experience of being sick. But it was Cheyne, especially, who embodied and popularised the notion of sensibility and a rhetoric of subjectivity in illness. The last decades of the century are represented, in Chapter 4, by the extensive correspondence of the Scottish Enlightenment physician William Cullen. With the Scottish Enlightenment there arrives a new sophistication in the idea of sensibility as it affects health and society; sensibility becomes less a consequence of overindulgence and more the gift of a highly civilised society whose members relate as an organic whole through 'sympathy'. This more positive attitude towards sensibility encourages greater freedom in self-expression and opens the door to increasingly dramatic subjectivity in medicine-by-post. In turn, the rhetoric of sensibility, which begins as a social fad, a style to communicate about illness, yields to an increasingly individual patient voice towards the close of the Enlightenment. The concluding chapter applies insights from the study of medicine-by-post rhetoric to the interpretation of eighteenth-century literary texts that represent the experience of disease and the doctor–patient encounter.

As in any serious study in history or literature, the author must acknowledge the limitations of his work. It would have been desirable to have been able to dedicate one's time to a yet broader base of source materials to support my thesis about changing doctor–patient rhetoric and its relation to prevailing medical concepts over the course of the eighteenth century. However, in the case of rhetoric much support for my thesis can be found readily in the eighteenth-century novel and other genres of letter writing which are most delightfully accessible and abundant. My hope is that this study encourages further work along this line and, also, that it validates the use of an interdisciplinary approach in the interpretation of eighteenth-century medicine and literature.

Steinke and Stuber, in a recent overview of the state of studies on medical correspondence, encourage more work on the letters 'as subjects to be studied on their own', a better definition of the actual 'function of the letters themselves' within the context of a particular place and historical period.[10] *Medicine-by-Post*, though begun some years back, was conceived in this spirit. And in 'Why, What and How? Editing Early Modern Scientific Letters in the 21st Century', Steinke considers the difficult challenge faced by the scholar in choosing which medical correspondence collections, and which letters in these collections, are likely to yield the most meaningful picture of an historical moment.[11] Steinke urges scholars to define precisely their purpose and authorial interest when considering a particular set of letters, as it is all too easy to let the letters – due to factors such as availability – select themselves!

While *Medicine-by-Post* is not an edition of a doctor's correspondence *per se*, I have had to deal with complex matters of choice as to which letters to represent. In this study, I have made a particular effort to define my focus and the purpose in my selection of particular physicians and doctor–patient correspondence. The doctors discussed in *Medicine-by-Post* are each distinguished by their separate medical theories representative of their particular decades. All are examined in the context of rhetoric in the doctor–patient correspondence. In the case of Dr William Cullen, I was faced with a collection of three thousand letters, to and from Dr Cullen, over a period of thirty-five years when he practiced in Edinburgh. I therefore selected volumes of Cullen's consultation letters and boxes of patient letters from different periods of Cullen's years in Edinburgh that would be representative over time; I focused on interchanges between Cullen and particular patients which were sustained (that is, a number interchanges resolving a particular illness) and also on those letters and consultation notes from and concerning his female patients in order to get a picture of women's patient voices and the physician's response to female concerns. All these letters were then examined for their rhetorical qualities and what this rhetoric reflected about the physician, the patient, and the pervasive academic and popular medical culture of the period.

I believe I have been able to select the letters in this book with a defined purpose that any reader can follow easily and will find to be consistent in purpose. However, I can also claim that I came to these letters without expectations, and let the letters speak to me and define their own themes and rhetorical character. If the interpretation of these letters seems too bold, I encourage others to proceed from here. I am content to have produced a starting place in how one might engage this fascinating world of eighteenth-century doctor–patient correspondence and its rhetorical practices, the likely significance of those rhetorical practices to the medical culture of the eighteenth century in England and Scotland, and to the literature of that period.

Wayne Wild

Notes

1. S. Pilloud, S. Hächler, and V. Barras, 'Consulter par Lettre au XVIIIe Siècle [Medical Consultation by Letter in the 18th Century], *Gesnerus: Swiss Journal of the History of Medicine and Sciences*, 61 (2004), 232–53.
2. D. Harley, 'The Social Construction of Sickness and Healing', *Social History of Medicine*, xii, 3 (1999), 411.
3. *Ibid.*, 421–2.
4. *Ibid.*, 423.
5. C. McIntosh, *The Evolution of English Prose, 1700–1800: Style, Politeness, and Print Culture* (New York: Cambridge University Press, 1998), Chapter 3, especially 160–8.
6. *Ibid.*, 144.
7. See R. Porter, *The Creation of the Modern World: The Untold Story of the British Enlightenment* (New York: W.W. Norton & Co., 2000), Chapter 7, 156–83; see also C. Fox, *Locke and the Scriblerians: Identity and Consciousness in Early Eighteenth-Century Britain* (Los Angeles: University of California Press, 1988).
8. A.J. Van Sant, *Eighteenth-Century Sensibility and the Novel: The Senses in Social Context* (New York: Cambridge University Press, 1993), 105–7.
9. The letters in this study contain a significant number of letters from patients to their physicians, thereby enlarging on the patient experience of illness. It was Roy Porter in 1985 who first urged a new perspective in medical historiography that tempered what had been the medical profession's 'progressive' account of medical history by a consideration of the patient's experience; see 'The Patient's View,' *Theory and Society*, 14 (1985), 175–98. This was followed by D. Porter and R. Porter, *Patient's Progress: Doctors and Doctoring in Eighteenth-Century England* (Stanford: Stanford University Press, 1989).
10. H. Steinke and M. Stuber, 'Medical Correspondence in Early Modern Europe: An Introduction', in *op. cit.* (note 1), 139–60.
11. H. Steinke, 'Why, What and How? Editing Early Modern Scientific Letters in the 21st Century', *ibid.*, 282–95.

1

Patients and their Doctors in Eighteenth-Century Britain: Etiquette, Eclecticism, and Ethics

I'll do what Mead and Cheselden advise,
To keep these limbs, and to preserve these eyes
(Alexander Pope, 'Imitations of Horace')[1]

Who shall decide, when Doctors disagree... ?
(Alexander Pope, 'Epistle to Allen Lord Bathurst')

Medicine-by-post, consultation with a physician by letter, was common in eighteenth-century Britain.[2] It was practicable because the hands-on physical examination was not to play an essential role in diagnosis until after the turn of the century. A narrative of current illness complemented by a detailed description of one's constitutional make-up was all that was required for most therapeutic decision-making. Medical doctors confined their physical observations to visual impressions of the face and the integument as well as the appearance of the urine. The eighteenth-century physician – in contrast to the surgeon and barber-surgeon – was primarily concerned with the internal organs, but he lacked the necessary instruments, reliable examination techniques, and the sophisticated anatomical–pathological correlation needed for the examination of those internal organs and the interpretation of physical findings. Such advances awaited the nineteenth century. So the Enlightenment physician, in the Galenic tradition, depended almost entirely on the patient's medical history to interpret the physical disturbances of the inner body. It was furthermore a matter of professional pride – and social nicety – that the physician distinguished himself from surgeons by the fact that he used his head rather than his hands.[3] Patients from the upper middle-class to the aristocracy employed medicine-by-post when it was inconvenient to visit their doctor in town, when they had retired to the country for the season, or if travelling abroad. The usual charge for a consultation-by-post was a guinea, the same as a visit to the doctor's office. Thomas Percival, author of *Medical Ethics* (1803), advised that a two guinea charge was reasonable for the initial consultation-by-post in that it required 'much more trouble and attention' than the standard office visit. However, the fee was not rigid, and the doctor might adjust the bill according to 'the circumstances of the case, or of the patient'.[4]

17

Medicine-by-post was a rapid and effective mode of communication – often accomplished within twenty-four hours – as well as convenient for doctor and patient alike. On an occasion when Samuel Johnson wished another 'letting of blood' to relieve his embarrassed breathing, he writes to Dr Thomas Lawrence (in Latin) that, 'I can scarcely come to you, nor is there any reason for you to come to me. You may say in one word, yes or no, and leave the rest to Holder and me.'[5] By letter, patients were able to apprise their doctor of the effects of a previously prescribed regime or recipe – as prescriptions were called – or else obtain reassurance from an established town physician that the local country doctor was managing their case correctly. Also, medicine-by-post encouraged patients to obtain expert advice from abroad; letters flowed routinely between the British Isles and the Continent, and doctors and patients in the American colonies often sought the expertise of European sages.[6] Sometimes 'second opinion' consultations were requested by patients directly, without the encouragement of their own physician or surgeon who might take offence; more often, however, the physician or surgeon collaborated with the patient in obtaining outside consultation in difficult cases.

The practice of medicine-by-post is exemplified in the fictional correspondence of Matthew Bramble with his physician and friend, Dr Lewis, in Smollett's *The Expedition of Humphry Clinker* (1771). In this epistolary novel, the irascible Mr Bramble has set off on a journey through England and Scotland in the hopes of restoring his health by engaging in typical eighteenth-century therapeutic manoeuvres: a change of scene, exercise in the form of riding in a coach, sea bathing, or trying out the waters of various spas. Bramble reports regularly to Dr Lewis on his therapeutic progress, mostly his disappointments with all prescribed treatments, ever more convinced that patients are their own best physicians:

Doctor,

The pills are good for nothing – I might as well swallow snowballs to cool my reins – I have told you over and over, how hard I am to move; and at this time of day, I ought to know something of my own constitution. Why will you be so positive? Prithee send me another prescription.[7]

Bramble's tone with his friend and family doctor might seem inappropriately brusque, but the patients who engaged in medicine-by-post were neither intimidated nor awed by their physicians. Eighteenth-century physicians in Britain were most unlikely to come from the aristocratic class – certainly not first-born sons – and medicine as a profession had not achieved the prestige that it would in the nineteenth century. The eighteenth-century physician's practice and reputation depended entirely on the patronage and favour of his clients. Minus the 'magic bullets' of modern medicine, the physician who attended the upper ranks of society would be most assured of gaining favour and professional success by catering to those views and treatments fashionable within the society he served.[8] The first decades of the century saw the British public became well-versed in medical matters, as the physician and social critic Bernard Mandeville portrays in the character of Misomedon in *A Treatise of the Hypochondriack and Histerick Diseases*.[9] There was a flood of popular literature on health matters and, as Roy Porter has shown in the case of the *Gentleman's Magazine*, laypersons were regular and confident contributors to this flow of published medical articles and controversies.[10] Patients were not only adept at keeping up with both the current state of medical knowledge but also with the fashionable jargon of their physicians. Thus, patients and their doctors shared a common rhetoric that facilitated medicine-by-post and which kept the profession from exercising authority through the power of an exclusive language.[11]

In 'The Doctor–Patient Relationship Through the Ages,' physician and medical historian Mark Altschule observes that while the 'content' of medicine is regularly expanding through new knowledge and technology, the 'process' – 'the interaction between doctor and patient' – has remained little altered in two thousand years. Altschule notes 'the persistence of the patients' complaints about the process of medicine' and the consistency of their concerns about the doctor–patient relationship.[12] In the eighteenth century, the 'content' of medicine changed dramatically in terms of medical speculation as to the underlying causes of disease, especially as the hydraulic concept of the body, iatromechanism, was replaced by theories of 'nervous sensibility'. Nevertheless, such changes in 'content' did not alter classic methods of treatment – bleeding, vomits, purgatives, horse riding, and so on. Rather, the efficacy of such treatments was newly explained through a new medical vocabulary. This is reflected in medicine-by-post letters that show no significant change in the therapeutic regimes or recipes advised to the patients but which evidences dramatic shifts in a medical rhetoric conforming to whatever the current fashionable medical theory.

Nevertheless, as Altschule claims, certain patient attitudes towards the 'process' of medicine remain predictably constant. From the Restoration and throughout all decades of the eighteenth century, the public's suspicion of the medical 'trade' finds regular expression in private letters and the merciless satire of physicians in plays, novels, and iconographic representations. The profession is exposed as heartless, secretive, avaricious, and arrogant. To guard against such abuse, patients wrestled for self-determination by arming themselves through avid reading about medical controversies, obtaining second opinions, and seeking alternative medicine options which included folk cures and remedies founded on superstitious beliefs. Eclecticism in the medical marketplace, combined with patient familiarity with current medical speculation and jargon, was the best defence against the tyranny of the medical profession. As the Alexander Pope lines at the head of this chapter suggest, one might trust in whatever was advised by one's physician, but 'When doctors disagree', when faith in one's doctors is less than complete, then the anxious patient had best shop around for a medical man who, by word of mouth, has had better luck.

Medicine-by-post itself served nicely as a wall against physician assault. Tobias Smollett, Scots-trained surgeon turned novelist, recounts in *Travels Through France and Italy* (1766) that while residing in Montpellier he decided to consult the famous Dr Fizes by post because:

> The account I had of his private character and personal deportment, from some English people to whom he was well known, left me no desire to converse with him: but I resolved to consult with him on paper. The great lanthorn of medicine is become very rich and very insolent; and in proportion as his wealth increases, he is said to grow more rapacious. He piques himself upon being very slovenly, very blunt, and very unmannerly; rather than to any superior skill in medicine. I have known them succeed in our own country; and seen a doctor's parts estimated by his brutality and presumption.[13]

Smollett, in addition to using medicine-by-post to distance himself from what he presumes would be a distasteful and expensive personal encounter, writes his letter to Dr Fizes in Latin as a test the French physician's credentials. But Carol Houlihan Flynn has suggested that Smollett is being somewhat disingenuous here, because 'as a practicing physician as well as splenetic patient' he is perfectly aware that he has the symptoms of consumption and wishes to deny his illness by turning 'medical consultation into a linguistic contest' over which Smollett, as patient, retains complete control. 'By refusing to see – and be seen by – his physician, Smollett hides behind words to remain free to invent his adversary's response to his condition.'[14]

Medicine-by-post letters offer us a front row seat in the arena where professional competence is tested by patient expectation and where professional pride may clash with patient anxiety. The patient's expectations centred on the doctor's skill, but even more on his manner and the interest he showed in the patient's particular medical problem. In the eighteenth century, as today, trust in one's own doctor coexisted with unreserved scepticism about 'doctors'. Confidence in the physician's moral judgment depended mostly on considerations of individual character.

Medical ethics today is considered institutional, a code to which the entire profession subscribes in the form of oath, and for which their behaviour is monitored by professional societies and the law. But in the eighteenth-century Britain, 'recommendations as to the proper behavior of doctors were often hard to distinguish from the much broader genre of *advice to gentlemen* purveyed in general conduct manuals.'[15] As Lisbeth Haakonssen explains in *Medicine and Morals in the Enlightenment*, 'one of the great obstacles to our understanding of eighteenth-century medical ethics is its constant inclusion of manners with morals, etiquette with ethics.'[16] The patient was the final judge of the physician's character, and medicine-by-post letters prove an invaluable barometer for revealing the alterations occurring in medical etiquette, hence, medical ethics as it existed prior to John Gregory's *Lectures on the Duties and Qualifications of a Physician* of 1772.

The letters of Samuel Johnson, whether to his own physicians or offering medical advice to his friends, provide a rich picture of some of the constants of eighteenth-century patient attitudes and experience. Although Johnson's erudition is famous and extends to a great interest in medical matters, his letters are surprisingly informal, even genial, and reflective of the general character of correspondence on medical matters in eighteenth-century Britain in terms of attitudes towards doctors, confidence in self-medication, and probing the spiritual meaning of illness as test of character. His letters, along with some of the observations and representations of private practice medicine by his contemporaries, such as James Boswell, Samuel Richardson, and Tobias Smollett, offer an essential backdrop against which the rhetorical changes this study considers took place, highlighting those changes and their significance within the context of usual patient experience.

The doctor: esteemed friend and satirised profession

While the established medical profession was regularly pictured as a conspiracy of charlatans who brandished Latinisms while their patients languished, such barbed criticism were much more readily meted out to the profession than to one's own doctor. Samuel Richardson, publisher and author, relied greatly on his doctor and friend George Cheyne, whose medical works were published by Richardson; in his epistolary novel, *Clarissa* (1747–8), a novel much approved by Samuel Johnson, Richardson gives us an unusually sympathetic portrait of Dr H., who attends the heroine in her final illness, and of whom Belford writes to Lovelace: 'Till now I always held it for gospel that *friendship* and *physician* were incompatible things.'[17] Alexander Pope also much admired Dr Cheyne whom he saw in consultation at Bath. Henry Fielding praised John Ranby, his friend and Sergeant-Surgeon to King George II, in pamphlets and in his novel *Tom*

Figure 1.1

Two doctors quarrelling whilst their patient deteriorates. Coloured engraving by I. Cruikshank, 1794. Courtesy: Wellcome Library, London.

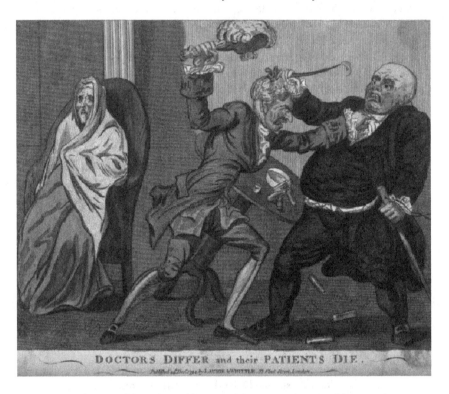

DOCTORS DIFFER and their PATIENTS DIE.

Jones (1749).[18] Although Fielding could pen scathing public attacks on individual doctors he suspected of charlatanism – such as the famous secretary of the Royal Society, James Jurin – yet in *Amelia* (1751) he says, 'Of all mankind the doctor is the best of comforters.'[19] Samuel Johnson, James Boswell, and Tobias Smollett each found fault – both comical and serious – with the profession, yet each of these authors equally appreciated and admired the particular humanity and skill of their own doctors (Thomas Lawrence, John Pringle, and John Moore respectively). Samuel Johnson wrote to Dr Thomas Lawrence in 1783, 'Since your departure I have often wanted your assistance as well as your conversation.'[20]

But admiration for one's physician still might be tainted by the prevailing stereotype of the money-minded medical profession. James Boswell, in a memoir describing a visit to his surgeon, Dr Andrew Douglas, typifies the ambivalent attitude patients held towards physicians. The reason for Boswell's urgent visit to Douglas was yet another attack of gonorrhoea. Boswell writes in his *London Journal* (1762–3) that, 'I thought of applying to a quack who would cure me quickly and cheaply. But then the horrors of being imperfectly cured and having the distemper thrown into my blood terrified me exceedingly.' He therefore decides to 'go to my friend Douglas, whom I knew to be skillful and careful; and although it should cost me more, yet to get sound health was a matter of great importance, as I might save upon other articles.'[21] The visit to the doctor, however, is disquieting, and Boswell remarks wryly:

> I joked with my friend about the expense, asked him if he would take a draft on my arrears, and bid him visit me seldom that I might have the less to pay. To these jokes he seemed to give little heed, but talked seriously in the way of his business. And here let me make a just and true observation, which is that the same man as a friend and as a surgeon exhibits two very opposite characters. Douglas as a friend is most kind, most anxious for my interest... But Douglas as surgeon will be as ready to keep me long under his hands, and as desirous to lay hold of my money, as any man. In short, his views alter quite. I have to do not with him but his profession.[22]

The temptation of eighteenth-century doctors to succumb to a growing medical consumerism was most pithily summed up in a remark of Henry Ballow, Esq. to Dr Akenside: 'My opinion of the profession of physic is this. The ancients endeavoured to make it a science, and failed; and the moderns to make it a trade, and have succeeded.'[23]

In similar ways, Smollett's fictional Matthew Bramble greatly values his close association with Dr Lewis but also finds he is irritated by the presumption of most of the profession:

> Between friends, I think every man of tolerable parts ought, at my time of day, to be both physician and lawyer, as far as his own constitution and property are concerned. For my own part, I have had an hospital these fourteen years within myself, and studied my own case with the most painful attention; consequently may be supposed to know something of the matter although I have not taken regular courses of physiology et cetera et cetera. – In short, I have for some time been of opinion, (no offence, dear doctor) that the sum of all your medical discoveries amounts to this, that the more you study the less you know. [24]

The image of the medical profession as unduly proud, as well as greedy, interfered with the best doctor–patient relationships. As in the experience of Boswell, patients harboured conflicted feelings about their doctor whose professional role too often upstaged the doctor as friend. As Bramble succinctly puts it to Dr Lewis:

Dear Dick,

You cannot imagine what a pleasure I have in seeing your handwriting, after such a long cessation on your side of our correspondence – Yet, Heaven knows, I have often seen your handwriting with disgust – I mean, when it appeared in abbreviations of apothecary's Latin.[25]

Samuel Johnson held his personal doctor, Dr Thomas Lawrence (1711–83) in the highest regard, an 'established' London physician who was president of the Royal College of Physicians. Still, Johnson most readily discovered the essential qualities of the 'good' physician character in the simple and unpretentious Robert Levet, an 'irregular' doctor, 'unqualified' by formal education but orthodox in practice, and whom Johnson had invited to live with him at his home from 1746 up to the time of Levet's death in 1782, a few years shy of his eightieth birthday.[26] He had remained, up to his last day, actively engaged in a peripatetic practice 'from Houndsditch to Marybone' tending London's less fortunate citizens.[27] In Johnson's eulogy, 'On the Death of Dr Robert Levet' (1783), Johnson describes a type of crude platonic ideal of that moral character most wanted in a physician, one rich in goodness and of great service to mankind even though unschooled in a gentleman's etiquette:

Yet still he fills Affection's eye,
Obscurely wise, and coarsely kind;
Nor, lettered Arrogance, deny
Thy praise to merit unrefined.

When fainting Nature called for aid,
And hovering Death prepared the blow,
His vig'rous remedy displayed
The power of art without the show.

No summons mocked by chill delay,
No petty gain disdained by pride,
The modest wants of every day
The toil of every day supplied.[28]

The qualities that Johnson eulogised in Levet were humility, an unpretentious manner, natural skill, compassion, and an unhesitating devotion to his calling. Absent in Levet was that egregious egotistism that

24

made the eighteenth-century physicians so regularly the butt of satire and suspect by their own clientele.[29]

Boswell described Mr Levet as Johnson's 'humble friend ...an obscure practiser in physick amongst the lower people, his fees being sometimes very small sums', but with an 'extensive practice that way.'[30] Boswell continues, 'such was Johnson's predilection for him, and fanciful estimation of his moderate abilities, that I have heard him say he should not be satisfied, though attended by all the College of Physicians, unless he had Mr Levet with him.'[31] Johnson communicated to Dr Thomas Lawrence news of the death of 'Our old Friend, Mr Levett', with the added reflection, 'So has ended the long life of a very useful, and blam[e]less man.'[32] For Johnson, the idea of being 'useful' was no small compliment. W. Jackson Bate says of Johnson's poem that 'the grief is sublimated to a general statement in which moral virtue, humble or great, walks in the midst of life, fulfilling the parable of the talents that always haunted Johnson: "The single talent well employed."'[33]

For Johnson, infirmity served as a reminder of one's moral duty to fulfil a meaningful and useful life; sickness, thus, was a test of personal character for the patient as well as the doctor. As Johnson writes to his friend, Hill Boothy, in 1755:

> This illness in which I have suffered some thing and feared much more, has depressed my confidence and elation, and made me consider all that I have promised myself as less certain to be attained or enjoyed. I have endeavoured to form resolutions of a better life, but I form them weakly under the consciousness of an external motive. Not that I conceive a time of Sickness a time improper for recollection and good purposes, which I believe Diseases and Calamities often sent to produce, but because no man can know how little his performance will conform to his promises, and designs are nothing in human eyes till they are realised by execution.[34]

Eighteenth-century doctors firmly believed that it was the patient's primary moral responsibility to be compliant with therapy in order to recover a sound state of health; but for the patient, the true moral obligation was more often to be found in the spiritual experience, in the test of one's fortitude, faith, and resolutions. It was George Cheyne's skill at combining these moral viewpoints, as we shall see, that distinguished his career and led to his immense popularity. Still, there was a reciprocal moral duty of doctor and patient to each other, for the doctor to provide his best services, and for the patient to follow his advice: this was the basis of an eighteenth-century 'practical ethics' – a tradition that combined Christian duties with classical teachings, in which there were three areas of moral responsibility: to God, to society, and to one's own self-improvement.[35] The patient's responsibility was to serve God through the preservation of God's creation, one's own physical body; the second responsibility was to recover health so as to return the service of one's society. For the physician, the third area of moral responsibility was particularly relevant, to improve one's mind and expand knowledge, which gave sanction to medical experimentation. This tradition of 'practical ethics' was fundamental to John Gregory's medical ethics in his *Lectures on the Duties and Qualifications of a Physician.*

Patient eclecticism and medical rhetoric in the letters of Samuel Johnson

Although Levet's credentials were a far cry from those of an established, Oxford-educated physician such as Dr Lawrence, Johnson had complete confidence in Levet's medical opinion. It seemed a curious relationship to Boswell, who described Robert Levet as an underqualified physician, of 'a strange grotesque appearance', austere, remote, and in no way typical of the erudite physician acquaintances included in Johnson's and Boswell's usual coterie of friends.

But Boswell himself saw no contradiction in seeking treatment outside of established medical circles for his recurrent bouts of gonorrhoea – a 'try-anything attitude', as Roy Porter describes it.[36] At one point, Boswell was especially concerned that he might pass on venereal infection to his intended bride, Montgomerie of Lainshaw, a first cousin. He therefore consulted several highly respected Scottish physicians, including John Gregory, professor of medicine at the University of Edinburgh, and his friend, the esteemed John Pringle.[37] However, not entirely reassured by the advice of these prestigious gentlemen, Boswell determined to go back to London and, based on the enthusiastic recommendations of a friend who claimed relief of his own venereal condition, called on Dr Gilbert Kennedy for his much-advertised Lisbon Diet Drink. Both Gregory and Pringle were highly sceptical of this proprietary concoction, but Boswell explains that although he found Kennedy to be a 'a gaping babbler', in whom 'I had no trust', still he 'made use of him as an engine to play upon and extinguish fire, which his decoction [*sic*] certainly does'.[38]

Before calling in a physician, it was not uncommon for the eighteenth-century patient first to experiment with home remedies or all-purpose proprietary mixtures proclaimed in bills and newspapers. Folk cures, empirical nostrums, and orthodox medical therapies were taken in succession or in combination, much to the frustration of the regular physicians who scolded their patients for 'irresponsible' self-medicating behaviour. For the suffering individual, however, there was no obvious advantage in the recipes of 'established' physicians over the much less costly remedies of 'vernacular' medicine. When one was sick, all ports in the storm were equally inviting.[39]

Samuel Johnson's learning and insatiable curiosity extended to medicine and might suggest that his letters on medical subjects would be exceptional. However, his correspondence is quite representative of lay medical attitudes towards eighteenth-century medicine among the upper classes and the literate upper-middle class in Britain.[40] Indeed, the eclecticism and empiricism that informs Johnson's letters on medical therapy, and his familiarity with contemporary medical opinion, is entirely in character for the period.[41] Johnson's letters to friends on medical subjects are filled with medical gossip and advice. While he often favours his own empiric cures, Johnson not infrequently supports his recommendations by citing reputable medical authorities or, with equal ardour, passes on remedies he has discovered in casual conversation with friends – often doctors – or through correspondence with medical acquaintances regarding a particular condition affecting one of his social circle.

In his efforts to assist Hester Thrale in finding a cure for her mother, Mrs Salusbury, who had breast cancer, Johnson first recommends a trial of the Malvern waters, forwarding the pamphlet by Dr John Wall entitled, 'Experiments and Observations of the Malvern Waters' (1756, 1763).[42] Then, after returning from a visit to his old schoolmate and close friend, the Birmingham surgeon Edmund Hector, Johnson writes to implore him:

> Yet perhaps I had not written so soon had I not had another favour to solicite. Your case of the cancer and mercury has made such an impression upon my friend, that we are very impatient for a more exact relation than I could give, and I therefore entreat, that you will state it very particularly, with the patient's age, the manner of taking mercury, the quantity taken, and all that you told or omitted to tell me.[43]

For his friend, Thomas Cummings, a Quaker merchant, the trustworthy Dr Levet serves as a medical resource for Johnson:

> I have been talking of your case with my Friend Mr Levet, who has had great practice, and of whom I have a very high opinion. He thinks you neither have nor ever had a proper dropsy. He says that your Lungs are much obstructed and inflamed, but he agrees with me that they are not ulcerated, and that the little flux of blood has nothing in it much to be feared. But as you are brought so low, he thinks your case out of the power of medicine, and to be helped only by proper diet, with occasional helps from slight emetics.[44]

But although Johnson's letters show him to be a repository of current medical knowledge from a variety of sources, they more significantly reveal an active mind with strong views as to the best remedies for ailments affecting his friends or himself. Johnson, for example, insisted on the benefits of vigorous phlebotomy. When troubled with asthma and dropsy, he complains to Hester Thrale in January of 1782, 'I was blooded on Saturday, I think not copiously enough, but the Doctor would permit no more.'[45] Then in March, again:

> Seven ounces! Why I sent a letter to Dr Lawrence, who is ten times more timorsome than is your Jebb, and he came and stood by while one vein was opened with too small an orifice, and bled eight ounces and stopped. Then another vein was opened, which ran eight more.[46]

Johnson was equally confident about the value of bleeding for many of his ill acquaintances, though he does not prescribe such treatment indiscriminately. He advises Mrs Thrale on her husband's condition:

> Gentle purges, and slight phlebotomies, are not my favourites, they are popgun batteries, which lose time and effect nothing. It was by bleeding till he fainted that his life was saved. I would now have him trust chiefly to vigorous and stimulating catharticks. To bleed is only proper when there is no time for slower remedies.[47]

Johnson wrote to the Reverend John Taylor that same year his opinion that 'The quantity of blood taken from you appears to me not sufficient', and that 'Thrale was almost lost by the scrupulosity of his Physicians, who never bled him copiously till they bled him in despair... and from that instant he grew better.'[48] Yet in 1784, the year of his own death, Johnson had advised Taylor quite differently:

> Your general distemper is, I think, a hectic fever, for which the bark is proper, and which quietness of mind, and gentle exercise, and fresh air may cure. Your present weakness is the effect of such waste of blood, as would weaken a young man in his highest vigour. It might be necessary, but it must sink both your courage and strength. Dr Nichols hurt himself extremely in his old age by lavish phlebotomy. Do not bleed again very soon and when you can delay no longer, be more moderate.[49]

Some two years earlier Johnson had jested with Hester Thrale that, 'I shall try to escape the other bleeding, for I am of the Chymical sect, which holds phlebotomy in abhorrence.' Johnson, thus, in a lighter vein![50]

Johnson's advice to his lady friend, Hill Boothby, is typical of the Chinese menu approach of the eighteenth-century layman. After expressing the sincere wish that God restore his 'Dear angel' to full health, Johnson feels obliged to offer his friend a nostrum to compliment her doctor's prescriptions. It is one of Johnson's personal favourite home remedies, a preparation consisting of dried Seville orange peels in a recipe which he teasingly refused to divulge to Boswell – who had been vexed by curiosity ever since he had first noticed his friend secreting orange peels into his coat pocket at their Club.[51] With Hill Boothby, however, Johnson is delighted to share his nostrum, which in nature and purpose might suggest to the modern gastroenterologist an eighteenth-century precursor of Metamucil with a chaser:

> Give me leave, who have thought much on Medicine, to propose to you an easy and I think a very probable remedy for indigestion and lubricity of the bowels.... Take an ounce of dried orange peel finely powdered, divide it into scruples, and take one Scruple [a twenty-fourth of an ounce] at a time in any manner; the best way is perhaps to drink it in a glass of hot red port, or to eat it first and drink the wine after it. If you mix cinnamon or nutmeg with the powder it were not worse, but it will be more bulky and so more troublesome. This is a medicine not disgusting, not costly, easily tried, and if not found useful easily left off.

He concludes, somewhat mischievously: 'I would not have you offer it to the Doctor as mine. Physicians do not love intruders, yet do not take it without his leave. But do not be easily put off.'[52]

Eighteenth-century physician authority was seriously limited in the eighteenth century in the face of such patient eclecticism, patients determined to decide the course of their treatment and who searched boldly for medical opinions that satisfied their own medical prejudices. Even the opinion of the esteemed Dr Lawrence is not sacrosanct, as evidenced in this letter to Hill Boothby:

> Dearest Dear,

> I am extremely obliged to you for the kindness of your enquiry. After I had written to you Dr Laurence came, and would have given some oil and sugar, but I took Rhenish and water, and recovered my voice. I yet cough much and sleep ill. I have been visited by another Doctor to day but I laughed at his Balsam of Peru.[53]

Johnson readily ignores both Lawrence's recommendations and the 'second opinion' of a consulting physician in favour of his own nostrums. He frequently shows the empirical side of his medical philosophy, another manifestation of eclecticism. Of 'alterative' medicines – those which have no immediate effect but work, gradually, through altering the humours – Johnson says to Bennet Langdon, 'My opinion... is not high, but quid tentasse nocebit? If it does harm, or does no good, it may be omitted.' This follows a detailed receipt of a medicine for the rheumatism that Johnson has tracked down for Bennet's use. One of the ingredients is root of lovage, and Johnson notes that this root, 'in Ray's Nomenclature is Levisticum', and 'perhaps the Botanists may know the Latin name'. He then adds, 'Of this medicine I pretend not to judge. There is all the appearance of its efficacy which a single instance can afford. The Patient was very old, the pain very violent, and the relief, I think, speedy and lasting.'[54] When Dr Lawrence suffers a stroke, Johnson writes to his wife, Elizabeth Lawrence, 'If we could have again but his mind and his tongue, or his mind and his right hand, we would not much lament the rest. I should not despair of helping the swelled hand by electricity, if it were frequently and diligently applied.'[55] What is remarkable in this letter is not Johnson's independent thought on health matters, so common to the period, but that Johnson had the temerity to suggest the use of such an empirical treatment – electrical therapy promoted by Methodist preacher and medico–religionist John Wesley – for use on the president of the Royal College of Physicians.

Yet, for all of Johnson's definite ideas on medical therapies, he retained great respect for members of the medical profession, and Boswell tells us that, 'Johnson had in general a peculiar pleasure in the company of physicians'.[56] Indeed, Johnson's esteem for the opinion of members of the established medical profession is illustrated by communications during his final illness in 1784. Levet had died two years earlier, and Johnson was under the care of Drs Heberden and Brocklesby. Although quite satisfied with his doctors, he did not discourage Boswell from consulting with some of the more prominent Scottish physicians about his condition. Boswell's personal doctor, Sir Alexander Dick, advised rhubarb, but also enclosed a *consilium medicum* from the learned Dr Gillespie. Writing to Boswell, Johnson praised Dr Gillespie for 'an excellent *consilium medicum*, all solid practical experimental , though he adds, 'I am at present, in the opinion of my physicians, (Dr Heberden and Dr Brocklesby,) as well as my own, going on very hopefully. I have just begun to take vinegar of squills.'[57] Following this communication, Boswell takes it upon himself to write a letter (in triplicate) requesting consultation from 'three of the eminent physicians who had chairs in our celebrated school of medicine at Edinburgh, Doctors Cullen, Hope, and Munro.' In this letter, Boswell reminds the physicians of Johnson's great respect for the moral integrity of the profession:

This, you see, is not authority for a regular consultation: but I have no doubt of your readiness to give your advice to a man so eminent, and who, in his Life of Garth, has paid your profession a just and elegant compliment: 'I believe every man has found in physicians great liberality and dignity of sentiment, very prompt effusions of beneficence, and willingness to exert a lucrative art, where there is no hope of lucre.'[58]

Boswell shifts into an entirely different rhetorical mode to describe Johnson's medical condition, a formal and objective case presentation resembling the kind of letter a physician might write to a consultant, a form common to the medicine-by-post of the early decades of the century:[59]

Dr Johnson is aged seventy-four. Last summer he had a stroke of palsy, from which he recovered almost entirely. He had, before that, been troubled with a catarrhous cough. This winter he was seized with a spasmodick asthma, by which he has been confined to his house for about three months. Dr Brocklesby writes to me, that upon the least admission of cold, there is such a constriction upon his breast, that he cannot lie down in his bed, but is obliged to sit up all night, and gets rest and sometimes sleep, only by means of laudanum and syrup of poppies; and that there are oedematous tumours on his legs and thighs. Dr Brocklesby trusts a good deal to the return of mild weather. Dr Johnson says, that dropsy gains ground upon him; and he seems to think that a warmer climate would do him good. I understand he is now rather better, and is using vinegar of squills. I am, with great esteem, dear Sir, Your most obedient humble servant.[60]

Despite this impressive array of consultants, it is certain that Dr Johnson would have been most grateful in his final hours to have had the presence of his 'old friend Mr Levet' also by his side. In a letter to Bennet Langton some three months after Levet's death, Johnson wrote:

I was musing in my chamber, I thought with uncommon earnestness, that however I might alter my mode of life, or whithersoever I might remove, I would endeavour to retain Levet about me, in the morning my servant brought me Word that Levet was called to another state, a state for which, I think, he was not unprepared, for he was very useful to the poor. How much soever I valued him, I now wish that I had valued him more.[61]

Johnson's rhetoric in his letters concerned with illness straddles the rhetorical forms that predominated throughout the eighteenth century in medicine-by-post. In his letters to acquaintances concerning medical matters, Johnson's familiar and conversational tone is remarkable in its great contrast to the formally structured and aloof rhetorical style for which he is famous. Bruce Redford, in his book on eighteenth-century familiar letters, *The*

Converse of the Pen, claims that Johnson's letters to Hester Thrale were unique among his epistolary output in terms of the rhetorical style. It was only in this interchange, says Redford, that Johnson shed his complex, often pompous, 'Ramblerian voice' and adopted a lighter tone of 'intimate conversation', consisting of 'the warm inconsequentiality, the private allusiveness, and the darting fragmentation of candid oral discourse'.[62] But this quality of informal conversation, of unpretentious coffee-table chat, clearly extended to the letters on medical subjects that Johnson wrote to Hill Boothby and numerous other acquaintances, and what is noteworthy is that even a compulsive stylist such as Dr Johnson modulated his rhetorical tone when addressing medical matters in the genre of the familiar letter.[63] The subject of illness in mid-century Britain invites a more intimate style, a rhetoric showing personal interest and concern, even urgency that supersedes usual formalities.

What is also clear from Johnson's correspondence is that personal illness is a legitimate topic of 'public' conversation, to be shared among a select group of friends. If patient confidentiality was necessary to physician etiquette, such decorum did not hold true for acquaintances within a circle of social equals.[64] That such private matters were topics of epistolary converse is not surprising if one accepts the public nature of the eighteenth-century letter as described by Habermaas, who explains that, 'the opposite of the intimateness whose vehicle was the written word was indiscretion and not publicity as such.'[65] The key word here is 'discretion', not privacy.[66]

In his written communications to Dr Lawrence, to request advice on acquaintances, Johnson uses a different rhetorical tone which, in its manner, falls somewhere between his austere, public voice and the informal, chatty quality of his familiar letters to Thrale and other friends regarding medical topics. In fact, he adopts the objective rhetorical mode that Boswell used to describe Johnson's own last illness to the Edinburgh consultants. When Johsnons applies to Lawrence for advice regarding an 'old Friend,' Mrs Chambers, whom 'I am extremely desirous to keep alive', Johnson details her case with studied objectivity:

> She is extremely heavy, and between the soreness and cumbrousness of her legs, and the weight of her body, is not able to cross the room.... She has now and then a fit of coughing, but not often, and is sometimes short breathed. Her Urine is thick and in a very large small quantity. On one leg she has several small ulcers, and one large ulcer on the other. The sores run little. The large ulcer is about the Shin, and that leg a little below the calf distils thin water through the cracks of the Skin.... She has sometimes pain in the side, and sometimes fetches involuntary sighs. [67]

Johnson offers no further description of the patient's suffering or discomfort, no words from the patient about her feelings, either physical or mental. His only addition to the plain facts is the opinion, based on his reading of Lawrence's treatise, *Hydrops*, that the patient suffers from 'a Dropsy in the Flesh'.[68] In a subsequent letter to Lawrence, Johnson is similarly scientific, adding apologietically that 'neither she nor her attendants are very good relators of a Case'.[69]

Yet, in describing his personal trials to Dr Lawrence, Johnson intersperses an objective narratives with surges of subjective feeling. The letters to Lawrence are written in Latin, certainly exhibiting erudition but also, perhaps, to borrow from a classical tradition that invited a certain degree of poetic and dramatic expression. It is paradoxical that Johnson should confide in one letter that although his difficulty in breathing 'is not painful, it is difficult to recount in Latin how much weariness it causes'.[70] One wonders what inhibited Johnson then from writing this part in English. Did he feel compelled to remain in a formal rhetorical mode for Lawrence? Nevertheless, Johnson persists in the classical language: 'Lying in bed, I must bear some part of that dire torture by which our ancestors overcame the stubborness of a silent defendant whose chest was piled high with weights'. Aware of the intimate relation of mind and body, Johnson adds that, 'I bear all these discomforts the more painfully, the more easily I am confident they can be relieved'. With great urgency he implores Lawrence, 'Therefore I beg and implore you, most learned of men, not to forbid the letting of blood.'

In a subsequent letter to Lawrence, the bleedings completed with good effect Johnson's rhetoric is a remarkable combination of the formal and the poetic – in fact the letter is written in verse form in the Latin:

> Now a relaxed spirit goes away and comes back to me with a freer movement; now less harsh coughing lacerates my chest and stomach.[71] So much good does bleeding at the right time accomplish, so much good the sweet poppy with its powerful juice. Now what remains? Provided only that I see how much warm baths might relieve tight skin, tomorrow I intend to go forth whither sweet Thrale recalls me. This too remains, that I express gratitude to the prince of doctors, and pray fervently that the skills that benefit all may not fail their master. Farewell.[72]

The discomfort experienced in March returns all too soon; and by mid-May Johnson complains (not in verse now) that 'Old diseases harrass me... such as I am scarcely equal to bearing. Sleep is brief, interrupted, and precarious. But I am overcome with sleepiness.' More bloodletting is sought, but the patient defers to Lawrence, 'But you, most learned man, will be the judge'. Johnson's rhetoric in his letters concerned with illness are truly representative of the rhetorical forms that predominated throughout the eighteenth century in medicine-by-post, a genre in its own right by virtue of the uniqueness of the doctor-patient relationship and the subject of personal infirmity. While Johnson's letters to physicians on medical subjects show the formality and a self-conscious effort at objectivity that predominated in the first third of the century, his letters also admit of a subjectivity and intensity of expression that begins to predominate from the mid-century. As I have suggested, Johnson's rhetoric looks forward, most particularly, to the medicine-by-post that characterises the final decades of the century – a rhetorical form that not only found a balance in objectivity and subjectivity, but that was also able to use that balance to escape the formulaic rhetoric of either iatromechanism or sensibility and achieve a more individualised patient voice.

Eclecticism in the medical marketplace: superstition and science, religion and class

Levet's humble practice, 'useful' and devoid of avarice and vanity, was indeed remarkable in what had become a competitive medical marketplace – a marketplace fuelled by the restless shopping around for medical miracle cures. But if patients were medical window-shoppers, it was in the spirit of 'caveat emptor'. Greed and quackery were intimately associated terms, but the epithet 'quack' did not actually serve to distinguish between 'established' physicians and any of the wide range of irregular doctors. All manner of healers routinely accused the others of dangerous practices, less out of concern for the actual welfare of the patient than to swell their own reputations in the medical marketplace. Even the most thoroughly established physicians were not exempt from the accusations of self-interest if they showed the slightest hint of advancing their practice through advertisements, or bills, which proclaimed some medication or surgical procedure unique to their practice. A physician was immediately suspect if overzealous in guarding the recipe of some private nostrum under the veiled excuse of public good, usually by claiming the necessity of preventing harm to the public through misuse of a new surgical technique by unscrupulous doctors or the inappropriate use of a potion by patients all too ready to be their own physicians.[73]

In Daniel Defoe's *A Journal of the Plague Year* (1722), a chronicle of the 1665 epidemic that, at its height, carried off some fifty thousand Londoners in a two-month period, the narrator expresses outrage at the many doctors who profited from the panic caused by the bubonic plague. 'Death was before their eyes, and everybody began to think of their graves', yet:

[W]holesome Reflections – which, rightly manag'd, would have most happily led the People to fall upon their Knees, make Confession of their Sins, and look to their merciful Saviour for pardon, imploring His Compassion on them in such a Time of Distress... had a quite contrary Extreme in the common People; who ignorant and stupid in their Reflections as they were brutishly wicked and thoughtless before, were now led by their Fright to extremes of folly; and as I have said before, that they ran to Conjurers and Witches, and all Sorts of Deceivers,.... So were they as mad upon running after Quacks, and Mountebanks, and every practicing old Woman, for Medicines and Remedies; storeing themselves with such Multitudes of Pills, potions, and Preservatives, as they were call'd; that they not only spent their Money but even poison'd themselves before-hand for fear of the Poison of Infection, and prepar'd their Bodies for the Plague, instead of preserving them against it. On the other Hand it is incredible, and scarce to be imagined, how the Posts of Houses and Corners of Streets were plaster'd over with Doctors Bills, and Papers of ignorant Fellows; quacking and tampering in Physick, and inviting the People to come to them for Remedies....[74]

While Londoners of means could flee the city, the poor were trapped in town and were especially vulnerable to those abuses enumerated by the journal's narrator. Defoe (in the voice of the journal writer) praises the dedication of many established physicians who, unlike the Anglican clergy, courageously remained in the city to minister to the sick. Still, a doctor's visit cost far more than a potion, and Defoe laments that even the brave example of qualified doctors could not stem the tide of a panicked and superstitious population rushing off to buy whatever ineffectual preventatives and cures were proffered by irregular healers.[75]

The attitude towards medicine taken by Defoe's narrator in the journal typifies the attitude of the more educated, middle-class Puritan at the turn of the century, and is also representative of a wider, educated public as well. The narrator's opinion on medical matters consists of a mix of respect for the new science with a healthy scepticism about what science alone has to offer. The narrator insists on self-determination in matters of health. Even as Defoe's journalist praises the 'College Physicians' for 'daily publishing several Preparations' at no charge to the public, he 'must acknowledge, I made use of little or nothing, except, as I have observ'd, to keep a Preparation of strong Scent to have ready, in case I met with any thing of offensive Smells, or went too near any burying place or dead Body' (290–1). And the observations of a doctor friend are noted: that despite the myriad of useful preparations offered by the physicians, they 'were in fact concocted from a small number of similar ingredients, made up in multitude of different formulations', and

35

that 'every Man, judging a little of his own Constitution and manner of his living, and Circumstances of his being infected, may direct his own Medicines out of the ordinary Drugs and Preparations.' Based on such advice, the narrator chooses to take Venice treacle, 'and thought myself as well fortified against infection as any one could be fortified by the power of physic' (291–2).[76] Defoe, like Johnson, was no more ready to become a sheep in the fold of established medicine than he was prepared to succumb to the commerce of quacks.

Defoe's Puritanism, mirrored in the narrator, must be appreciated as contributing in a crucial way to how the journal writer sees disease as a spiritual test and a test of self-reliance during illness. Of the many novel treatments offered to plague-ravaged Londoners, whether from established physicians or charlatans, none were effective. That the plague comes to an end, insists the narrator:

> [I]t was evidently from the secret invisible Hand of him [sic] that had at first sent this Disease as a Judgement upon us; and let the Atheistic part of Mankind call my Saying what they please, it is no Enthusiasm; it was acknowledg'd at that time by all Mankind; the Disease was enervated and its Malignity spent, and... let the Philosophers search for Reasons in Nature to account for it by, and labour as much as they will to lessen the Debt they owe to their Maker; those Physicians, who had the least Share of Religion in them, were oblig'd to acknowledge that it was all supernatural, that it was extraordinary, and that no Account could be given of it. (300)

This Providential account of the plague is joined, in Defoe's hands, with rigorous empirical analysis of the causes and spread of the pestilence – including observations that resemble current modern notions of an incubation period and a period of infectivity – and the narrator addresses, in precise detail, the awful consequences of enforcing a quarantine on a family touched by the infection – the likelihood of spreading disease to uninfected members of a household who are forced to remain indoors with the first victim. What seems a most paradoxical blend of superstition and science in Defoe's journalist shows how misleading it is to assume medical beliefs are predictable based on social class alone or the level of education of the patient.

Jonathan Barry, in *Piety and the Patient: Medicine and Religion in Eighteenth Century Bristol*, effectively challenges the notion that eighteenth-century patient medical preferences neatly break down along class or religious lines. Certainly the poor, especially the rural poor, of necessity favoured less costly vernacular cures and readily obtainable proprietary medicines. In contrast, the aristocratic patient, influenced by the growing prestige of new science, 'was prepared to pay large sums' for the services and pills of established practitioners, partly 'as a symbol of... membership of the affluent classes', and partly to distinguish himself or herself from practices identified with religious enthusiasts. Yet, argues Barry, middle-class patients seem to have straddled these extremes of medical definition.[77]

Through the diary of William Dyer (b. 1730), a Bristol accountant, Barry uncovers the wide range of medical beliefs of middle-class Bristol society. Dyer at age fourteen had spent only several months apprenticed to an apothecary, but throughout his life Dyer gave frequent medical advice and pharmacological services to fellow Bristol citizens. Like Samuel Johnson, he had broad intellectual pursuits, including medicine, and he entered into his diary a great variety of medical treatments which had been administered to people in his social circle and which he found worthy of note. Dyer was actively involved in humanitarian activities in Bristol and conversed with some of the more notable representatives of Enlightenment intellectual society. He was a 'loyal Anglican' but also attended Dissenter gatherings in Bristol and was close friends with many Methodists, including John and Charles Wesley. Barry characterises Dyer's religious practice as an 'ecumenical pietism' representative of many in the Bristol community, and Dyer's medical eclecticism reflects the influence of Methodist and Dissenter ideas in fashioning medical therapies which acknowledged the inextricable ties between physical and spiritual health.

The prescriptions Dyer took for his own needs, as well as those he dispensed, ranged from standard medications and proprietary nostrums to folk remedies. He was a strong proponent of the electrical therapy advanced by John Wesley, a therapy which, Barry explains, 'in Bristol remained most firmly associated with amateurs, including both Methodist and Anglican ministers'.[78] Dyer not only administered electrical treatment to patients but even developed a reputation as a respected consultant in this form of therapy. As Barry explains, Dyer's use of the machine was clearly empirical and primarily of medical interest – as it was for Wesley. He used his electrical apparatus, purchased from London, to treat primarily chronic musculo–skeletal, joint, and neurological complaints, as well as hypochondria and melancholy, conscientiously recording efficacy and treatment failures. Yet it was also true that electricity was for many pietists, including Dyer, evidence of the Behmenist contention that fire was the omnipresent force in creation, the force responsible for the union of the spiritual and material worlds.

Also as part of his belief in the link between the physical and spiritual body, Dyer advised treatment with spa waters which, as Barry reminds us, 'were traditionally associated with saints' and with dreams.[79] Dyer's medical philosophy encompassed a belief in the association of disease and 'a bad life', the effects of the imagination on illness, and even witchcraft and 'possession'.[80] In placing Dyer well within the mainstream of Bristol society, Barry shows that Dyer is not an anomaly but representative of the attitudes of a large segment of British society in combining the most up-to-date ideas of established medicine with religious, superstitious, and vernacular traditions.

In Samuel Johnson's correspondence as we have seen the same readiness as Dyer to seek cures from a broad range of medical options, including electricity. In subsequent chapters, medicine-by-post letters provide strong additional evidence to support Barry's contention by illustrating that upper-class patients showed the same tendency as middle-class patients to combine orthodox with vernacular medicine.[81] The enormous popularity of Dr George Cheyne (discussed in Chapter 3) was based on his ability to appeal to a public that naturally responded to his blend of morality and spirituality with the speculations of natural philosophy.

Finding the ideal doctor

Bernard Mandeville warned of the dangers of affectation and vanity, both in physician and patient, in *A Treatise of the Hypochondriack and Histerick Diseases* (1711):

> 'Tis Pride that makes the Physician abandon the solid Observation of never-erring Nature, to take up with loose Conjectures of his own wandering Invention, that the World may admire the Fertility of his Brain; and it is Pride in the Patient, that makes him in love with the Reasoning Physician, to have an Opportunity of shewing the Depth of his own Penetration.[82]

Some forty years later, Tobias Smollett richly illustrated all the pretensions of the medical profession in *The Adventures of Ferdinand Count Fathom* (1753). The eponymous villain, of low birth, first passes himself off as a count but, when this masquerade fails, he decides that posturing as a physician might prove the perfect charade to restore his funds and introduce oneself to young ladies of wealthy families:

> He wisely came to the resolution of descending one step in the degrees of life, and of taking upon him the title of physician, under which he did not despair of insinuating himself into the pockets of his patients, and into the secrets of private families, so as to acquire a comfortable share of practice, or captivate the heart of some heiress or rich widow.[83]

Fathom realises that superficial effect and appearance are particularly important for his plan (as Smollett appreciated from his own knowledge of the ways of medical colleagues). The protagonist is well aware that 'the success of a physician, in great measure depends upon the external equipage in which he first declares himself an adept in the healing art' (241). Fathom, therefore:

> [R]epaired to Tunbridge with the first of the season, where he appeared in the uniform of Aesculapius, namely, a plain suit full trimm'd, with a voluminous tye perriwig; believing that in this place, he might glide, as it were, imperceptibly, into the function of his new employment, and gradually accustom himself to the method and form of prescription. (241)[84]

The new doctor explains to his prospective clients that he studied in Padua but only 'for his amusement' and now practices his skills as a 'gentleman', without expecting compensation. Although Fathom's medical education consists only in the perusal of a few medical texts, this proves no obstacle to developing a flourishing practice:

> Being but little conversant with the Materia medica, the circle of his prescriptions was very small: his chief study was to avoid all drugs of rough operation and uncertain effect; and to administer such only as should be agreeable to the palate, without doing violence to the constitution. Such a physician could not but be agreeable to people of all dispositions; and as most of the patients were in some shape hypochondriac, the power of imagination cooperating with his remedies, often effected a cure. (165)

In such manner, Fathom easily becomes a popular 'novelty' at Tunbridge: 'There was something so extraordinary in a nobleman's understanding medicine; and so uncommon is a physician's prescribing gratis' (243). The author explains that any 'illiterate pretender' can make an impression through the eloquent display of 'common notions, and superficial observation' which 'will be more agreeable, because better adapted to the comprehension of the hearers.' Rhetorical skills are critical to Fathom's success; he is 'blessed with a flow of language, an elegant address, a polite and self-denying stile of argumentation' that make him seem 'infinitely superior' in argument with other physicians who, although they might have 'more solid learning', were sure to lose in a contest of popularity (165).

But just as the reader of this history is prepared to respond with amusement and astonishment at the success of pseudo–medico Fathom, Smollett complicates our judgment of what it means to be a medical man of good character. A young woman who is happily treated by Fathom in the absence of her personal physician is shocked when her own doctor returns and behaves in a rude manner that makes Fathom seem by far the more desirable 'doctor'. Dr Looby is at first blind to Fathom's hoax but not to the young doctor's threat to his own practice; and instead of gratitude for the care Fathom has provided his patient, or taking an interest in treatment that has revived her, the doctor stages a dispute directly in front of the recovering patient. He looks at the vials by the bedside, and categorically pronounces them 'trash'. The young woman's mother is upset at this rough behaviour, especially after the kind Dr Fathom has produced such a 'happy and surprising effect'. Dr Looby chastises, 'Effect! (cried this offended member of the faculty) pshaw! stuff, who made you the judge of effects or causes?' (248). The doctor then snubs Fathom and ignores the tactful suggestion that the two men remove from the bedside to pursue their discussion. 'I am resolved... never to consult with any physician who has not taken his degrees at either of the English universities,' insists Dr Looby. Fathom's response must be taken as giving voice to Smollett's own strong sentiments about the exclusivity and arrogance of the established English doctors, 'Upon the supposition (replied our adventurer) that no person can be properly educated for the profession at any other school.'[85] He continues:

> How far you are in the right... I leave to the world to judge, after I have observed, that in your English universities, there is no opportunity of studying the art; no, not so much as a lecture given on the subject: nor is there one physician of note, in this kingdom, who has not derived the greatest part of his medical knowledge, from the instructions of foreigners. (249)

The key word here is 'art'. But Dr Looby now suspects that he may be dealing with 'one of those... who graduate themselves, and commence doctors, the Lord knows how: an interloper, who without license or authority, come hither to take the bread out of the mouths of gentlemen, who have been trained to the business in a regular manner.' Fathom's reply makes clear what he intends by the 'art' of medicine:

> Never was money laid out to less purpose:... for it does not appear, that you have learned so much as the basis of medical acquirements, namely, that decorum and urbanity which ought to distinguish the deportment of every physician: you have even debased the noblest and most beneficial art that ever engaged the study of mankind, which cannot be too much cultivated, and too little restrained, in seeking to limit the practice of it, to a set of narrow-minded illiberal wretches, who, like the lowest handicraftsmen, claim the exclusive privileges of a corporation. (249)

Fathom's words smart, especially coming from a medical impostor – and pretend gentleman – but one who, to his credit, recognises the inherent value of assuming the appropriate professional manner with his patients, intuitively conveying concern – even if feigned – for the patient's well-being over self-interest. 'Decorum and urbanity', as discovered in proper rhetoric, and a show of sensitivity, is what Smollett advises the good physician. It would seem that the deportment of a true gentleman signals more who should be trusted with one's health than the degree on the wall, though the two together would be best. Gentility combined with gentle remedies, as fathom discovers, is the prescription for patient trust and a successful medical career. This was ethical behaviour, even for an impostor!

Indeed, Dr Samuel Bard, in his commencement address to the graduating class of doctors at King's College in New York City in 1769, 'A Discourse on the Duties of a Physician', instructs: 'In your intercourse with your Fellow Practitioners, let integrity, Candour, and Delicacy be your Guides.' He admonishes, 'Never affect to despise a Man for the want of a regular Education, and treat even harmless Ignorance, with Delicacy and Compassion, but when you meet with it joined with foolhardiness and Presumption, you must give it no quarter.'[86] In the wings we imagine Dr Levet with Dr Johnson nodding in agreement.

Yet, it would be a Procrustean interpretation of Johnson's eulogy of Dr Levet, to say that Levet, whatever his virtues, is the complete representation of the ideal eighteenth-century physician. Finally, we would be forced to share in Boswell's reservations for this gentle man who is not, finally, a 'gentleman' in the eighteenth-century meaning. 'Politeness' – and all the word implies – and 'learning' are essential qualities of moral character in the complete eighteenth-century physician – qualities not fully expressed in Dr Levet. His humanity is a sign of a 'moral sense', but Levet lacks the requisite delicacy and refinement associated with the more privileged classes who measured individual worth and character on the exquisite scales of sensibility.

In Samuel Richardson's epistolary novel *Clarissa*, the admirably 'paternal' Dr H. personifies those qualities Johnson admired in Levet – usefulness, extreme compassion, modesty, and absence of self-interest – but Richardson also dramatises the social obligations of physician and patient to each other based on an ideal of sensibility.

After Belford has removed Clarissa from the intolerable surroundings of the Roland apartments, and out of the hands of an egregious apothecary, a 'shocking fellow, of a profession tolerably genteel', Belford is grateful to report to Lovelace that Clarissa is now attended by a new apothecary, Mr Goddard, who is:

[A] man of skill and eminence; and conscience too; demonstrated as well by general character, as by his prescriptions to this lady: for pronouncing her case to be grief, he ordered for the present only juleps by way of cordial; and as soon as her stomach should be able to bear it, light kitchen-diet; telling

Mrs Lovick that that, with air, moderate exercise, and cheerful company, would do her more good than all the medicines in his shop.

This has given me, as it seems to it has too the lady (who also praises his modest behaviour, paternal looks, and genteel address), a very good opinion of the man; and I design to make myself acquainted with him; and if he advises to call in a doctor, to wish him... my worthy friend Dr H. – whose character is above all exception, as is his humanity.[87]

Dr H. is consulted, and Belford writes to Lovelace of the doctor that he 'paid his respects to her, with the gentlemanly address for which he is noted'. The doctor advises Clarissa, with great modesty, 'Indeed madam, you are very low... But give me leave to say, that you can do more for yourself than all the faculty can do for you.' He concurs with Mr Goddard's diagnosis of 'A love case', adding, 'My good young lady, you will require very little of our assistance. You must, in great measure, be your own doctress' (1081). The medical men win Clarissa's confidence. Both the apothecary and the physician, in painful contrast to either Clarissa's father or Lovelace, show respect for her authority over her own body, and in showing such sensitivity, and 'paternal' kindness, take on the social and moral obligations that properly belonged to Clarissa's nouveau riche family and her suitor.

In showing fortitude and patience in illness, and in expressing gratitude towards her caregivers, Clarissa fulfils her role as model patient in an idealised doctor–patient relationship. The benevolent attention of Dr H., Clarissa's acknowledgment of his care, and her resignation to her trials of illness, are elements of an implied moral contract between patient and doctor – the acting out of the code of 'practical ethics'. The physician's duty is to act out of a sympathetic concern for the sufferer and out of considerations of humanity; the patient's obligations are to attend to the doctor's advice and do what is necessary to recover health – so as to return to one's role in family and society. Also, the patient is expected to demonstrate gratitude for the attentions of the physician, most commonly – as part of an implied contract – by payment. Clarissa insists on paying Dr H. despite his protestations. This is partly out of pride – 'I will not be under obligation, she explains' – but also Clarissa is keenly aware of her responsibilities within a larger social context: 'I suffer this visit, because I would not appear ungrateful to the few friends I have left, nor obstinate to such of my relations as may some time hence, for their private satisfaction, inquire after my behaviour in my sick hours' (1081).

The significance of the rhetoric in the doctor–patient relationship here is still more evident in a later interchange between Dr H. and Clarissa, in which he urges her to accept his services without payment, Dr H. explains that as her malady 'was rather to be relieved by the soothings of a friend, than by the prescriptions of a physician, he should think himself greatly honoured to be admitted rather to *advise* her in the *one* character, than prescribe her in the *other* .' Clarissa's response is that:

> [S]he should be always glad to see so humane a gentleman: that his visits would *keep her in charity with his sex*: but that, were she to *forget* that he was her *physician*, she might be apt to abate of the confidence in his skill which might be necessary to effect the amendment that was the end of his visits. (1082)

As mentioned earlier in this chapter, the role of doctor as friend and doctor as professional are always in precarious conflict, even though ideally they are one. In this case, the physician, Dr H., would truly become 'friend', but Clarissa reminds him that it might diminish his effectiveness as a professional. The scene also makes clear the fine line between the professional distance that instils patient 'confidence' and that arrogant aloofness which assumes authority over the patient.

In this doctor-patient interchange, Richardson is anticipating a matter of great concern to medical ethicists in the latter part of the century – how to conjoin the qualities of exquisite sympathy and compassion without unmanning the physician and making him unable to act decisively for the benefit of the patient. John Gregory, in his *Lectures on Duties and Offices of a Physician* (1772), modelled his ideal physician on the man of sensibility:

> I come now to mention the moral qualities peculiarly required in the character of a physician. The chief of these is humanity; that sensibility of heart which makes us feel for the distresses of our fellow-creatures, and which of consequence incites us in the most powerful manner to relieve them. Sympathy produces an anxious attention to a thousand little circumstances that may tend to relieve the patient; an attention which money can never purchase: hence the inexpressible comfort of having a friend for a physician.... If the physician possesses gentleness of manners, and a compassionate heart... the patient feels his approach like that of a guardian angel ministering to his relief.[88]

But Gregory also explains that such physicians who are regularly exposed to 'scenes of distress' are able to 'feel whatever is amiable in pity, without suffering it to enervate or unman them.' Gregory feels obligated to assure his students that 'The insinuation that a compassionate and feeling heart is commonly accompanied with weak understanding and feeble mind, is malignant and false. Experience demonstrates, that a gentle and humane temper, so far from being inconsistent with vigour of mind, is its useful attendant.'[89]

It is in no way incongruous with the times that Gregory was also the author of *A Father's Legacy to His Daughters* – published posthumously in 1774 – a conduct book of great popularity. As Lisbeth Haakonssen explains, 'the poignant last words of a dying man to his soon-to-be orphaned daughters appealed to a public taste shaped by the sentimental literature of Rousseau, Richardson, and Henry Mackenzie.'[90] In common to both the conduct guide for his daughters and his lectures on the duties of a physician, Gregory is distilling ethics from manners. Ethics are associated with 'sincerity' and are immutable, whereas manners are transient and artificial, a product of contemporary civilisation and customs. Mary Fissell points to Gregory's stress on the 'importance of sincerity and the evils of artifice', which for medical professionals distinguished the true 'ingenuous' and 'liberal' gentleman–physician from the 'coxcomb'.

Thomas Percival, in his *Medical Ethics* (1803), was also very anxious to distinguish true compassion from 'that unmanly pity which enfeebles the mind'.[91] As Lisbeth Haakonssen explains, Percival is striving to encourage a 'genuine sympathy' cultivated by education and training which replaces 'turbulent emotion' with a 'calm principle' that 'enabled the physician to transcend the paralysing effects of pity.'[92] The Humean influence is apparent; indeed, Hume used the word 'sentiment' to mean those 'calm passions' that allow us to control the more 'violent passions'.

The 'paternal' attention which Clarissa receives from Mr Goddard and Dr H. models the conjoining of masculinity with tenderness that is the ideal in the man of sensibility and, equally, the perfect caring physician. The word 'paternal' must not be taken in the pejorative sense of assumed authority or condescension. Clarissa writes to Miss Howe: 'Indeed, I am very weak and ill: but I have an excellent physician, Dr H., and as worthy an apothecary, Mr Goddard – Their treatment of me, my dear, is perfectly *pater-nal* !' (1088). Richardson uses italics to set off the word on each occasion it is used, drawing the reader's attention to this quality as especially admirable in members of the medical profession. Clarissa 'really looked upon him [Dr H.] and Mr Goddard, from their kind and tender treatment of her, with regard next to filial', writes Belford to Lovelace (1090). When Clarissa's condition has significantly deteriorated, Belford recounts the following words that Clarissa addresses to her medical men:

> I am inexpressibly obliged to you, sir, and to you , sir (curtsying to the doctor and to Mr Goddard) for your *more* than friendly, your *paternal* care and concern for me. Humanity in your profession, I dare say, is far from being a rare qualification, because you are gentlemen *by* your profession: but so

much kindness, so much humanity, did never desolate creature meet with, as
I have met with from you both. (1248)

Finally, Clarissa, approaching the end of her illness, wants to be assured
by the doctor that she has met her obligations as patient, and she desires that
her friends be assured that she has 'omitted nothing which so worthy and so
skilful a physician prescribed'. Yet, being her 'own doctress', Clarissa
challenges Dr H.'s advice that she go into the country to take the air. This
prescription seems to her merely a futile 'last resource', and she chides Dr H.
for playing at 'the *true* physician', offering placebo cures in a hopeless case
(1276). Clarissa, with all due respect for her physician, retains ultimate
responsibility for her body and determines the course of her medical care. It
is, finally, the patient who engages the services of the doctor and the
apothecary, and in the end these men are subject to her whims. Percival
instructed, in his *Medical Ethics*, that:

> The *feelings* and *emotions* of the patients... require to be known and to be
> attended to, no less than the symptoms of the disease.... Even the *prejudices*
> of the sick are not to be contemned, or opposed with harshness. For though
> silenced by authority, they will operate secretly and forcibly on the mind,
> creating fear, anxiety, and watchfulness.[93]

Thus, Richardson's medical tableaux in *Clarissa* are the literary model of
a new medical ethics of doctor–patient relationship, an ethics germinating
within a society striving to live the values of sensibility.

In a letter dated June 1762 to Dr John Moore, Tobias Smollett, then
forty-one years of age and suffering severely from asthma and consumption,
expressed sentiments very reminiscent of the fictional Clarissa. Smollett
addresses his doctor with kind regard and much gratitude – very different
from his tone with the haughty Dr Fizes – but at the same time announces
his resignation to his illness and his clear intention to retain final decision-
making power over his treatment:

> I am much affected by your kind concern for my health, and I believe the
> remedy you propose might have a happy effect; but it must be postponed. To
> tell you the truth, I have a presentiment that I shall never see Scotland
> again.... I might retrieve my constitution by a determined course of exercise
> and the cold bath; but neither my indolence nor my occupation will permit
> me to persevere in these endeavours.[94]

Smollett's confession to Dr Moore acknowledges what Percival was to
state so clearly in his *Medical Ethics*, that the mind has a profound influence
on therapeutic outcome, and that the patient is most acutely aware of his or

her own mental state and must, therefore, take personal responsibility for maintaining a healthy state.

While Smollett's resigned and rather gentle tone in his letter to his doctor is in no way characteristic of his novelistic style, the protagonist of *The Expedition of Humphry Clinker*, Matthew Bramble, communicates in his own testy manner that he is fully conscious how a troubled mood can undermine physical well-being as well as the interest to pursue those measures necessary for cure:

> I find my spirits and my health affect each other reciprocally – that is to say, every thing that discomposes my mind produces a correspondent disorder in my body; and my bodily complaints are remarkably mitigated by those considerations that dissipate the clouds of mental chagrin.... It must be owned, indeed, I took some of the tincture of ginseng, prepared according to your prescription, and found it exceedingly grateful to the stomach; but the pain and sickness continued to return, after short intervals, till the anxiety of my mind was entirely removed, and then I found myself perfectly at ease.[95]

Therefore, Bramble instructs his physician to be a good listener, appreciating fully the therapeutic value of a 'writing cure':

> Dear Doctor,

> If I did not know that the exercise of your profession has habituated you to the hearing of complaints, I should make a conscience of troubling you with my correspondence, which may truly be called the lamentations of Matthew Bramble. Yet I cannot help thinking, I have some right to discharge the overflowings of my spleen upon you, whose province it is to remove those disorders that occasioned it; and let me tell you, it is no small alleviation of my grievances, that I have a sensible friend, to whom I can communicate my crusty humours, which, by retention, would grow intolerably acrimonious.[96]

We shall see, from medicine-by-post letters, that the difference in the rhetorical tone of the fictional Clarissa and Matthew Bramble, in writing about their respective illnesses, reveals more than just the personal style of authors Richardson and Smollett, or even the nature of the protagonists of the novels, but reveals an underlying and pervasive difference in the rhetoric that was encouraged by society and the medical community at the time each of these novels was written. What is similar, however, is the appreciation of how mind and body interact and that the patient must remain the final judge of his or her own medical needs – the acknowledgment that the physician must finally defer to the patient's judgment regarding their own body.

Practical ethics and medicine

There is good reason to expect eighteenth-century doctor–patient correspondence to be revealing about both medical etiquette and medical ethics. As Lisbeth Haakonssen writes in *Medicine and Morals in the Enlightenment*, 'The aim of medical ethics was to portray the role of the medical man and the roles of those with whom he interacted.' For this reason the genres of character sketch – one should include Johnson's poem on Dr Levet – and conduct book were 'closely related' to writings on medical ethics; and it is no coincidence that Gregory and Percival considered their works as modelling moral behaviour for young men who aspired to a medical career.[97]

What becomes evident in reading medicine-by-post letters is that doctor–patient correspondence proved an welcome opportunity for the physician to display his moral character. This fact is most obvious in the letters of Drs George Cheyne and William Cullen to their patients, but it is a pervasive quality discovered in the medicine-by-post genre. The written interchange between doctor and patient also describes the moral responsibilities of the patient, and established physicians strictly admonish their clients to follow instructions and to be especially wary of bedside gossip – from well-meaning friends – that might tempt them to try frivolous cures and to seek perilous advice from empirics and other unscrupulous doctors. Indeed, the patient is to blame for any consequences of such imprudence and moral laxity! Patients equally write to their physicians to affirm that they have followed instructions to the letter, or else to apologise for moral lapses in attending to their health – either by omission, such as failing diet or other changes in habit, or for taking cures from other than their own physician.

In their introduction to *The Codification of Medical Morality*, Robert Baker, Dorothy Porter, and Roy Porter have written, 'It is today acknowledged that the eighteenth century constituted a crucial epoch in the crystallisation of medical ethics.' Among the significant reasons for this, they suggest, were the 'rising demand for medicine, the emergence of a more literate, more demanding public in the age of Enlightenment, the advent of a better-trained medical profession, many of whom had undergone a philosophically-oriented university education; the growth of new medical institutions, and so forth.'[98] But the authors, along with other contributors to this same volume on medical ethics, find more subtle changes in eighteenth-century society that resulted in the impulse to conceive a distinctly modern medical ethics.

Important among these societal changes was the breakdown of the trust in the gentleman's code of conduct. With the rise of the bourgeois power and prestige, and the rise of Puritan and dissenting religious groups, aristocratic mores were questioned. The aristocratic code of honour that required duelling was condemned as especially barbaric. For Thomas Percival the custom of duelling was not only repugnant to him personally but a subject worthy of inclusion in his *Medical Ethics*.[99] As Mary Fissell explains, 'It was [Lord] Chesterfield's letters to his son, published in 1774, which revealed what many already knew and accepted – that good manners were not so much a sign of innate virtue as the indicator of social expedience.... [The] manipulative quality of politeness was denounced.'[100] Fine manners, as exemplified by the aristocracy and upper classes, was no longer, of itself, a sufficient assurance of professional integrity.

Such changes were important in terms of medical ethics because in the early part of the century it was the popular literature on manners and courtesy that had served to instruct medical apprentices how to behave with patients – and with others within the profession – and which had provided guidelines for physicians who wanted to present themselves as gentlemen to their aristocratic patrons. There was no such instruction specifically designed for medical practitioners. What finally came to replace the obsolete 'gentleman's code' was the model of the 'man of feeling', a model of sincerity which encompassed the ideals of the Scottish Enlightenment philosophers and influenced ethicists and medical moralists.

The philosophical idea of a 'moral sense' – a term originating with Lord Shaftesbury – was expanded upon by the Scottish philosopher Dr Frances Hutchinson (1694–1746), and it was then taken up by David Hume and Adam Smith. Their descriptions of the highly valued qualities of 'sensibility' and 'sympathy', manifested in polite society, corresponded with medical descriptions of the function of the nervous system as taught by prestigious medical lecturers at the University of Edinburgh, professors such as Robert Whytt (1714–66) and William Cullen (1710–90). It was on these principles that John Gregory based his *Lectures on the Duties and Qualifications of a Physician*.[101] When Gregory, addressing Edinburgh students from diverse religious and social background, described 'the moral qualities peculiarly required in the character of a physician', he used a rhetoric derived from philosophy and from the novel of sensibility: 'Sympathy produces an anxious attention to a thousand little circumstances that may tend to relieve the patient.'[102]

In keeping with an important segment of Scottish Enlightenment thinking, Gregory's medical ethics is based on a philosophy that esteems motivation over action, and believes that 'true moral sentiments would make themselves apparent in those of merit.'[103] Gregory, in his condemnation of pretentious dress and other insincere artifice, is gendering the profession of medicine as masculine in contrast to the perceived effeminate manners of a dying aristocracy.

Haakonssen has argued compellingly that late-eighteenth-century medical moralists (Gregory, Percival, Gisborne, and Benjamin Rush) were developing a modern medical ethics derived from a longstanding tradition of 'practical ethics,' which conjoined Christian duties with the Hippocratic–Galenic–Baconian ideal of the moral physician and natural philosopher. 'Practical ethics' was concerned with the application of theoretical ethics to the duties of daily life and to professional obligations. The concentration of interest in this form of medical ethics in Scotland, and its dissemination by those associated with the study of medicine at the University of Edinburgh, is explained by the origins of 'practical ethics' in a Protestant natural law tradition prevalent in Scotland since the seventeenth century.[104]

It was this foundation of 'practical ethics' for medical ethics that invited non-medical writers to have a voice in describing the moral obligations of physicians. Among the most prominent of these conduct books for physicians was Thomas Gisborne's *An Enquiry into the Duties of Men in the Higher and Middle Classes of Society in Great Britain, Resulting from their Respective Stations, Professions and Employments* (1794). Gisborne (1748–1846) was a renowned divine in the Church of England who took as his model for the ideal physician the Christian gentleman.[105] It was such merging of Christian medical values, of generosity and gentleness, with classical medical ethics, that characterises the latter decades of the eighteenth century.

Classical medical training, as perpetuated at Oxford and Cambridge, instilled the idea that the moral character of a physician was not innate but cultivated only by long years of study and experience. This translated, in modern England, into moral integrity being the reserve of those privileged, Church of England physicians who had trained at Oxford and Cambridge, with all others being suspect intruders and unethical physicians (as illustrated earlier in this chapter by the interchange between Dr Looby and Count Fathom in Smollett's *The Adventures of Ferdinand Count Fathom*). The established English physician was concerned with his practice, the individual patient, and maintaining the 'guild' exclusivity of the Royal College of Physicians. In contrast, the traditions of Christian medicine, and the Paracelsian tradition, emphasised charity towards the sick and needy and provided care to the larger community, preferred gentler cures over the harsh purges and emetics of classical medicine, and encouraged patient self-help. The Christian ethic deplored the severity of modern treatments and the apparent greed and secrecy of the established medical brotherhood, which it judged immoral for those very reasons.[106]

What Haakonssen and others do not explain fully is why the established British medical profession, so firmly based in classical teaching, and for so long resistant to Christian tenets of healing, should be ready to adopt 'practical ethics' into the education of doctors during the final decades of the eighteenth century, and to make 'sensibility' and 'sympathy' the model qualities of the Enlightenment physician. To argue that this was the culmination of a philosophy of 'practical ethics' in Scotland seems insufficient. First, as will be seen in the medicine-by-post of mid-eighteenth century, there already was, in England, clear indications of a new ideal of physician character being formed, with doctors who wished to distance themselves from the image of the classically-trained, insensitive and aloof, physician. Second, the effects of Scottish influence passed readily outside of Scotland, showing this was not a local phenomenon. It seems much more persuasive that a broader effect on medicine in Britain had readied the profession for adopting 'practical ethics' and for incorporating Christian medical values as well – such as the expanding physician interest in the community, in city and town, hygiene and military and hospital health.[107]

The study of medicine-by-post shows that established medicine was able to accommodate the idea of a new medical ethics because of two critical developments, the speculative system of 'nervous sensibility' replacing the iatromechanical model of human physiology, and the dramatically new rhetoric that this paradigm shift engendered – a rhetoric that simultaneously, and with circularity, infected both medical and lay consciousness. The language of doctor–patient communication experienced a metamorphosis that redefined the ideal of physician character and the profession's moral obligations to both individual patient and to society. Indeed, Thomas Gisborne eloquently defined the moral contract between physician and those he served in a manner that would profoundly influenced Percival in writing his *Medical Ethics* at the turn of the century.

In this setting, it is hardly surprising that established doctors, to achieve professional recognition and authority, were ever diligent in renewing their efforts to satisfy their patron–patients by fully adopting fashionable philosophical trends and social refinements. Such pressures not only influenced the ideal of physician character but also shaped the character of medical knowledge itself, as described in the seminal work of N.D. Jewson.[108] In the following pages, I expand on Jewson's observations by showing how those societal tastes that modulated physician behaviour were themselves shaped by prevailing medical speculation on human physiology. The reciprocal influence of the rhetoric of the eighteenth-century medical and social worlds, as exposed in the changing rhetoric of medicine-by-post, explains the urgency of a reconceived modern medical ethics.

Notes

1. Richard Mead (1673–1754), an eminent London physician, and William Cheselden (1688–1752), a famous surgeon. Cheselden was a remarkable technician who was able to remove a bladder stone in under a minute – no small virtue in an age without anaesthesia!

2. D. Porter and R. Porter, *Patient's Progress: Doctors and Doctoring in Eighteenth-Century England* (Stanford: Stanford University Press, 1989), 76–8.

3. Please note that I use the pronoun 'he' for physicians because in this period the physicians were, in fact, all male. Women were active in midwifery and alternative ('unorthodox') medicine. On the state of physical examination in the eighteenth century, see Porter and Porter, *ibid.*, 74–5; R. Porter, *The Greatest Benefit to Mankind: A Medical History of Humanity* (New York: W. W. Norton and Company, 1997), 257; and, I. Loudon, *Medical Care and the General Practitioner 1750-1850* (Oxford: Clarendon Press, 1986), 18–19. An example of the slow adoption of instruments to assist in medical examination is the fact that Auenbrugger (1722–1809) described the technique of percussion of the chest in the late eighteenth century, but it was not adopted till the nineteenth century after Laennec (1781–1826) published his famous treatise on the use of the stethoscope in 1819. Such instruments and definitive hands-on examination techniques, only had meaning when conjoined with an understanding of pathological anatomy, also developed at the turn of the century.

4. T. Percival, *Medical Ethics: Or a Code of Institutes and Precepts Adapted to the Professional conduct of Physicians and Surgeons* (Manchester, 1803), 45. See Chapter 4 for examples of the variable fees received by Dr William Cullen in his extensive medicine-by-post practice in Edinburgh.

5. Johnson to Dr Thomas Lawrence (1711–83), 1 May 1782, in *The Letters of Samuel Johnson*, 6 vols., B. Redford (ed.), (Princeton: Princeton University Press, 1992), IV: 34 (Latin) and V: 53 (English translation). All subsequent references to the letters of Samuel Johnson in this chapter are from this collection and will be cited as *Letters*.

6. Eminent American doctors (such as Benjamin Rush) often had received some part of their medical training in Europe, especially at Leyden or Edinburgh. Rush, for example, had attended lectures at Edinburgh and regarded William Cullen as his most influential mentor. See J.M. O'Donnell, 'Cullen's Influence on American Medicine,' in *William Cullen and the Eighteenth Century Medical World* (Edinburgh: Edinburgh University Press, 1993), 234–46. American doctors not only resorted to consulting with their European teachers and colleagues but also depended on European medical journals. Rush was greatly upset when the flow of European medical journals

51

to America was interrupted by the British blockade during the American
Revolution. He wrote Cullen in 1783: "One of the severest taxes paid by our
profession during the war was occasioned by the want of a regular supply of
books from Europe." From R.J. Kahn and P.G. Kahn, 'The *Medical
Repository* – The First U.S. Medical Journal (1797–1824)', *The New
England Journal of Medicine,* 337, 26 (December 25, 1997): 1926.

7. T. Smollett, *The Expedition of Humphry Clinker*, R.R. Preston and O.M.
    Brack, Jr. (eds), (Athens: The University of Georgia Press, 1990), 7. 'Reins'
    are the kidneys.

8. See N.D. Jewson, 'Medical Knowledge and the Patronage System in 18th
    Century England', *Sociology,* 8 (1974), 369–85

9. B. Mandeville, *A Treatise of the Hypochondriack and Histerick Diseases*
    (1711); Second Edition: Corrected and Enlarged by the Author (1730), in
    Volume 2 of *The Collected Works of Bernard Mandeville* (Facsimile Editions),
    (New York: Verlag, 1981).

10. R. Porter, 'Laymen, Doctors and Medical Knowledge in the Eighteenth
    Century: The Evidence of the *Gentleman's Magazine,*' in *Patients and
    Practitioners,* R. Porter (ed.), (Cambridge: Cambridge University Press,
    1985), 283–314. On the proliferation of medical printed matter, see also
    G. Holmes, *Augustan England: Professions, State and Society, 1680-1730*
    (Boston: George Allen & Unwin, 1982), 167.

11. Physicians might exercise their knowledge of Latin to impress patients or
    consult amongst themselves, but this practice was satirised in almost every
    late seventieth and eighteenth-century play that represented the medical
    profession. Examples of doctors ridiculed for their pretentious use of
    Latinisms include Aphra Behn's *Sir Patient Fancy* (1678) and *Three Hours
    After Marriage* (1717) by Alexander Pope, with John Gay and Dr John
    Arbuthnot. Samuel Johnson, however, felt quite at home writing to his
    physician and friend, Dr Robert Lawrence, in Latin.

12. M. Altschule M.D., 'The Doctor–Patient Relationship Through the Ages,'
    Alabama Journal of Medical Sciences 21, 4 (1984), 438. Altschule was
    president of the Boston Medical Library, 1976–9, as well as curator of prints
    and photographic materials in the rare books department of Countway
    Library of Medicine, Harvard Medical School, 1970–88.

13. T. Smollett, *Travels Through France and Italy* (1766), F. Felsenstein (ed.),
    (New York: Oxford University Press, 1979), 89.

14. C. Houlihan Flynn, 'Running Out of Matter', in *The Languages of Psyche:
    Mind and Body in Enlightenment Thought,* G.S. Rousseau (ed.), (Berkeley:
    University of California Press, 1990), 147–85.

15. R. Baker, D. Porter, and R. Porter (eds), *The Codification of Medical
    Morality: Historical and Philosophical Studies of the Formalization of Western
    Medical: Volume 1, Medical Ethics and Etiquette in the Eighteenth Century*

(Boston: Kluwer Academic Publishers, 1993), 6.

16. L. Haakonssen, *Medicine and Morals in the Enlightenment: John Gregory, Thomas Percival and Benjamin Rush* (Amsterdam-Atlanta, GA: Rodopi, 1997), 34.

17. S. Richardson, *Clarissa: Or The History of a Lady*, A. Ross (ed.), (New York: Viking, 1985), 1277. Perhaps the character of Dr H. was inspired by Dr Cheyne, but there are no allusions to any physical similarities to Cheyne as one might expect if Richardson intended any direct comparison with his own doctor.

18. H. Fielding, *The History of Tom Jones, A Foundling*, F. Bowers (ed.), (Connecticut, CT: Weslyan University Press, 1975), VIII, xiii, p. 468.

19. H. Fielding, *Amelia* (1751), D. Blewett (ed.), (London: Penguin Books, 1987), III, ii, p. 98. *Amelia* is discussed in more detail here in Chapter 5. Also in Chapter 2 there is a full description of Fielding's vicious satirical attack on physician James Jurin, in which Fielding took John Randy's side in a heated pamphlet war over the treatment of Sir Robert Walpole's bladder stone.

20. Johnson to Dr Thomas Lawrence, 16 April 1783; *Letters*, IV: 123.

21. J. Boswell, *London Journal: 1762–1763*, F.A. Pottle (ed.), (New York: McGraw-Hill, 1950), 156.

22. Boswell, *ibid.*, 157–8. W. Ober refers to this episode to illustrate the 'ambivalence of the doctor–patient relation' in 'Boswell's Clap', in *Boswell's Clap and other Essays: Medical Analyses of Literary Men's Afflictions* (Carbondale: Southern Illinois University Press, 1979), 7.

23. A quotation from Sir John Hawkin, *Life of Johnson*, in J. Boswell, *The Life of Samuel Johnson*, 6 vols., G.B. Hill (ed.), (New York: Bigelow, Brown & Company, 1921), 3, 25, footnote.

24. Smollett, *op. cit* (note 7), 25.

25. *Ibid.*, 324.

26. By 'established physicians', I am specifically referring to those English doctors, Anglican, who had trained at Oxford or Cambridge, and were accepted as members and fellows into the Royal College of Physicians in London – an elite group. 'Regular' or 'qualified' physicians refers to a broader group of doctors who followed accepted 'orthodox' medical practices and usually had some basic medical training, though not at Oxford or Cambridge. 'Irregular' doctors consisted of a mix of those who were considered 'unqualified' by any formal medical education and who often employed 'unorthodox' alternative medical treatments and advertised their own proprietary elixirs and cure-alls. As such, there was an array of 'irregular' practitioners, ranging from 'unqualified' but orthodox practitioners to itinerants, empiricists, and faith healers. Except for 'established' physicians, the terms are not precise and there is great overlap in the types of medical

practice that were available to the public. These terms were appropriated indiscriminately by doctors to cast aspersions on one another, and the terms quack and charlatan were used freely to attack rivals in the healing profession. See Loudon, *op. cit.* (note 3),11–28. Also, the relation between regular and irregular doctors in Britain is examined in W.F. Bynum and R. Porter (eds), *Medical Fringe and Medical Orthodoxy 1750-1850*, (London: Croom Helm, 1987).

27. Boswell, *op. cit.* (note 23), 1: 281–2; Robert Levet, or Levett (1704–82).

28. S. Johnson, 'On the Death of Robert Levet (1783)', in D. Greene (ed.), *The Oxford Authors, Samuel Johnson*, (New York: Oxford University Press, 1984), 35–6.

29. See J. Wiltshire, *Samuel Johnson in the Medical World: The Doctor and the Patient* (New York: Cambridge University Press, 1991), 195–222, for a detailed analysis of this poem in the light of eighteenth-century medical practice.

30. According to Johnson biographer W. Jackson Bate, Levet came from a poor Yorkshire family. After working in London, most likely in the capacity of servant, he became a waiter in Paris. His medical education consisted of attending some medical lectures in anatomy and pharmacy at the University of Paris on the invitation of some surgeon patrons of the place where Levet waited on tables; see W. Jackson Bate, *Samuel Johnson* (New York: Harcourt Brace Jovanovich, 1975), 271. D. Porter and R. Porter have described Levet as good example of those 'empirics and itinerants providing cheap, if unqualified and unreliable, medical services to the lower classes, to those who could afford medicines costing no more than a glass of ale....', *op. cit.* (note 2), 11.

31. Boswell, *op. cit.* (note 23), 1:282.

32. Johnson to Dr Lawrence, 17 January 1782; *Letters*, IV, 6. Thomas Lawrence (or Laurence) was Oxford trained and was president of the London College of Physicians from 1767–74.

33. Jackson Bate, *op. cit.* (note 30), 563.

34. Johnson to Hill Boothy, 30 December 1755, *Letters*, 1:117. Miss Hill Boothby, 1708–56, is described in the *Dictionary of National Biography* as 'a woman of considerable ability', whom Johnson befriended only a few years before her death. That Johnson developed much affection for her is evidenced by the warms epithets he uses to address her in the letters, such as 'my sweet angel' and 'Dearest Dear'.

35. Haakonssen, *op. cit.* (note 16), 27–35.

36. R. Porter, *Health for Sale: Quackery in England 1660–1850* (New York: Manchester University Press, 1989), 54.

37. Pringle was renowned for his contribution to military hygiene.

38. J. Boswell, *In Search of a Wife, 1766–1769*, F. Brady and F.A. Pottle (eds),

(London: McGraw-Hill Book Co., 1956), 290. See also, Ober, *op. cit.* (note 22), 16. The Lisbon Diet Drink was a 'tonic diet drink', a concoction of sarsaparilla, sassafras, guaiac, glycerrhiza (root of liquorice) and mezereum (bark of root of spurge laurel). See J.W. Estes, *Dictionary of Protopharmacology: Therapeutic Practices, 1700–1850* (Canton, MA: Science History Publications, 1990).

39. See M.E. Fissell, *Patients, Power, and the Poor in Eighteenth-century Bristol* (New York: Cambridge University Press, 1991), ch. 2 and 3; J. Barry, 'Piety and the Patient: Medicine and Religion in Eighteenth-Century Bristol', in R. Porter (ed.), *Patients and Practitioners: Lay Perceptions of Medicine in Pre-Industrial Society* (New York: Cambridge University Press, 1985), 145–76. See also Porter and Porter, *op. cit.* (note 2), 79–81.

40. For a discussion of what constituted the middle class in eighteenth-century Britain, see P. Langford, *A Polite and Commercial People: England 1727-1783* (New York: Oxford University Press, 1989), 61–8.

41. However, on the particulars of Johnson's knowledge of medicine, see Wiltshire, see *op. cit.* (note 29), Chapter 2.

42. Johnson to Hester Thrale, 15 June 1771; *Letters*, I, 361–2.

43. Johnson to Edmund Hector, 12 December 1772; *Letters*, I, 416.

44. Johnson to Thomas Cummings, 25 May 1774; *Letters*, II, 140–1.

45. Johnson to Thrale, 28 January 1782; *Letters*, IV, 7.

46. Johnson to Thrale, 14 March 1782; *Letters*, IV, 19. In this case, Johnson was phlebotomised the equivalent of a pint of blood in modern blood bank units. What Johnson calls asthma and dropsy, and which has been interpreted as 'bronchitis' by twentieth-century doctors, according to Redford, *op. cit.* (note 5), to me suggests congestive heart failure, in which case phlebotomy would serve to relieve symptoms of shortness of breath and fluid overload. In a letter to Hester Thrale, Johnson writes, 'my nights are bad, very bad' (17 June 1784; IV, 334), a typical complaint of patients with congestive heart failure who experience worse symptoms when recumbent. In January of 1782, Johnson wrote to Thrale that after a surgeon was called to draw out sixteen ounces of blood, 'I... had an Elysian night compared to the nights past' (6 January 1782; IV, 6).

47. Johnson to Thrale, 24 August 1780; *Letters*, III, 304–5.

48. Johnson to Thrale, 20 April 1780; *Letters*, III, 242.

49. Johnson to Rev. John Taylor, 19 June 1784; *Letters*, IV, 335.

50. Johnson to Thrale, 8 May 1782; *Letters*, IV, 38. The 'chymical sect' refers to followers of Paracelsus.

51. Boswell, *op. cit.* (note 23), Vol. 2, 378.

52. Johnson to Hill Boothby, 31 December 1755; *Letters*, I, 120–1.

53. Johnson to Boothby, 3 January 1756; *Letters*, I, 122–3.

54. Johnson to Bennet Langdon, 17 April 1775; *Letters*, II, 200–1.

55. Johnson to Elizabeth Lawrence, 26 August 1782; *Letters*, IV, 71.

56. Boswell, *op. cit.* (note 23), Vol. 4, 338.

57. Johnson to Boswell, 2 March 1784; in Boswell, *op. cit.* (note 23), Vol. 4, 303. Bulb of squill, or sea onion, was used as a diuretic; see under 'Scilla' in Estes, *op. cit.* (note 38), 174.

58. Boswell to Edinburgh physicians, 7 March 1784, *op. cit.* (note 23), Vol. 4, 304. The reference is to Johnson's portrait of Samuel Garth (1670?–1718/19), physician and poet of 'The Dispensary' and other works, in *Lives of the Poets* (1777), (New York: E.P. Dutton & Co., 1925); quotation is found on 315 (1961 reprint).

59. As subsequent chapters will show, this formalised mode of medical writing predominated in the earlier part of the eighteenth century as an extension of the 'new science' rhetoric prescribed by the Royal Society (see Chapter 2). Over the century, this deliberate, objective style of medical history persisted within medicine-by-post, but intermixed, as here, in a letter that also referred to the subjective concerns of the patient and the correspondent writing on the patient's behalf.

60. Vinegar, called 'acetum,' was used for medicinal compounds. It served as a mild diuretic and refrigerant (a medicine which decreases body temperature by reducing the force of circulation, used for inflammation and fevers); see note above re: squills. For more details, see under 'Acetum' and 'Refrigeration' in Estes, *op. cit.* (note 38).

61. Johnson to Bennet Langdon, 20 March 1782; *Letters*, IV, 23.

62. B. Redford, *The Converse of the Pen: Act of Intimacy in the Eighteenth-Century Familiar Letter* (Chicago: University of Chicago Press, 1986), 217. See also C. McIntosh, *The Evolution of English Prose* (New York: Cambridge University Press, 1998), 131–7.

63. In the concluding chapter of this book, I reconsider Johnson's rhetorical style in some of these same letters, and also in his letters composed in Latin to Dr Lawrence, in the context of the changes in rhetorical style in medicine-by-post over the course of the century.

64. As will become evident in later chapters, physicians might take extraordinary liberties in regard to patient confidentiality, as Cheyne did in his correspondence and popular medical works (see Chapter 3). Patient confidentiality did not become formalised as an obligation of medical ethics until the last decades of the eighteenth century, in the works of John Gregory and Thomas Percival (see Chapter 4).

65. J. Habermaas, *The Structural Transformation of the Public Sphere: An Inquiry into a Category of Bourgeois Society*, translated by T. Burger (Cambridge, MA: The MIT Press, 1989, paperback edition 1991), 49. This topic is taken up in much greater detail in Chapter 3.

66. See also L.W.B. Brockliss, *Calvet's Web: Enlightenment and the Republic of*

Letters in Eighteenth-Century France (New York: Oxford University Press, 2002), 96–104, especially 102–3. Brockliss illustrates that even within the republic of letters, the 'savant' correspondence dedicated to natural history and antiquary matters, there was an expectation of sharing local gossip with circles of 'mini-republics'.

67. Johnson to Dr Lawrence, 17 June 1767, Litchfield; *Letters*, I, 282–3.
68. T. Lawrence, *Hydrops* (1756). Dropsy is a fluid collection presenting in any part in the body.
69. Johnson to Dr Lawrence, 20 June 1767, Litchfield; *Letters*, I, 284.
70. Johnson to Dr Lawrence, 21 January 1782; *Letters*, IV, 7 (Latin), V, 51 (English translation).
71. 'Spirit' is here used in the Latin sense, meaning 'breath'.
72. Johnson to Dr Lawrence, 20 March 1782; *Letters*, IV, 24–5 (Latin), V, 52 (English prose translation by B. Redford).
73. H.J. Cook, in *Trials of an Ordinary Doctor: James Groenevelt in Seventeenth-Century London* (Baltimore: The Johns Hopkins University Press, 1994), recounts a dramatic case of a Dutch physician, Joannes Groenevelt, whose career in England was destroyed largely because of his repeated efforts to commercialise his practice. He not only advertised a group medical practice through the mail, but also published his own specialised surgical technique to remove bladder stones, and later claimed he had a secret formula for dissolving stones. Groenevelt was not only a foreigner, but also a substantial threat to the business of other physicians, and he thereby made himself a highly vulnerable target for the College of Physicians of London, whose leaders had reinvigorated their efforts to regain a tight control over all medical practice in the city limits. When a patient complained she had suffered grave consequences from taking Groenevelt's pills for the stone, the Censors of the College of Physicians of London were especially aggressive in pursuing the case.
74. D. Defoe, *A Journal of the Plague Year* (1722); A. Burgess and C. Bristow (eds), Shakespeare Head edition (Oxford: Blackwell, 1928), 35–6. Subsequent page references in text, in parentheses.
75. Andrew Wear lists the 'diverse range of practitioners' of the seventeenth century as including, in addition to regular physicians, iatrochemists (followers of Paracelsus), 'patients and their families, neighbours, charitable gentlewomen or noblewomen, clergymen and their wives, wise-women, uroscopists, astrologers, herbalists, and empirics'. See 'Medicine in Early Modern Europe, 1500-1700', in L.I.Conrad, M. Neve, V. Nutton, R. Porter and A. Wear (eds), *The Western Medical Tradition* (New York: Cambridge University Press, 1995), 321.
76. Venice treacle consisted of opium, scilla (bulb of sea onion) and some fifty-seven other ingredients; see Estes, *op. cit.* (note 38).

77. Barry, *op. cit* (note 39), 145–76.

78. Barry, *ibid.*, 153–4.

79. *Ibid.*, 151.

80. *Ibid.*, 159.

81. See, for example, the correspondence between Dr James Jurin and Bishop Cari in Chapter 2.

82. B. Mandeville, *A Treatise of the Hypochondriack and Histerick Diseases*, iv.

83. T. Smollett, *The Adventures of Ferdinand Count Fathom*, J.C. Beasley (ed.), (Athens: The University of Georgia Press, 1988), 241. Subsequent page references in text, in parentheses.

84. Sir John Hawkins, in his *Life of Johnson*, comments that, 'The physicians in Hogarth's prints are not caricatures: the full dress with sword and a *great tye-wig*, and the hat under the arm, and the doctors in consultation, each smelling [*sic*] to a gold-headed cane... are picture of real life in his time.' See footnote in Boswell, *op. cit.* (note 23), 327. Tunbridge Wells was a major health spa and an ideal choice for Fathom.

85. Smollett, like most other Scottish and foreign physicians, would have been denied the study of medicine at Oxford or Cambridge, where enrolment was restricted to members of the Church of England. Smollett's medical training consisted of an apprenticeship, in 1736, to the Glasgow surgeons William Stirling and John Gordon. It seems likely that he had attended classes at Glasgow University prior to the apprenticeship but never matriculated. In 1740 Smollett became surgeon's second mate in the Royal Navy. In 1744 he opened a surgical practice in London, in Downing Street. Only in 1750 did he purchase an MD (not an uncommon practice) from Marischal College, Aberdeen, for £28. The fact that the London medical establishment was unwelcoming to Scottish physicians would seem to account only in small part for Smollett's limited success in the London medical scene.

86. S. Bard, *A Discourse on the Duties of a Physician* (1769) first published by A. & J. Robertson of New York in 1769 (Bedford, MA: Applewood Books 1996), 19.

87. S. Richardson, *op. cit.* (note 17), 1075. Subsequent page references in parentheses are in text. Unless otherwise specified, all letters are from Bedford to Lovelace.

88. J. Gregory, *Lectures on the Duties and Qualifications of a Physician* (London, 1772), 19–20. A student of Gregory's had published an unauthorised version of the lectures in 1770, prompting Gregory to produce his own 'New Edition, corrected and enlarged' in 1772.

89. *Ibid.*, 19–20.

90. Haakonssen, *op. cit.* (note 16), 52–3.

91. Percival, *op. cit.* (note 4), 125–6.

92. Haakonssen, *op. cit.* (note 16), 153–4.

93. Percival, *op. cit.* (note 4), 10–11.
94. *The Letters of Tobias Smollett*, L.M. Knapp (ed.), (Oxford: Clarendon Press, 1970), 105–7. The term asthma is used in the eighteenth century to represent the same symptoms that we describe today, shortness of breath with wheezing.
95. *Ibid.*, 151.
96. *Ibid.*, 33–4.
97. Haakonssen, *op. cit.* (note 16), 35.
98. Baker, 'Introduction', *op. cit.* (note 15), 3.
99. Percival, *op. cit.* (note 4), 138.
100. M. Fissell, 'Innocent and Honorable Bribes: Medical Manners in Eighteenth-Century Britain', in Baker, *op. cit.* (note 15), 19–45. For a very complete picture of the discrediting of the aristocratic ideal coincident with the rise of the middle class, and the 'sentimental revolution,' in eighteenth-century Britain, see Langford, *op. cit.* (note 40), Chapters 3 and 10. Langford describes the advantages to middle-class social mobility, and hence the enormous appeal, of adopting a 'code of genteel conduct' based on sensibility over the more rigid requirements of landed property and wealth which had dominated until the mid-eighteenth century (464).
101. T. Beauchamp, 'Common Sense and Virtue in the Scottish Moralists', in Baker, *ibid.*, 99–121. See also L.B. McCullough, 'John Gregory's Medical Ethics and Humean Sympathy', in Baker, Porter and Porter, *op. cit.* (note 15), 145–60. Christopher Lawrence provides detailed insight into the relationship of 'The Nervous System and Society in the Scottish Enlightenment', in *Natural Order: Historical Studies of Scientific Culture*, B. Barnes and S. Shapin (eds), (Beverly Hills: Sage Publications, 1979), 19–40.
102. J. Gregory, *op. cit.* (note 88), 19. For more on Gregory and the University of Edinburgh, see Chapter 4.
103. Fissell, *op. cit.* (note 100), 34–6. Later in the century, physicians such as Thomas Beddoes and James Makittrick Adair were particularly critical of the influence of fashion on the public's attitude towards health and disease and on the behaviour of physicians: see R. Porter, '"Expressing Yourself Ill": The Language of Sickness in Georgian England', in *Language, Self, and Society*, P. Burke and R. Porter (eds), (Cambridge: Polity Press, 1991), 276–99; also R. Porter, 'Civilisation and Disease: Medical Ideology in the Enlightenment', in J. Beach and J. Gregory (eds), *Culture, Politics, and Society: Britain 1660–1800* (Manchester: Manchester University Press, 1991), 154–83.
104. Haakonssen, *op. cit.* (note 16), 27–35.
105. Gisborne's *An Enquiry into the Duties of Men* went through six editions between 1794 and 1811. See R. Porter, 'Thomas Gisborne: Physicians, Christians and Gentlemen', in A. Wear, J. Geyer-Kordesch and R. French,

(eds), *Doctors and Ethics: The Earlier Historical Setting of Professional Ethics*, Clio Medica 24 (Amsterdam-Atlanta, GA: Rodopi, 1993), 252–73.

106. See A. Wear, 'Medical Ethics in Early Modern England', *ibid.*, 98–130.

107. M. Foucault, 'The Politics of Health in the Eighteenth Century' (1976) in C. Gordon (ed.), *Power/Knowledge: Selected Interviews and Other Writings, 1972–1977* (New York: Pantheon Books, 1980), 166–82. Foucault argues in this essay that the eighteenth-century physician gained a 'politically privileged position' in his role as 'the great advisor and expert' in matters of hygiene rather than in his role as therapist. It would be only in the nineteenth century that, according to Foucault, the doctor would base his political power on his wealth and social status.

108. Jewson, *op. cit.* (note 8).

2

New Science Rhetoric in Medicine-by-Post:
The Private Practice Correspondence of Dr James Jurin

I am very sorry to find that you are in so indifferent a State of health, & it
would be a matter of exceeding pleasure to me, if I could be any way
instrumental in amending it; but you know Sir, how difficult it is to give
proper directions at so great a distance, especially when the case is not very
particularly & exactly stated.

James Jurin to Paul Dudley,
Attorney General of Massachusetts[1]

The rhetoric of medicine-by-post modulated in character over the course of
the eighteenth century in close accord with the ideology and language of
medicine and natural philosophy fashionable to particular decades of the
Enlightenment. The efforts of the Royal Society of London, from the late-
seventeenth century, to establish a rhetoric suitable to the goals of the 'new
science' – the empirical science of Bacon galvanised by Newtonian
mathematics – strongly influenced doctor–patient correspondence in the
first three decades of the eighteenth century. The patient and doctor voice in
this period was configured in a distinct manner by the prescriptions and
proscriptions of the new science rhetoric which modelled a detached
objectivity in all scientific-related observation; subjectivity was actively
discredited, even in respect to one's body in time of illness. However, by the
close of the fourth decade one can discern the introduction of subjectivity in
the narration of the case history in medicine-by-post: the first hints of a
medicine of sensibility (based on the nervous system) replacing the
iatromechanical (hydraulic) medical theories favoured by the doctors who
practiced in the shadow of Newton.

Dr James Jurin (1684–1750), secretary to the Royal Society from 1721
to 1727 (during the presidency of Sir Isaac Newton), was representative of
the elite physicians associated with the new science. He was an 'established'
physician, part of that exclusive club of physicians who had received their
medical degrees from Oxford or Cambridge and were licensed by the Royal
College of Physicians of London to practice medicine in London and its
immediate environs.[2] Furthermore, Jurin was strongly identified with the
proponents of iatromechanical medicine, those physicians who were
attempting to apply Newtonian mathematics and physics to human

physiology and who were immensely influenced by the medical empiricism of the influential Leiden physician and teacher Hermann Boerhaave. Iatromechanical medicine was not only a major influence on speculative medical thought during the first third of the eighteenth century but largely shaped its rhetoric.[3]

Jurin's biography, as detailed by Andrea Rusnock in her edition of Jurin's correspondence, provides a valuable example of the social background and educational experience of an accomplished physician of the early-eighteenth century.[4] To begin with, it is evident how much a career in medicine owed to patronage and influential family contacts in addition to one's natural abilities. Jurin was born in London in 1684. His father was a member of the Dyer's Company and his maternal uncle, Caleb Cotesworth, was an eminent physician. Through the influence of a relation, John Houblon, Lord Mayor of London and first Governor of the Bank of England, Jurin entered the Royal Mathematical School at Christ's Hospital. His success there led to a full scholarship at Trinity College, Cambridge, where he received a BA degree in 1705, became a Fellow in 1708, and earned a Masters degree in 1709. That same year, in common with many young men who aspired to the study of medicine and natural philosophy, Jurin went to Leyden to attend the lectures of Boerhaave. He was accompanied by his close college friend, Mordecai Cary, who was to become the Bishop of Cloyne and Killala (and whose medicine-by-post letters to Jurin are detailed later in this chapter). Jurin did not get a medical degree while at Leyden but returned to England to take the position of Head Master of the Newcastle-upon-Tyne Public School, a position he acquired through the patronage of Richard Bentley, classicist and Master of Trinity College.[5] At Newcastle, Jurin 'offered a series of courses on mathematics and mechanics to the general public, making him one of the first to lecture publicly outside of London on Newtonian natural philosophy.'[6] He remained in Newcastle till 1715 when a dispute with the town over money and friction with various citizens resulted in his departure to Cambridge to seek a medical degree, now made possible by the 'considerable sum' of funds he had accumulated while lecturing and teaching in Newcastle.[7]

Jurin's interest in medicine may have followed from time spent at Leiden, but Rusnock also suggests that 'the promise of financial security and a successful life in London cannot be dismissed as factors in his decision' to turn to a medical career.[8] Therefore, Jurin returned to Cambridge to get his M.D. in 1716 and, with the help of his physician uncle, established a successful practice. In 1724 he married the well-to-do widow of a Northumbrian landowner. Jurin became Secretary to the Royal Society in 1721, his tenure lasting till Newton's death in 1727. He was highly regarded for his knowledge of natural philosophy as well as medicine, and he made

Figure 2.1

Portrait of James Jurin (1684–1750) by James Worsdale.
© The Royal Society.

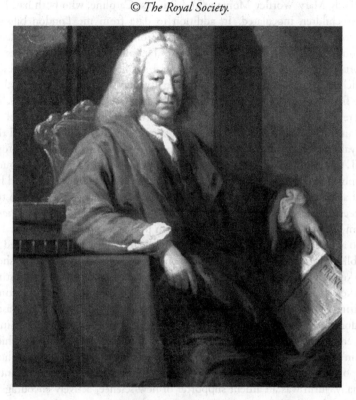

Signature of James Jurin.
Courtesy: Wellcome Library, London.

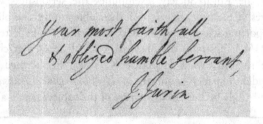

impressive intellectual contributions in the areas of capillary and fluid dynamics, the force of the heart as pump, optics, and meteorology, especially as applied to health. Jurin was recognised most in his own time for establishing the safety and benefit of smallpox inoculation through the use of comparative mortality statistics. In the early 1720s, smallpox inoculation was still quite controversial despite the very public advocacy of the procedure by Lady Mary Wortley Montagu and Princess Caroline, who both had had their children inoculated. In addition to data from the London bills of mortality, Jurin collected case reports from physician correspondents throughout Britain and New England. He published yearly updates of mortality ratios (inoculated versus natural smallpox deaths) in pamphlets which were praised for their 'strict neutrality' and which were influential in the final acceptance of inoculation by the medical community (22–7). As Secretary to the Royal Society, Jurin reinvigorated epistolary communications with scientists in Europe and America and established the Royal Society as the premier clearing house for scientific inquiry in Europe and America. Jurin's facility with English, Latin, and various foreign tongues, combined with his scientific, mathematical, and medical knowledge, and his tact as critic of papers submitted to the Royal Society, all contributed to the success of his tenure as Secretary. As editor of the *Philosophical Transactions*, from 1720–27, he popularised Newtonian principles and breathed new life into a dying publication. He was also a public figure who readily engaged in public controversies. On two occasions Jurin refuted works by Bishop Berkeley: once defending the validity of the new calculus and protesting Berkeley's assertion that modern mathematics led to atheism; another time writing a satirical critique in response to Berkeley's overly-enthusiastic endorsement of tar water as a panacea. Jurin also became embroiled in a vehement pamphlet war concerning the death of Robert Walpole for which Jurin's recipe for dissolving bladder stones, *lixivium lithontripticum*, was held responsible by several of the Earl of Orford's other medical consultants.[9] Finally, Jurin was an ardent supporter of new science, actively encouraging empirical methodology.

The following letter to Mr James Handley from Jurin, in his role as Secretary to the Royal Society, exemplifies the seriousness with which representatives of the new science took their obligation to be objective and precise in reporting scientific or medical observations. The letter, dated 30 January 1723/4,* illustrates the obsessive clinical detail that characterised new science rhetoric, what Frederick N. Smith has termed a 'nervous factuality' evident in papers submitted to *The Philosophical Transactions of the Royal Society*.[10] Only because of the nature of the subject here – a case report

---

*In England, until 1752, both the Julian (Old Style) and Gregorian (New Style) calenders were in use. The Roman year began in March (December was the tenth month), and thus, a letter written in January was dated according to both systems.

on a man who has vomited up a live caterpillar – does Jurin's response to Handley seem to verge on Swiftian parody of the new science and its rhetoric:

Sir,

Both your Letters came safe to my hands. The first read some time ago to the Royal Society, & I am to return you their thanks, as I likewise do my own in particular, for your readiness to communicate so extraordinary a case, for such indeed it appears to be. But give me leave, Sir, to mention to you a Scruple, that was made by some Gentlemen present at the reading of your Letter, who made it a Question, concerning that you were not present at vomiting up of Insect, whether it really came from the Stomach, or might happen to have lain unobserv'd in the Vessel, into which the Patient vomited. That such Insects are to be found at that time of year, especially in mild Winters, is certain, as I have more than once seen myself; so that if the Insect came from the Stomach, it might have been swallow'd a few days before in a Sallad, & might , as you may say, have fix'd it self upon the inside of the Stomach, & by its vellication might occasion the pains which the Patient complain'd of.[11] Such a Stimulus upon so sensible a part as the Stomach must undoubtedly affect the neighbouring parts, by what we commonly call the Consensus Partium, or Nervorum, the effects of which are well known, tho the means of its Operation is difficult to explain. The Organs of Respiration being hereby provoked to more frequent contractions, it is easie to see that an Asthma might be occasion'd, to which perhaps the presence of the Diaphragm upon the Stomach now inflamed & painfull, with the disturbance hereby given to the Insect, which must prompt it to take faster hold, & consequently to vellicate the nervous wall of the Stomach more strongly might greatly contribute. For the pain hereby occasion'd would hinder the Patient from using a full inspiration, & would by that means make the frequency of it more necessary. The Diarrhoea might be produced by the communication of the Stimulus upon the Stomach, to the Intestines, & likewise to all those canals, that discharge any liquors into the one or the other, particularly the Ductus Choledochus: & possibly the quality of the Animal it self & the Excrements might contribute to this Effect, some of these Insects being as I remember, said to be of a venomous nature. You have, Sir, my hasty thoughts upon a Subject, which I have not time to consider more particularly: such as they are, they are entirely submitted to your Judgement by,

Sir,
Your most obliged
humble Servant
J. Jurin Secr.
R.S.[12]

Although Jurin's letter must strike the modern reader as comical, it nonetheless exemplifies the very serious ideals of new science and its rhetorical prescriptions as set forth by the Royal Society. Those guidelines had been clearly expressed in 1667 by Thomas Sprat in *The History of the Royal-Society of London, for the Improving of Natural Knowledge*.[13] Brian Vickers, in 'The Royal Society and English Prose Style: A Reassessment,' has described this work as an 'official, quasi-commissioned document' authored by a young clergyman (later, Bishop of Rochester) who 'was not a scientist, and had a limited understanding of the nature of scientific research'. Yet, explains Vickers, Sprat did have a 'sufficient knowledge of, and sympathy with, the program formulated by Francis Bacon for the reformation of science, which had indeed swept through virtually all social, political, or religious groups in the seventeenth century.'[14] Sprat was representative of the widespread obsessive interest in scientific matters by the general population of England from the Restoration through to the early-eighteenth century. The public's exposure to the new scientific rhetoric came through several sources. Among those publications popularising the new science was *The Philosophical Transactions of the Royal Society*, which Frederick N. Smith explains 'contained the latest news on that science – were widely read, and not only by scientists – although just who and who was not a scientist at this time is itself problematic – but by well-read laymen generally'.[15] As mentioned in the previous chapter, contributions to *The Gentleman's Magazine* (founded in 1731) prove the linguistic comfort with which the educated layman could discuss natural philosophy and medical matters with scientists and physicians. The magazine appealed to a broad reading public without compromising scientific terminology or detail, and without an evident hierarchy of regard for the opinion of expert over layman.[16]

What did these publications transmit about proper rhetorical style? Sprat, in his history, explains that the society (incorporated in 1662) had been forced to respond to the dangerous proliferation of 'Fancy' and 'Passions' in scientific discourse, manifested 'by the luxury and redundance of *speech*,' and 'the ill effects of this superfluidity of talking' which has 'already overwhelm'd most other *Arts* and *Professions*'. Sprat asks, 'Who can behold, without indignation, how many mists and uncertainties, these specious *Tropes* and *Figures* have brought on our Knowledge?' The Society's response to this threat is the concerted effort to condemn all such 'extravagance' of speech:

> [T]o reject all amplifications, digressions, and swelling of style: to return to the primitive purity, and shortness, when men delivr'd so many *things*, almost in an equal number of *words*. They have exacted from all their members, a close, naked, natural way of speaking; positive expressions; clear senses; a native easiness; bringing all things as near the Mathematical plainness, as they can: and preferring the language of Artizans, Countrymen and Merchants, before that, of Wits, or Scholars.[17]

The last comment signifies a preference for words with English roots over the use of polysyllabic Latinisms.

These rhetorical goals were adopted by the established medical profession to achieve the prestige and authority associated with natural philosophy. Prominent Augustan physicians were attracted to a Newtonian-based iatromechanical theory of medicine which attempted to describe states of health and disease as reducible to mathematics, especially the measurement and calculation of hydraulic pressures in the human body.[18] Iatromechanical physiology produced numerous papers and scientific controversies, but in everyday medical practice even the most ardent physician followers of the iatromechanical school still depended primarily upon the verbal representation of symptoms by the patient. Similarly, medical therapy remained based on the classical teachings of Galen, modulating the six non-naturals: exercise, food and drink, evacuations (including sexual), air, sleep, and the state of mind (the passions).[19] It was the doctor's work to restore health through vomits, cathartics, bleeding, exercise, change of scene, and alteration in diet. Medical treatment, in short, remained unaffected by iatromechanical speculation even though physicians now explained the benefit of such long familiar treatments on the basis of fashionable hydraulic physiology.[20]

If iatromechanical philosophy failed to alter medical practice in any significant manner, the new science rhetoric was adopted by medical practitioners and by their more sophisticated patients, both of whom incorporated the essentials of Sprat's prescriptions for the writing of natural philosophy into the writing of personal medical history and consultation. Physicians and patients – and family members or acquaintances who wrote on behalf of a patient – strove to write about illness in a dispassionate, unadorned prose, eschewing fanciful metaphor or simile, but with that 'nervous factuality' that becomes, in medicine-by-post, a matter of obsessive clinical detail. In what Smith calls 'the neutral jargon of the new science', there is the display 'of a certain methodology: the meticulous accumulation of physical evidence, the citation of only the most credible witnesses, and an extremely cautious approach to argument from "matters of fact" to hypothesis or opinion.'[21] There is, furthermore, 'a desire... to stick to what are perceived as facts; an avoidance of anything beyond the scientifically observable; and a willingness (at least implicit) to let others offer hypotheses, opinions and judgments.'[22] The obligation of the patient writing to his or her doctor in the early eighteenth century was, similarly, to represent the factual details of an illness: symptoms, quality of pulse, menstrual history, description of the urine, any abnormalities of the integument such as colour, rash, or inflammation. These facts, if possible, should be corroborated by a reliable witness, a family member or the local doctor. The language of the patient's letter should aim for a direct style, one in which similes are reserved to amplify upon factual description and should refer only to things in nature. A physician provided with such predictable information might, with some confidence, venture diagnosis and treatment by post.

The new science character of medical discourse is well illustrated in a series of consultation letters in which the Northumberland Presbyterian minister John Horsley (1685–1732) consults Jurin about a case of diplopia (double vision). Jurin's explication of Horsley's detailed observations in this case displays Jurin's great medical acumen but, more importantly, the letters demonstrate the power of a rhetoric that is available to both non-physician and professional, allowing them to communicate about illness with unusual facility. Although Horsley was an occasional lecturer on natural science, the new science rhetoric, as mentioned previously, would have been equally familiar to any literate person who read magazines and kept up with the popular press.

In a letter, dated 1 July 1723, Horsley describes the accident which he believes is responsible for the visual disorder now suffered by Thomas Brown of Shawden Esq., a Justice of the Peace, who:

> [D]id lately by a violent Fall from his Horse receive some Hurt upon his Breast & one of his Shoulders, some Part of his Forehead just above his Eye & his Temple being also hurt by the Fall. Since this happened, if he looks wth both his Eyes open, his Sight is obscure and confus'd, and the Objects appear double: But if he closes one Eye & looks wth the other alone (even wth that which was affected by the Fall;) his Sight is Single, clear, & distinct.[23]

From the same letter we learn that Mr Brown has already seen a physician who determined that the 'Optic nerve was disorder'd or contorted by ye Concussion'. Horsley, however, recollects that a volume of *The*

Philosophical Transactions had contained a case of 'Duplicity of Vision' associated with headaches and seizures, which was 'suppos'd to proceed from ye Distorting of ye Fibres of ye Optic Nerves from their Natural Parallelism'. In exemplary Royal Society form, Horsley proceeds to offer Jurin the following anecdotal account of the case, but certified by witnesses and subjected to proper scientific observation:

> When I first saw Mr Brown after he had met with this misfortune, I observ'd that he look'd very much asquint with one Eye especially, which before he us'd not to do. And upon my acquainting him with it, he told me that all his other Friends had remark'd ye same thing.

> I was willing to try how far the Apparent & Real Object were separated from one another when his Eye was plac'd at a certain Distance, and found upon Trial that at the Distance of 16 Feet they were about 4 Feet remov'd from each other.

> I ask'd him if he could so order his Eyes as to see but one Object; He told me he could: And after some Endeavours so fix'd his Eyes upon a Glass that stood on a Table before him, as to see it single. I narrowly observ'd his Eyes at this Time, and it was very manifest (both to myself & others too who were present) that in this Case he look'd much asquint wth the one Eye, but pretty direct wth the other. (MS 6146)

Horsley twice assures the reader that the reported abnormalities were witnessed by others. In addition, he conducts formal experiments on the extremely cooperative Mr Brown, and then presents his observations in the plainest language possible, ready-made for publication in *The Philosophical Transactions*. Horsley goes on to conjecture that the 'Chrystalline Humour, or the Eye it self or it's Axis was some way or other distorted & had chang'd it's former Natural Place or Position; or at least... The Fibres of the muscles or of the *Procossus Cibares*' have lost their tone secondary to the 'Shock in the Fall'. However, he will defer to Jurin, and the letter concludes with the obligatory apology for any incompleteness:

> It was but a little Time that I was with Mr Brown, and therefore cou'd not make all the Enquiries that might be proper & needful in such a Case: But I hope to see him again very shortly, and then I shall inform my Self farther, he being very obliging & ready to make any Trials or answer any Questions that may be propos'd. (MS 6146)

Jurin's reply indicates the depth of his consideration of the case and, unlike the case of the vomited insect, here his explanation, though speculative, is right on the mark in explaining the ophthalmologic phenomenon of diplopia:

> Being now return'd from Tunbridge Wells, where I spent the three last Months, I sit down to consider your two obliging Letters of the 1st & 16th of July.
>
> Mr Brown's seeing double & sometimes squinting, seems to me to depend rather on the inability of some one, or more, of the Muscles of the Eye to perform their office, than upon any distortion of the Fibres of the Optick Nerve.
>
> By your Experiment, when that Gentleman endeavor'd to fix his Eyes upon a Glass, so as to see it single, it appears that he pointed the Axis of one Eye directly towards the Glass, but turn'd the other Eye another way, so as to look visibly asquint. If he had had the natural command of the Muscles of both Eyes, so as to point both their Axes directly to the same place, the Object must have appear'd Single: if he had not that command of the Muscles of one Eye as to make them act in concert with those of the other, the Object must have appear'd double, because both Axes were not directed to the same point, & he could not possibly see the Object single, unless by turning one Eye quite another way, so as to receive no Image at all of the Object.
>
> This I imagine you will be farther satisfy'd in, if, in repeating the Experiment, you find that, when the Gentleman sees double, he looks a little asquint, & looks much more asquint, when he sees the Object single.[24]

The case of Mr Brown becomes, through new science rhetoric, elegantly metamorphosed into both observed phenomenon and experiment. Whether the subject be an insect in the gut or seeing double, and whether the correspondent be a doctor or gentleman scientist, a patient, or his relative, the rhetoric of new science is the fashionable rhetoric of the more sophisticated early-eighteenth-century medicine-by-post correspondent.

Adherence to proper scientific rhetoric, and its accoutrements, serves substantially to validate the narrative of illness. This can be seen in the case of Henry Shafto, a gentleman of Whickham, who asked his surgeon, Jacob Johnson from Newcastle-upon-Tyne, to consult Jurin on a medical disorder. This series of letters additionally provides insight into the etiquette of medicine-by-post.

Although Shafto has previously been a patient of Jurin, he prefers that Johnson initiate communication with him. Johnson obliges in a letter of 10 December 1727 addressed 'To Doctor Jurin to be Left att Batsons Coffee House over against ye Royall Exchange, London':

Sir

I am order'd by a Gentillman, who once had the honour to be under your
care when att Newcastle; to desire the favour of your advice, he is often
troubl'd with deliriums, butt more especially after Drinken, he was formerly,
when att London under the Care of Doctor Strother and friend, he
frequently has intervalls which Continues a Considerable time, as upwards
of three or four Months, I have nott been Concern'd with him above two
days, In which time I have Blister'd and bled him, and findes him much
More Compos'd butt will nott presume to proceed any farther without your
advice, so if you please to take the trouble of Enquiring into the particulars
of his mallady of one of the above mentioned Gentillmen, [I] shall take itt as
a Singular favour, he is a Man of Fortune and would thankfully pay any Sum
of Money. In order for his recovery, he Committs himself solely to your Care,
his name is Henry Shaftoe of Whickham near Newcastle, he also desires you'l
send him down your Prescription as often as you think Nessasary, & order
him his propper Regimen and draw a Bill upon him payable att sight, when
ever you please; the answering of these at first post, will very much obblige
Sir

> Your Most obbedient
> Humble Servt Jacob Johnson[25]

Two days after Johnson's introductory letter, Shafto finds it appropriate to
appeal to Jurin directly:

Sir

Last Post Mr Jacob Johnson Surgeon in Newcastle did by my order write to
you desiring the favour of a prescription from you on my account his
acquaintance with you being but small.... My distemper, I call a confirmed
Leprosy, it affects the head, nerves and spirit, in short the whole man is out
of order. It concerns me, not a stranger to you, not a little to think that I
should live so long in London without your advice[.] a Return to your favour
shall not be wanting and a Line from you to me will be almost a Cure.... (MS
6139)

Although a respectable professional intermediary is available in the person of
Mr Johnson, Jurin invites the patient to provide him with more specifics of
his illness, as we can deduce from this response of Shafto from 24 December:

Sir

I received your Letter in answer to mine, satisfactorily, and in obedience to
your request to send to you the symptoms of the Leprosy to the best of my

judgmt; and with Mr Johnsons approbation. The skin is rough, and has red and scaly spots, on several parts. The head when a plaister is applied, as has been, scabs all over. I had Mr Horsher of Newcastle before Mr Johnson, who blooded me in the neck, and gave physick by way of pills and several Cephalick mixtures for the head as well as the whole Disease, yet the same symptoms appear.[26] I am sorry, I had not the good fortune to be your patient, before I left London, whither in my fancy, I shall be obliged to journey in the end for your immediate Care. I do not expect an answer, apprehending Mr Johnson a properer Correspondent, it being his business and not mine, besides a double Correspondence will give you a needless trouble[.] You sho'd have had an answer Past post if Whickham had afforded fitt paper. I doubt not your further direction and assistance and crave Leave to Subscribe. (MS 6139)

In this epistolary relationship, Shafto, though now in direct communication with Jurin, defers to Johnson as the 'properer Correspondent'. Indeed, on 12 January 1727/8 Johnson writes to Jurin to apprise him of Shafto's response to the treatment plan. However, Johnson also introduces some important facts that contradict Shafto's narration of events, providing a tension in this medicine-by-post triangle:

[I] suppose by this time you have got a Letter from him, where he mentions his Mallady to be More a Leprosy than anything Else for he does not Care to have itt said that he has any disorder in his head, I have already been along with those Gentillmen that were Concern'd for him formerly and they never observ'd the Least symptom Immaginable, he has one small scorbuticall spott in his arm butt itt seems to me to be no more then Cuticular. Last week he was as much disorder'd in his head as Ever, and was much Confus'd with strange Phantoms.... (MS 6139)

Jurin has received varied accounts of the medical history from patient and doctor. Johnson has discredited Shafto's report of a skin condition, and furthermore claims the patient is in a state of denial, that he 'does not care to have itt said that he has any disorder in his head'. From the initial consultation request, Johnson has alluded to Shafto's drinking problem and suggests that the 'deliriums' are from alcohol. Which account is Jurin to believe? Jurin's request for a description of symptoms from the patient may indicate a preference for the firsthand report from the sufferer, or at least he may want this to supplement Mr Johnson's history for completeness. Jurin may have been catering to the patient's ego, a show of interest meant to satisfy an apparently well-to-do client. But the question remains, in the face of such contradictory information, how would the patient's account weigh against the local surgeon's report in Jurin's estimation of the case?

Shafto might have scored some points with Jurin on the basis of class and educational background. A striking feature of these letters is the contrasting level of education displayed by the correspondents. Jacob Johnson writes very ungrammatically, with almost no punctuation marks and frequent misspellings. Shafto, on the other hand, shows considerably more polish in his writing, and one suspects his educational background is probably somewhat closer to that of Jurin. Jurin, then, may have felt a greater natural affinity for the patient than for a provincial surgeon. There are no extant letters from Jurin that definitively reveal his opinion on the case, but a postscript in a brief note from Johnson, dated 27 February 1727/8, indicates that Jurin also felt Johnson to be the 'properer Correspondent':

Sir,

Have punctually observ'd your Orders to Mr Shaftoe, & he has had a Relapse since you heard from me, but is now in a Tolerable Way, and resolves if the Weather will permitt, to be at London about Easter....

P.S. Mr Shaftoe is very uneasy to have a Letter from you (MS 6139)

The fact that Jurin maintains communication with Johnson while apparently neglecting to write Shafto strongly suggests that Jurin favoured Johnson's account of events over the patient's. That preference, I would argue, is based less on social or professional status than on Johnson's more proper observation of the prescriptions of medical communications. While neither Shafto nor Johnson is meticulous is recording clinical details, Johnson – whose grammar may be wanting – yet manages to establish professional authority. His epistolary style is direct and unpretentious and he names corroborating witnesses to his own medical observations. Furthermore, Johnson demonstrates a proper restraint in proffering diagnoses or treatments that are best left to the consultant: 'I have Blisterd and bled him... butt will not presume to proceed any farther without your advice'. Such professional deference from doctor to consultant, or respect from patient to an established medical authority, continues well into the latter part of the century. In a letter dated 28 July 1789 and addressed to Dr James Wood, Dr William Cullen, the distinguished Edinburgh professor of medicine, scolds his medical colleague for presuming to recommend his own diagnosis before Cullen has had a chance to interpret the clinical information for himself. Cullen is also critical that Wood has omitted details in the case of a Mrs Mercer:

I am not satisfied with any opinion you have given concerning the seat of disease, nor can I venture to ascertain it.... You perhaps have not mentioned the circumstances because they had no influence upon your judgement, but you should have allowed me to have mine also.[27]

Johnson, therefore, in seeking consultation from Jurin, adheres to the formula and gestures of new science rhetoric, including his deference to authority for the interpretation of his own clinical observations. Compare this with Shafto's rather presumptuous and subjective conclusion that 'My distemper I call a confirmed Leprosy, it affects the head, nerves and spirit, in short the whole man is out of order.' Shafto's complaint is dramatic but vague. To declare that 'the whole man is out of order' is not very precise or useful information for one's physician. Johnson had also informed Jurin that Shafto is 'disorder'd in his head' and 'Confus'd with strange Phantoms'; in short, the patient is prone to fantastical ideas and, by implication, must be regarded as suspect as a interpreter of his own symptoms. It should also be noted that Shafto, although a man of considerable fortune – so we are informed by both Johnson and the patient himself – commits a singular breach of doctor-patient etiquette in his letter by the rather brazen attempt to bribe Jurin into taking his case. Shafto should have been aware of the impropriety of a man of his standing offering remuneration to Jurin in such a direct manner. As Judith Schneid Lewis has explained in her study of the eighteenth-century accoucheur (the male-midwife) and their aristocratic patients, 'It was simply not considered appropriate for one gentleman to pay another for services rendered.... Fees usually were not discussed.'[28] At some point after treatment a sum would be received by the doctor – a guinea was standard for a doctor's visit, and a larger payment for a prolonged service – but 'the direct transfer of money from one hand to another was especially frowned upon' among gentlemen.[29] Johnson does convey to Jurin that Shafto is a 'Man of Fortune and would thankfully pay any Sum of Money,' but one senses that Shafto advised Johnson to include such a remark in his introductory letter, especially as Shafto echoes the same offer in his subsequent letter to Jurin. If, in the end, neither Shafto nor Johnson are model correspondents, I believe that Johnson must have seemed, to Jurin, the more proper and credible of the two correspondents largely by virtue of his greater observance of new science rhetorical form.

Despite the noble rhetorical aspirations of the community of natural philosophers, Brian Vickers has shown that Royal Society members regularly transgressed their own guidelines, peppering their written works with Latinisms and various figures of speech.[30] Even Sprat's *History* 'is written in a straightforward English prose, but with a free use of rhetoric, both of figures... and tropes.'[31] Nonetheless, despite this regular bending or outright violation of their own rhetorical rules, natural philosophers and medical practitioners vigorously distinguished themselves from those enthusiasts who, in Sprat's words, employed a 'vicious abundance of Phrase, this trick of Metaphor, this volubility of Tongue, which makes so great a noise in the World'.[32] Such contradiction is explained largely, says Vickers, by appreciating that the mission of Sprat's history was to align the Royal Society squarely with the Church of England, thereby reinforcing the Anglican church's anxiety over the dangerous 'noise' of Nonconformists and Dissenters. By extension, all forms of enthusiasm, alchemy, and quackery, become associated with religious dissension and were condemned fordisseminating falsehoods in rhetorical sheep's clothing. In other words: by their rhetoric ye shall know them!

Through membership in the Royal College of Physicians, and by association with the Royal Society, physicians hoped to establish their credentials as scientists deserving of the trust and respect of the public. The plain, objective rhetoric claimed by Jurin's colleagues was a sign of veracity, opposed to the hyperbole of quacks and mountebanks and all those irregular practitioners of medicine who were seen to be eroding the public's trust in the medical marketplace through language meant to deceive. The response of irregular and fringe medical practitioners, such as the seventeenth-century political radical and religious dissenter Nicholas Culpepper, was to use the same ammunition as Sprat had employed but to join battle with the established physicians. Culpepper, for example, charged the medical profession with propagating Latinisms and professional jargon solely for the purpose of confounding the average citizen and keeping patients in the dark in matters that might make them more independent and self-reliant. If Sprat and the established scientific community argued that Latinisms and polysyllabic words were evidence of the corrupting influence of foreign tongues on the purity of English language and science, Culpepper and other fringe medical practitioners claimed Latinisms and professional jargon were intentionally propagated by the established professions solely for the purpose of exclusivity. Thus, medical rhetoric was a two-edged sword wielded by persons on opposite sides of the religious fence, and of diverse educational background, for their own political and socio-economic interests as much as for any philosophic ideology or linguistic purity.[33]

Pamphlet wars

The significance of rhetoric in medicine as a tool of authority and a weapon of contention is illustrated dramatically in the pamphlet war between James Jurin and a distinguished surgeon, John Ranby, on the occasion of the death of Sir Robert Walpole. John Ranby, 'Principal Serjeant Surgeon to His Majesty, and FRS,' was Walpole's personal physician. When Walpole suffered from a bladder stone but refused surgery, Ranby called in consultants Sir Edward Hulse (First Physician to King George II) and Jurin.

They all agreed on trying Jurin's stone-dissolving elixir, *lixivium lithontripticum*. Walpole responded to this mixture, passing a large stone and multiple stone fragments, but his health rapidly deteriorated thereafter. Despite increasing pain from urinary obstruction, he still refused lithotomy, even by the extraordinarily skilled William Cheselden who could extract a bladder stone in under three minutes. Walpole wrote to his son that, 'This Lixivium has blown me up. It has torn me to pieces. The affair is over with me. That it be short is all I desire'.[34] The contents of this letter became public, and Jurin became embroiled in a public debate about his treatment of Walpole. Ranby, Hulse, and Cheselden, all blamed Jurin's concoction for Walpole's death, and Ranby published 'A Narrative of the Last Illness of the Right Honourable the Earl of Orford,' which held Jurin's *lixivium* to be specifically responsible for Walpole's painful demise.[35] To make matters still worse for Jurin, Henry Fielding, a great admirer of Ranby, contributed his own scathing satirical pamphlet, 'The Charge to the Jury, or the Sum of the Evidence on The Trial of A. B. C. D. and E. F., All MD For the Death of one Robert at Orfud, at a Special Commission of Oyer and Terminer held at Justice-College, in W___ck-Lane [*sic*], Before Sir Asculapius Dosem, Dr Timberhead, and Others, their Fellows, Justices, etc.' In this squib, Fielding refers to the '*deadly instrument*, called a Lickliverum Lithoskipticum,' and Jurin becomes emblematic of a 'Reconciliation' of the established and quack physician.[36]

Jurin response to this public challenge to his reputation appeared in a pamphlet entitled *Expostulatory Address to John Ranby Esq*. It is a remarkable document for the modern reader who is familiar with Jurin's impressive credentials – for not once does Jurin offer a single medical justification for the use and safety of his elixir, but instead he attacks Ranby's credibility solely on the grounds of his deficient and illogical rhetoric. It is an often embarrassing performance, but we should not miss the frequent invocation of those very same rhetorical ideals so dear to the proponents of new science rhetoric.

The portion of Jurin's pamphlet that addresses Ranby's account of Walpole's 'last illness' follows a critique of Ranby's rhetorical shortcomings in the 'Treatise on Gunshot-Wounds': 'Let us now see, how much you have improved in the Art of Writing, by examining your *Narrative of Orford's Last Illness*, with the same Freedom we have hitherto used.'[37] Jurin begins his attack on Ranby by questioning his motives for writing his narrative and performing the autopsy on Walpole's body. He undermines the historical tradition on which Ranby justifies his public rehearsal of Walpole's last illness and the post-mortem findings:

You begin your Preface by acquainting the present World with a Maxim of the past, which I can scarce believe was so universal as you represent it: namely, *That fulfilling the Will of the Dead, as ever, even among the most uncivilized Nations, esteemed an indispensable Obligation and sacred Duty ; and that a man who could transgress in this essential Point, was looked upon as capable of violating his Father's Ashes, and committing the most execrable Enormity....* Was there never a fanatical or unreasonable Will in all Antiquity? And if there was, did the Executor always think it prudent to perform it? – Had the late *Earl of Orford* desired that *your Bladder* should be explored instead of his own, would you have made no Objection to the Operation? (32–3)

Further aspersions on Ranby's purpose for publishing his 'Narrative' follow later in the pamphlet: 'By the by, this is the third time *Mr Ranby* is honourably mentioned by himself, in a Page and an [*sic*] half; which discovers the profound Veneration he has for the third Person when it stands for the first – as well as the small Deference he pays to it in its own Place' (43).

Jurin's defence is essentially a page-by-page analysis of Ranby's rhetorical faults exposed in a scathing and sarcastic tone:

You declined Quotation in your first Performance [the 'Treatise on gunshot-Wounds']: I wish you had declined it here too, or at least quoted more to the Purpose. In the name of Wonder! what Affinity is there between a Woman's Care in gathering her Robe about her, that she might fall decently, (which is the meaning of your Quotation) and a Man dying peaceably in Bed, who desires his Bladder may be opened after his Decease, for the Benefit of his Fellow-Creatures? (33)

Elsewhere Jurin finds much fault with Ranby's casual use of metaphor. He objects to the description of Walpole arriving in the country and '*taking a little Air*' as 'an Expression no Man of common Sense ought to be indulged in' (36). Worse is Ranby's tendency to hyperbole. When Ranby describes Walpole's extreme discomfort on travelling as '*enough to fill one's Mind with Horror,*' Jurin remarks, 'Did his Lordship see an Apparition on the Road? Or do those Circumstances raise *Horror* in you, that create Compassion and Sympathy in other People?' (37). For Jurin this is not only a matter of hyperbole but sloppy semantics, as when Ranby refers to the '*preternatural Irritation* 'of the bladder which causes Jurin to ask, 'Pray, what is preternatural in an Irritation to make water, when the Bladder is diseased?' (34-5). Jurin loses all patience remarking on Ranby's use of the word 'Rest' at one point in the text:

I should have been obliged to you likewise if you had given the Word Rest a little more *Rest*: which in one or two pages you have harrassed quite out of its meaning. – As, *absolute Rest* – *On Rest* – *Rest naturally, seldom failed to remedy*. – notwithstanding all the *Rest* imaginable; with many more unnecessary *Rests*, thro' the rest of your *Narrative*. (36)

Also under frequent attack is Ranby's inconsistency and imprecision in details, such as the lax description of the bladder dissection as showing a crisscrossing of 'Ridges'. Jurin tries to upstage Ranby in a show of erudition, suggesting that 'Perhaps you mean Fleshy *Fasciculi* disposed like the *Carneæ Columnae* in the Ventricles of the Heart; your Words at least convey this Idea' (48). The strain of Jurin's critique of Ranby's rhetoric shows itself all too often, frequently with embarrassing results: 'Sir Edward Hulse *thought his left Hand warm again, and his Thigh warmer*. He only thought so. Did he feel his Hand and Thighs, or only *think* he felt them? Whether were his Thighs*warmer* than his left Hand, or *warmer* than *themselves?*' (40). Or again, '*At Eight this Evening Mr Ranby with his Hands* (no body could imagine it was with his Feet) *pressed the bottom of his Belly, and the Water gushed out...*' (42). Jurin stoops even to this *ad hominem* attack on Ranby:

> Thus ends your *Historical Detail of my Lord Orford's last illness*: and I dare venture to affirm, that *sagacious Statesman* could not have given a more manifest Proof of the Alteration wrought in his Intellects, by the Violence of his Disorder; than his assigning you a Task, which by this time, I hope you are satisfied, you was altogether unqualified for. (46–7)

That a physician of Jurin's intellect and stature should be writing a piece of this character seems inconsistent with the dignity of his public persona as established physician and Secretary to the Royal Society. Yet, as Anita Guerrini has shown, medical pamphlets of the early-eighteenth century which dealt with medical controversies – as opposed to informational pamphlets – typically adopted the *ad hominem* rhetoric of political debates, and were 'aiming at persuasion rather than proof'. Furthermore, Guerrini observes that although:

> [Q]uestions of scientific theory were, at least on the surface, the topic of medical pamphlet debates, the rhetorical nature of the pamphlet genre served to subvert its very expression. Medical pamphleteers abandoned all vestiges of objectivity even while they argued for their superior learning. They resorted to every rhetorical device known to Grub Street, from metaphors and emotional appeals to irony and satire.[38]

The crux of the pamphlet debate was what kind of 'specialised knowledge' was necessary to identify the medical practitioner as a 'gentleman physician'; and the aim of established physicians in England was to secure their identity, in the public eye, as the elite among medical professionals through their association with natural philosophy and the currency of new science rhetoric. Underlying the rhetoric of individual medical pamphlet skirmishes was a war of professional status based on educational and social background. The battle over what constituted proper medical rhetoric was, flagrantly, a public rather than professional debate. Geoffrey Holmes has described early-eighteenth-century medicine as:

> [B]eyond comparison the most pamphlet-ridden of... professions. From the avalanche of writings issuing from the leading polemicists among the physicians, apothecaries and surgeons of Augustan England, one might well conclude that the pen was considered to be far mightier than the prescription, the powder and the poultice.[39]

This proliferation of medical pamphlet debates, suggests Guerrini, came out of physician insecurity as to what constituted professional authority, but Guerrini also points out that bringing such a debate into the public arena only further loosened the moorings of medical authority. Such internecine warfare usually turned on personality and created a circus atmosphere of *ad hominum* verbal abuse. Furthermore, the welter of divided medical opinion fed into the Augustan literary Zeitgeist: a preoccupation with the unravelling of societal structure and morality and the general dumbing-down of intellectual taste. In recent work, Carey McIntosh has detailed the anxiety and low 'literary self-esteem' of early-eighteenth-century English writers, particularly in the first two decades. McIntosh contrasts this intellectual worry about language with the ongoing 'battle of the books' between ancients and moderns. In the latter case, argues McIntosh, at least 'the moderns could point to contemporary achievements in natural philosophy to justify their optimism. But not even the cockiest of them could argue that the language and literature of early-eighteenth-century England outshone the language and literature of Homer and Virgil.'[40]

To build on Guerrini and McIntosh, I would like to suggest that the unsettled state of medicine in the Augustan age was much more analogous to the transitional state of English literary style than it was to the established position of natural philosophy, and that this insecurity persisted well beyond the earliest decades of the century. Medicine did not hold the prestige or the promise of progress that was associated with such disciplines as mathematics, physics, or chemistry. In this cultural milieu, physicians were greatly motivated to find ways to hitch their wagon to the natural philosophy star in order to bolster their own authority and gain respect as a profession. The adoption of new science rhetoric to medicine was the most immediate –

and, possibly, the only available – stratagem for physicians to take to associate themselves with the exciting progress going on in other sciences.

Meeting the mark: patients and medical rhetoric

Educated patients were as enthusiastic as their physicians to adopt the rhetoric of new science in describing their own symptoms. This may have come about, for many, as an unconscious imitation of the language of science which had become so ubiquitous in the popular press. Even if some patients, such as Mr Shafto, missed the mark in conforming to the new fashion in medical rhetoric – through ignorance, lack of interest, or sheer contrariness – enough medicine-by-post from this period bears witness to a general conformity to the rhetorical model promulgated by the Royal Society.

Dr Jurin appears to have had definite expectations as to how patients should write their medicine-by-post (see the epigraph to this chapter). In his letter to the Attorney General of Massachusetts, Jurin complains of Mr Dudley's lack of precision in delineating his symptoms, a fault particularly irksome and limiting to medical consultation 'at so great a distance'. The more complete text follows:

> I am very sorry to find that you are in so indifferent a State of health, & it would be a matter of exceeding pleasure to me, if I could be any way instrumental in amending it; but you know Sir, how difficult it is to give proper directions at so great a distance, *especially when the case is not very particularly & exactly stated* [italics mine] For this reason I dare not give you any more than one piece of advice, & that is to use constant riding, as much as your strength will permit.... [I]f any great benefit is expected from this Exercise, a Man ought to ride 20 or so miles a day for 2 or 3 Months together, till he has got rid of the complaint. I heartily wish that [by] this or any other means you may recover the desired state of health, & am with the greatest respect & esteem....[41]

However, patients could take their physicians to task for lack of clarity also. Thomas Worsley, Esq., writes to Dr Jurin in November 1746, regarding Jurin's regimen for bladder stone: 'I give you the trouble of this chiefly to desire you would be a little more explicit as to my taking your palliative Prescription. Should I take it constantly every eighth hour whether I have much pain upon me or not? Will not that be rather too much for my Stomach?'[42]

Clearly, both patients and their doctors had an obligation to be very precise if medicine-by-post was to work effectively. The physical examination was of limited use in eighteenth-century medicine, as mentioned previously, but, consequently, the exactness in description of symptoms and constitution was paramount to a meaningful medical dialogue by post. Educated patients seem to have been not only familiar with the expectations in content, form, and vocabulary for such communications, but seem to have been remarkably self-confident in their ability to satisfy the demands of consultation by letter. In fact, patients not infrequently trusted their own capability in this regard over that of their local physician. Mordecai Cary, Bishop of Clonfert, who corresponded in great detail with Jurin about his wife's medical condition, only reluctantly complied with Jurin's request for a note from the local physician:

Dear Doctor

Underwritten I send my wifes case as stated by our Physician. I was unwilling to omit anything which You thought of any use; but to be plain, I do not see any great light You can receive from it. I am very sensible of Your kind meaning in requiring such a state of her case taken by a Physician but I am afraid You will find Yourself disappointed.[43]

Local physicians might anticipate that their patients would provide consultants with written personal accounts of an illness to supplement their doctor's own consultation request; indeed, patients were not infrequently invited to do so by their own physician. Once patients had described their symptoms to a consultant, they might defer subsequent communications to the regional doctor as the 'properer Correspondent' as in the case of Mr Shafto. Examination of letters from this period indicate, however, that it was by no means unusual for a simultaneous correspondence to occur, with both patient and doctor writing to the consultant about the progress of an illness. In such cases the patient might well play off one doctor against the other or hope to monitor the appropriateness of locally prescribed therapy by reporting adverse affects of treatment to the physician consultant in town.

A series of eight letters written by Bishop Mordecai Cary to James Jurin between the years 1733–34/5 are concerned with a prolonged period of ill health for the bishop's wife. Though only the bishop's half of the correspondence is extant, these letters are among those few precious examples of an extended private-practice medical correspondence in the first third of the eighteenth century. As such, this correspondence offers a generous sampling of the character and particulars of medicine-by-post from the first third of the century. Yet more relevant, the letters show consistently, and unmistakably, the profound influence of new science rhetoric on the layperson who had need, or the desire, to write to a physician for medical advice.

In the instance of the Cary–Jurin correspondence, we have letters written to Jurin by a friend and a man of similar level of education. Mordecai Cary (d.1751) had attended Trinity College at Cambridge where he was introduced to Jurin by Richard Bentley. Jurin became Cary's tutor from 1708 to 1709, and the two men became lifelong friends and shared many intellectual interests. For example, they travelled together to Leyden to attend the medical lectures of Herman Boerhaave. In 1731, Cary became Bishop of Clonfert, and then in 1735 Bishop of Cloyne and Killala. Jurin and Cary maintained an active correspondence which included scholarly discussions about classical literature and the finer points of Greek and Latin translation and interpretation. Indeed, most of the letters that Cary sent to Jurin during his wife's illness are divided between extraordinarily deliberate clinical descriptions of Mrs Cary's condition and, in sharp contrast, a much more natural and relaxed prose in which Cary argues fine points on interpretation of Homer, Euripides, and Demosthenes. Cary's discussions are liberally peppered with quotations in Greek, and he makes frequent reference to the works of modern scholars. Cary does not hesitate to criticise, often with humour, Jurin's translation and interpretation of classical works; and while he readily defers to the doctor on medical matters, he is a stickler for precision:

> But heark you, Dear Doctor, (*ut caedam tua vineta*) [so that I may cut back your vineyards], what do You mean by using the word *parum* in Your own Prescriptions? You mean *paullum* or *pauxillum*, not *parum*. A little is *paullum*: the true English of *parum* is too little. I question whether Tom Bentley would take Physick prescrib'd by such a word: tho for my self & my wife I assure You we are quite of another mind.[44]

Cary, himself, strives for the greatest exactness, and completeness in communicating to Jurin the details of his wife's ailments. Cary's first letter about this matter, dated June 1733, provides a splendid example of the kind of obsessive detail that a patient, or in this case a spouse, might feel necessary to provide the doctor for consultation by post:

> Dear Doctor

> Above a month ago my wife took cold by going into new rooms where the walls were damp, after a walk that had heated her. Thereupon her left breast, which You may remember to have been lanced by Mr Cheselden 16 years ago, has been ever since in great pain with little intermissions or rather removals of the pain, as sometimes into her hands sometimes into one hip sometimes into her right breast & right armpit: but her most constant complaint is of the bone under the left breast & of her back bone betwixt the scapulae and thereabouts. The breast has been much swelled, then abated, & now it is a little bigger than the other whereas when she is well, it is less than

the other. We find no lump, nor sign of inflammation. It has been poultised by advice of a Physician, 12 days together with white bread & milk & a little brandy. This poultise has been discontinued now a fortnight. She has been purged four times & once blouded [*sic*]. Her menses have been regular; her urine thick & troubled, till after standing some time it has let fall a gross sediment that looks to me like Cremor Tartari at the bottom of a dish of tea. Her wandring pains into her arms & hips, & shoulders as other parts we are apt to think Rheumatick. That gnawing pain in the breast it self, which as she complains draws down from the neck, & hinders the free use of her left arm & goes to the bone under the breast & to the back-bone & sometimes to the left breast & to her armpits & sides I suppose proceeds from some contraction or affection of the nerves of the left breast. She has complained of the pains running about & under her breast like some living creature; but that complaint is much abated: or as she expresses it, the mouse that us'd to run up & down is much lessen'd.

She keeps within doors, lives very low in meal & drink. Her pain excepted, she is not sick.

Now, Dear Doctor, I have told you the case, I must beg your advice by the next post directed to me at Eyrecourt in Ireland. At the same time, if You have any news, it will be obliging to send it. I dare say You would take it amiss if I made any Apology for this freedom, and therefore I will say no more but that I am

Your old friend
Mordecai Clonfert[45]

The bishop adds as an afterthought: 'The pain in her left breast she sometimes compares to that of forks or darts stabbing the part. This complaint indeed she has made at times, these 16 years; as often as she has got cold, or almost before every rain.'

Several elements of this epistle should be remarked. First, is the compulsive detail of Cary's report, a quality found in all his subsequent letters to Jurin regarding Mrs Cary. He reminds Jurin of a remote surgery performed by the famous William Cheselden upon Mrs Cary's left breast for a cyst or abscess some sixteen years earlier, information that might be significant to Jurin. With great exactness Cary renders the sequence of events, describing the environmental factors which might have precipitated the cold from which he marks the onset of his wife's present illness. Cary has supplied Jurin with a precise map of the radiation of pains out from the area of the breast and observed the size of the inflamed breast in relation to the normal breast. Relevant treatments that have been administered to date are recorded, including the inevitable purging and bleedings. Cary has also noted the limitations in range of motions that the condition has imposed on the patient's ability to move her left arm. He completes his medical history with the obligatory description on the state of the patient's menses and appearance of her urine.

Bishop Cary's description of the standing urine as 'a gross sediment that looks to me like Cremor Tartari at the bottom of a dish of Tea' is the first subjective element of the letter, and it is presented in the form of a simile. However, this is a simile that would be acceptable in new science rhetoric, justified by its very precision, by the allusion to something very material, and by the evident need to convey a qualitative description to a consultant who is physically absent and unable to perform his own analysis.[46] In a letter of June 9, Cary describes his wife's urine as now appearing 'like the grounds of a small yeasty beer' and 'leaves a white sediment on the sides of a large glass from top to bottom: which sediment to the eye looks white and greasy, but to the finger feels gritty & indeed when rubbed along the glass you hear the sound of sand.' Cary allows space in his letter to include his wife's own colourful but scientifically less rigorous similes: 'She has complained of the pains running about & under her breast like some living creature; but that complaint is much abated: or as she expresses it, the mouse that us'd to run up & down is much lessen'd'; and the postscript notes: 'The pain in her left breast she sometimes compares to that of forks or darts stabbing the part.' It is only through these similes, which the husband–editor has considered worthy of inclusion, that we get to hear the patient's own voice. In a letter of 28 July, he writes:

> [I]n the lower part of the same breast she complains too of pain as if the part were stitching up with a needle and thread.... [A]t times she has pains in all parts of her body which she likens to broken-pointed needles pricking her lightly in some parts, & in other parts to a living creature of the bigness of a fly moving quickly up & down. (MS 6140)

Cary makes certain that Jurin understands these precise but rather literary and somewhat 'fanciful' descriptions are attributed to the patient and not to him. Perhaps the bishop was just humouring his wife by including her similes in his letter, but much more likely such inclusiveness is but another manifestation of the effort to be objective in reporting illness: communicating the patient's own observations, however fanciful, for the sake of completeness.

Although Cary ventures interpretation of some of his wife's symptoms, he does so only tentatively and deferentially: 'her wandring pains into her arms & hips, & shoulders as other parts *we are apt to think* Rheumatick,' and 'that gnawing pain in the breast itself... *I suppose* proceeds from some contraction or affection of the nerves of the left breast' [italics mine]. Contrast this wording with the presumption of Henry Shafto's self-diagnosis, that the 'distemper, I call a confirmed Leprosy'. Cary leaves the diagnosis to Jurin; his suggestions for possible aetiologies of his wife's complaints are more descriptive than diagnostic. The bishop closes his letter by acknowledging Jurin's authority in diagnosis: 'I have told you the case, I must beg your advice by the next post'. How different in tone is this from the audacity of Shafto who writes that 'a Return to your favour shall not be wanting' (MS 6140).

While the bishop awaits Jurin's recommendations by post, Mrs Cary, we learn, has welcomed advice from women at Clonfert who do not defer to any consultant from London. In the second letter in the series, dated 9 June, Cary writes:

> Now I must beg pardon for this second trouble. I told you in my last that the menses have been regular. As to time indeed they have been so; but not so much in quantity as they used to be. To this want of due quantity & to bad blood & to wind & to gravel the good women impute the flying pains. For flying pains My wife has at times in most parts of her body.... She has been blouded [*sic*] in the left foot. She poulticed the breast with an herb bruised and fryed in Lard, by which she has softened it, & she thinks it something easier. The herb I believe is Herb Robert, a solid shining round hairy stalk & red small flower.
>
> She has drunk a Chalybeate Water these 3 or 4 days about a quart in the morning before breakfast.[47]

Evidently Mrs Cary has begun to take vernacular cures while her husband becomes more frustrated at not receiving a response from Jurin after three letters.[48] A third letter to Jurin from Cary, dated 12 June, shows evidence of some anxiety and, perhaps by way of prodding Jurin to respond, Cary amplifies on the alternative medical advice to which Mrs Cary has seen fit to apply:

> She takes Millipedes: has left off chalybeate waters. An old woman has been to see her today, who they say has cured many sore breasts; she makes very light of my wifes ailing, & pretends to cure it without fail by an Oyl made of white Lily roots and butter.[49]

In the letter of 12 June, the bishop expresses concern about his wife's condition, but it is evidence of the prescriptions of rhetorical objectivity that Cary retains a tone of aloof objectivity even while expressing his deep concerns. Also remarkable in this letter is that the bishop faithfully records his wife's own factual observations about her breast lesion even when her clinical description diverges significantly from his own physical examination:

> The place aggriev'd of my wifes breast is close to the bone in the very highest part of it in a perpendicular dividing the breast into two equal parts right & left. There is not an acute pain in it, nor swelling or hardening I can perceive (for I felt it very freely this morning) but my [wife] says there is a little hardness and a constant tugging as she calls it. – The great vein of her left arm which comes to the back of the hand & distributes veins to the fingers, is often very remarkably full & quite astrut,[50] and then her arm is in pain till she holds up her hand above her head, & then the vein sinks & the pain abates. Pray, Dr, is there any reason to fear a Cancer? and if it should prove a Cancer, what must we do? (MS 6140)

It is tempting to read Bishop Cary's questions here as a moment in which the veneer of objective reporting breaks down, but the context suggests otherwise. The bishop's questions are not only preceded by precise clinical descriptions but followed by an entirely scientific inquiry: 'Did you ever know Salivation practis'd in such a Case? For a Cancerous humour in lips and nose I have known a boy salivated with good success'.[51]

Cary is clearly open to empiric cures, and he is even receptive to the vernacular treatments. Perhaps the 'old woman… who they say has cured many sore breasts' is right, that there is no cancer but only an inflammation and that she can 'cure it without fail' with home remedies. Such cures, we have seen, were as much at hand to the early-eighteenth-century patient as in the seventeenth-century world of Robert Burton, who observed in *The Anatomy of Melancholy:* 'Cunning men, Wizards, and White-witches, as they call them, in every village, which if they be sought unto, will help almost all infirmities of body and mind.'[52] Burton was addressing 'Lawfull' versus 'Unlawfull' cures, and Jurin, we can be sure, would have felt similarly about folk cures dispensed by irregular practitioners. Cary, however, demonstrates typical eighteenth-century eclecticism in seeking various cures for his wife, though he is careful, whatever his anxieties for her, to remain within the boundaries of new science rhetoric to frame his empirical inquiry on salivation to Jurin.

A letter of 28 July is exuberant in its expression of relief and gratitude for the receipt of a reply from Jurin: 'A thousand thanks to You from Your patient and myself for Your three letters of 12, 19, & 21th [*sic*] June'. This confirms one's sense that the bishop and his wife had become, indeed, quite anxious while anticipating a reply from Jurin – at least some receipt (a prescription containing the ingredients of a medication) – which had not yet arrived. The 12 June letters must have crossed in the mail; after 12 June, Mrs

Cary has begun on the treatment plan advised by Jurin. Although the 28 July letter is full of appreciation for Jurin's recipes, this same letter – composed after a month of adhering to Jurin's treatment plan – also conveys the independence of patients from blind adherence to physician authority:

[The] Prescription we follow'd, only that we added the Emplast [plaster] & Cumin & Camph.[53] Our reason was what you say 19 June viz that if once the Menses come in a proper quantity, she may then at once leave off the Emmenagogues[54] & make use only of the Prescription in my last. – The menses came in due quantity & the Urine came to be right so that we left off the use of the Chalybeate Water also. But why, perhaps, You will ask, did we not use your Prescription of 21 ult? The reason was this. I sent the Prescription to the Apothecary & told him what You had sd on 19th ult & that the menses and urine were right & so left it to his discretion to follow which Prescription he thought best. And what Did he? he left out the Emmenagogues, but put in twenty grains of mercury for Morning & as much for Evening, whereas Your prescription gave only 20 grains in the Evening & None in the Morning. Therefore as I thought this dangerous, we follow'd Your Prescription of the 12th. Tho the Apothecary says he has known 30 grains of Mercury taken every morning, & as much every Evening for 3 months together without danger of Salivation. Well, but what has been the effect of the Medicines? Why, on this day three Weeks my wife thought her self perfectly well. But afterwards she took a little cold, & hereupon the old Symptoms returned together with some new ones.... The new Symptoms were a sore mouth, & pain in the right part of her neck & in the right ear. The Symptoms both new & old are all very considerably abated, and she hopes may wear off by time. She wears a Plaister on the left breast, a Plaister that is recommended by some Neighbouring Ladies who have been in [*sic*] her Case.... She dreads more Physick this season but what You think proper she will do. She will begin Monday to sit with her window open, keeping as far as she can from the wind. This is in order to get abroad & be us'd to the Air before the Warm season is quite spent. She is brought very low in flesh, drinks nothing but Tea & Whey, eats white meats. She is no way sick she says; & imputes her want of Appetite only to want of Air.

You will please to send us Your Orders as to Victuals, Drink Air & Medicines: tho she prays You to send no more Medicines, this season if you can help it. (MS 6140)

This letter demonstrates some of the difficulties encountered with medicine-by-post, including a jostling for authority over the patient's body. In addition to Jurin's definitive prescriptions (which Jurin copied onto the back of Cary's letters for future reference), there is the intervening advice of the apothecary, the reluctance of the patient to endure more harsh medications, and the continued use of vernacular remedies. The bishop attempts, in his letter, to represent this welter of cures and personal preferences by the patient as some kind of ultimate rational compromise reached through a process of objective deliberation. If Cary and his wife refuse the apothecary's formula, neither do they happily invite continuation of Jurin's therapeutic plan. Cary's wife is reluctant to endure any more unpleasant medications after a month on a harsh regimen: 'She dreads more Physick this season' and 'she prays You to send no more Medicines, this season if you can help it'. Although the bishop tells Jurin that 'what you think proper she will do,' Mrs Cary seems to have a mind of her own on these matters. She has not hesitated, to continue with the treatment of a 'Plaister on the left breast... recommended by some Neighbouring Ladies who have been in on her Case'. Several chefs appear to have been invited to cook Mrs Cary's therapeutic broth, and it is unclear how certainly Jurin's authority prevails in reality. We can only observe the written assurance of the

Figure 2.2

Example of corrections on the letter dated 28 July 1733, from Mordecai Cary to James Jurin. Courtesy: Wellcome Library, London.

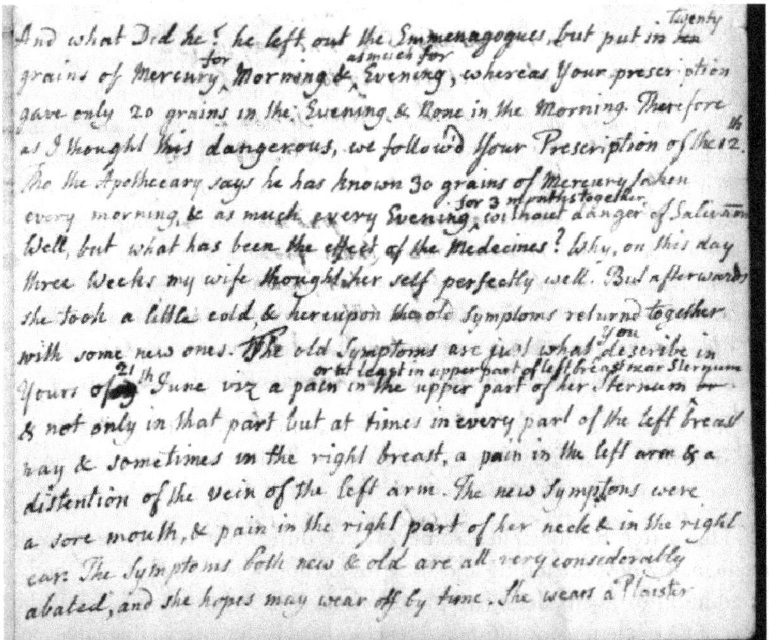

bishop, who would not wish to insult a respected consultant and good friend, that Jurin's medical opinion reigns supreme: 'What you think proper she will do'.

Cary is compulsive about recording his wife's symptoms with extreme accuracy over the ensuing months. Visual inspection of the July 28 autograph is exceptionally revealing in this respect. There is an abundance of corrections – words crossed out and additions or emendations squeezed between lines – which occur only in those sections of the epistle where the bishop acts as recorder of his wife's many symptoms. Such emendations are totally absent from the rest of the autograph which moves on to matters unrelated to Mrs Cary's health. It is only in the medical portion of the letter that 'nervous factuality' is made visible through superscriptions and cross-outs; perhaps this also betrays the bishop's frustration at trying to record such a multiplicity of vague complaints. In contrast, the second half of the letter, concerned with friends, politics, and scholarship, is not only free of corrections but conveys a distinct air of relaxed conviviality, a relief from the rhetorical obligations of the first half of the letter: 'Dr Tom Bentley I suppose if his manuscripts are not burnt and if any body else will trust him with a lodging, will plod on in pursuit of Fame by publishing Homer, & not be discourag'd by his loss of a pair of Breeches and a couple of Guineas....' This abrupt change of tone in Cary's letter, between the 'nervous factuality' of the medical report and the unencumbered epistolary freedom associated with non-medical matters, is a striking feature throughout the correspondence and accentuates the fact that medicine-by-post had its own special, often arduous, rhetorical expectations.

Whatever epistolary pains it may have cost him, the bishop, as mentioned earlier in this chapter, clearly prefers his own detailed account of his wife's condition to the local doctor's assessment. In a communication to Jurin on 1 August 1733, Cary encloses the local doctor's report on Mrs Cary, as requested by Jurin, but with a disclaimer: 'I am very sensible of Your kind meaning in requiring such a state of her case taken by a Physician but I am afraid You will find Yourself disappointed.' The doctor's history of Mrs Cary's case is then appended within the body of the letter – although the handwriting seems to be Cary's (see Figure 2.2) – and the bishop immediately adds his own remarks, amplifying significantly on what the doctor has written:

The Drs State of My wifes Case.

Mrs Cary has the same pains all over her body especially under the Omoplatae[55] that she feels in her breasts. – She complains of a Twitching of her Nerves & fibrous Contractions – There seems to be a great Sizyness

Figure 2.3

Letter of 1 August 1733, from Mordecai Cary to James Jurin.
Courtesy: Wellcome Library, London.

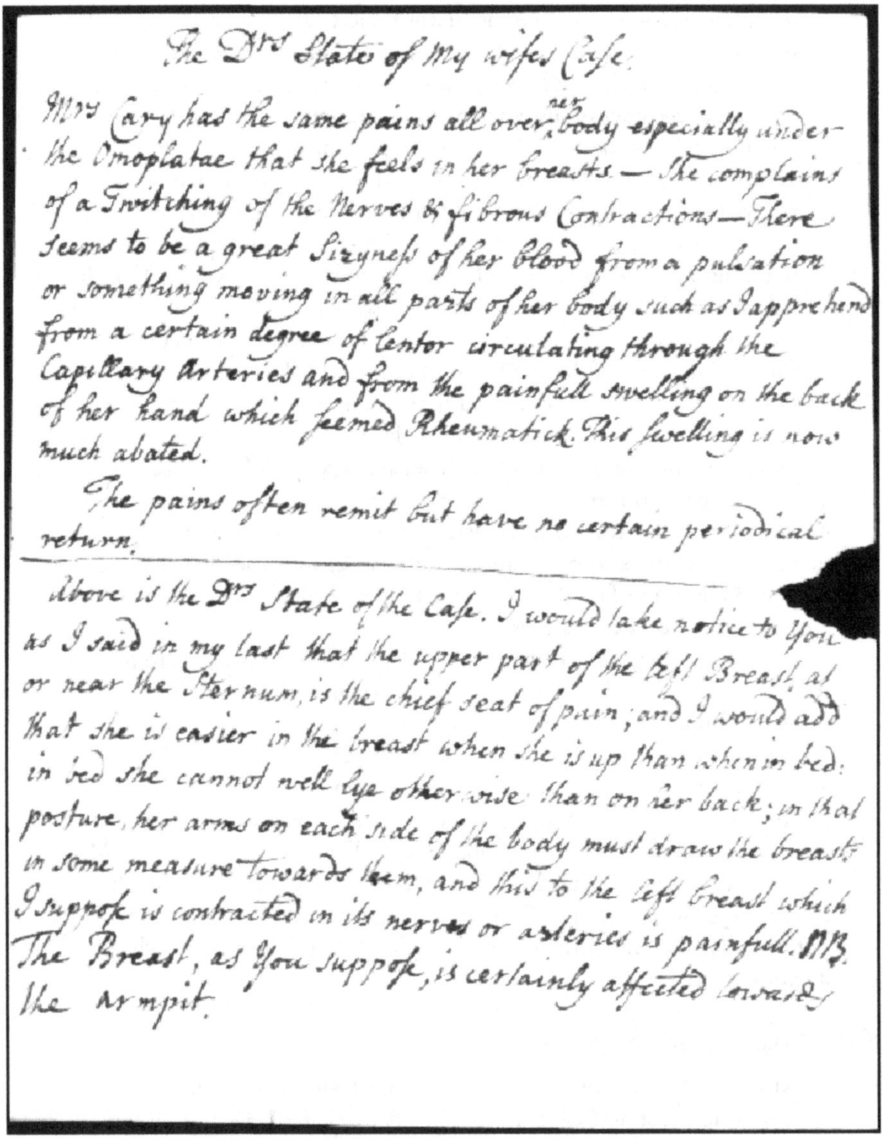

The Dr's State of my wifes Case.

Mrs Cary has the same pains all over her body especially under the Omoplatae that she feels in her breasts — She complains of a Twitching of the Nerves & fibrous Contractions — There seems to be a great Sizyness of her blood from a pulsation or something moving in all parts of her body such as I apprehend from a certain degree of lentor circulating through the Capillary Arteries and from the painfull swelling on the back of her hand which seemed Rheumatick. This swelling is now much abated.

The pains often remit but have no certain periodical return.

Above is the Dr's State of the Case. I would take notice to You as I said in my last that the upper part of the left Breast, at or near the Sternum, is the chief seat of pain; and I would add that she is easier in the breast when she is up than when in bed: in bed she cannot well lye otherwise than on her back; in that posture, her arms on each side of the body must draw the breasts in some measure towards them, and this to the left breast which I suppose is contracted in its nerves or arteries is painfull. NB. The Breast, as You suppose, is certainly affected towards the armpit.

[thickness or viscous property] of her blood from a pulsation or something moving in all parts of her body such as I apprehend from a certain degree of lentor[56] circulating through the Capillary Arteries and from the painfull swelling on the back of her hand which seemed Rheumatick. This swelling is now much abated.

The pains often remit but have no certain periodical return.

[line drawn on page]

Above is the Drs State of the Case. I would take notice to You as I said in my last that the upper part of the left Breast, at or near the Sternum, is the chief seat of pain; and I would add that she is easier in the breast when she is up than when in bed: in bed she cannot well lye otherwise than on her back; in that posture, her arms on each side of the body must draw the breasts in some measure towards them, and this to the left breast which I suppose contracted in its nerves or arteries is painful. NB. The Breast, as you suppose, is certainly affected towards the armpit. (MS 6140)

The bishop is confirmed in his preference for his own observations over those of this local physician which are, indeed, disappointing. The doctor provides nothing here to improve on the bishop's own thorough medical report. The doctor's statement of the case only substantiates that early-eighteenth-century medicine was a medicine of symptoms, and that proximity to the physician added little to what could be conveyed in a letter.

Following the August letter, there is now an interval of several months before Cary updates Jurin on his wife's condition. The letter is addressed to Jurin at his home in Austin Friars. Although Mrs Cary seems unimproved, Cary reasserts the great faith both he and his wife have in Jurin's medical knowledge and a readiness to comply with renewal of previously prescribed medical regimens. However, Mrs Cary has been on mercurials and now presents with a new problem: she is passing worms in her stool. In reference to this matter one is particularly struck by the absence of subjective elements in Cary's note:

After her Mercurial course, she voided at 2 or 3 different times, many worms, two of 'em large size I should rather say of great length, i.e. above half a yard in length, the rest small ones. Her menses have been regular enough; whenever they have not been so, she has been uneasy. Her food has been very low; her drink nothing but Barley-water. I could not persuade her to come to Town: there's no Physician she can trust in, but Dr Jurin. (MS 6140)[57]

Cary shares no alarm and he makes no mention of Mrs Cary's mental or physical state in consequence of this disturbing turn of events. Instead, a discussion of Euripides follows: 'Now will you take down Your little Euripides,' writes Cary, 'the same I dare say you had at School....' The letter concludes: 'But I beg pardon for these *minutiae Grammaticae*. However, if an author be worth reading, it is worth while to understand him'. Jurin, however, requests more detail about the passage of parasites from Mrs Cary's bowels, and in the next communication of 20 November 1734 Cary replies:

> In your last you desir'd to know whether the Worms she had voided were round or flat. The first of the Two she thinks was round; the second as well as she remembers was flat; but the flatness she imputes to its being dead.
>
> You are pleas'd to allow my explication of Euripides....(MS 6140)

The first part of the November letter taxes the Bishop with new complaints to detail. Mrs Cary has developed a rash and an irregularity in her menses. The opening of the letter provides a picture of the rigours of eighteenth-century therapy and suggests the firmness of resolution necessary on the part of the patient to be compliant with such prolonged and uncomfortable treatments:

> I beg leave to acquaint You with the state of my wife's health and to desire your directions thereupon. In March last she went thro her Spring Course of Physick, which she continued 40 days: in Sept. last she went thro her Autumn Course which continued 30 days. In Sept. the Purges, tho increas'd in the last 2 doses, had no effect at all upon her. She finds her breast better than she expected ever to find it: tho in sharp weather or upon taking the least cold, she feels the return of her old pains. But now she has a new complaint, that is of an intolerable Itching in back, belly & thighs; in which parts upon the least scratching or even rubbing (though she forbears as much as possibly she can) there riseth and remaineth a red scurfy spot, as broad as her thumb.[58] This complaint is about a week old. Now I think it necessary to let You know next February she will be 46 years old; that before her last Course of Physick she found the menses not so regular as they should be; that on 26 July last they came & continued 5 or six days, that on 15 Aug. upon riding they appear'd again but in very small Quantity, only a drop or two as if she had pricked her finger, & nothing more till 10th October last & then they continued five or six days in a very large quantity. Since sd 10th October she has seen nothing of 'em, tho by her breath I perceive 'em to be in her body. Upon these Symptoms we beg you advice. (MS 6140)

For the resolution of the breast inflammation, Dr Jurin is given full credit in a postscript of the above letter: 'My Wife presents her best respects to yours a million of thanks for the Benefit she has rec'd by Your Prescription'. But even with the relief of this most worrisome symptom,

92

Cary remains tireless in his role as narrator of his spouse's evolving medical complaints. He details a newly-developed skin condition and then follows this with a log of menstrual alterations, including a vivid simile of small menses being no more than 'if she had pricked her finger' – a simile, it should be noted, both quantitatively precise and entirely of the physical, scientific world.

In a final letter concerned with Mrs Cary's health, dated 8 February 1734/5, it would seem that Mrs Cary's complaints have turned to some of the more familiar complaints of middle age:

> She is quite clear of the itching scurfy spots which she says were chiefly on her thighs where from the breadth of a silver penny they use'd to spread into that of a Crown piece. All her complaint Now is, that she grows very fat....

> She desires to know, first prefacing that she is pretty well, whether she is to go into her Spring Course for her breast: she almost thinks she needs not; but will follow your direction. (MS 6140)[59]

While direct responses of Jurin to Cary's medical inquiries do not survive, we can judge the character of his responses in part by what is missing. Jurin, as we have mentioned, was an ardent proponent of the application of Newtonian principles to medicine. His regimens for Mrs Cary were evidently harsh, iatromechanical descendants of classical methods, meant to keep the 'pipes' open. There is no evidence from any of Cary's letters that Jurin modified his prescriptions out of consideration for the distresses caused by his prescriptions, though her desire to stop treatment is often voiced through her husband. Nor do we have any suggestion that Jurin deigned to respond to the alternative treatments mentioned by the bishop; he seems rather to have ignored them. Not once in any letter does Cary acknowledge that Jurin either has rejected or acquiesced to any of the several proposed changes, or additions, to therapy offered by the local healers, apothecary, women neighbours, or the old lady with her folk cures.

The letters from Bishop Cary to Jurin might be considered a special case for several reasons. Cary's education (including attending lectures at Leyden) and his close ties to Jurin might predispose him to a heightened attention to medical details and proper rhetorical nuance in communicating on medical matters. However, it could equally well be argued that the close friendship of Cary and Jurin would prompt the bishop to dispense with rhetorical formalities and to express his concern about his wife's condition with greater freedom and greater expression of feeling. The fact that Cary is describing the symptoms of his spouse rather than some medical problem of his own, and that the patient is a female, might have influenced the form and tone of the Cary's letters to Jurin, but similar rhetorical character pervades other letters sent to Jurin, letters that concern male patients.

The same quality of remarkable objectivity and emotional restraint consistent with the influence of new science rhetoric is seen, for example, in the letters to Jurin from Shallett Turner (1692?–1762), a professor of modern history at Cambridge and also a personal friend of Jurin. Turner describes his phthisical symptoms in a letter from 29 May 1726 as if he were a doctor standing at his own bedside:[60]

> Since I saw you Sir I have used the cold Bath, and the medicines you prescribed, and have rode out every day; but I think my illness grows upon me, and I observe my self to waste and fall away in flesh very much wch is the thing that discourages me the most, and makes me think my case dangerous You may be sure sir I have a great many Doctors here, some will have me go to Montpelier [*sic*], and others to Edinburgh.... You will be so good as to be very particular in your directions and I shall punctually observe and follow them.... I have generally a fit of low spiritedness attended with pains in my neck and shoulders every day; I do not sleep well at nights, always with some uneasiness and sweating upon my first going to sleep.... I shall only beg leave to ask you whether my blister may not run too much, I have it dressed twice a day and it makes a great discharge.[61]

The attempt at objectivity levels the hierarchical importance of one symptom over another. Even Turner's concern about his wasting becomes just another part of the medical report; 'low spiritedness' is not addressed separately from the rheumatic complaints which accompany it. Part of this derives from the complete association of mind and body with which eighteenth-century patients and doctors viewed health and illness.[62] The importance of mental state may be the basis of Turner's query if the waters at Tunbridge Wells – recommended by Jurin, who spends the summer months there – 'be good tho' the season for company be not till June'.[63] The mind-body connection remained strong throughout the century. However, as the century wore on, patients would more clearly distinguish their purely physical symptoms from their subjective experience of being sick. In contrast to Turner's very deliberate exposition of his ailments, the patients of later generations would likely describe not only wasting and rheumatism, but would elaborate on the discomfort and fears attending that condition, and in a dramatic narrative intended to enlist not just the medical opinion of their doctor but his active sympathy.

Hints of a new epistolary patient voice

The beginnings of this new epistolary voice, albeit a very limited personal voice, can be seen to enter into letters written to Jurin after 1740. For example, when the architect Thomas Worsley (1710–78) wrote to Jurin in 1746 about bladder stones, he inquired:

> I should also be glad to know whether in case I enter upon a strict Course in order for a Cure whether the Remedy are not so rough and forcing as to be dangerous, & whether it would not put me to great pain, for I must also acquaint you that the Frame of my Body and my Constitution are rather delicate and too sensible. I should willingly undergo a Course of Remedy and observe any rule in Diet etc.... if I was not discouraged from it by the thoughts of Pain and Danger.[64]

Worsley, as we know, had good reason to express anxiety in taking Jurin's stone-dissolving preparation since this letter was written shortly after the death of Walpole and the publicity surrounding Jurin's *lixivium lithontripticum*. But Worsley conveys his hesitation in proceeding with this potentially harsh medication on the basis of what he judges to be his delicate and too sensible constitution. Weak constitutions are not new, but what was previously a descriptive fact in the medical history now appears as a bargaining chip in the negotiation between patient and doctor for modifying therapy.

When John Huxham (1692–1768), a physician friend of Jurin, consulted him about his wife's illness in 1742, he voiced personal concerns not found in Bishop Cary's letters:

> Dear Sir!
>
> I beg Leave to desire your Advice on my poor wife's present threatening Disorder – as she is an exceedingly good Woman her death wou'd be no small Loss to ye neighbour hood [*sic*], but to my & my poor Children absolutely irreparable.... She is about 46, of a thin & tender Constitution, of weak nerves & a bilious scorbutic Habit [etc.]... I have vomited & purged Her frequently & She bears it well; but ye very drastic Purges greatly hurt Her....[65]

In both Huxham's and Worsley's letters, the patient's constitution is not merely another medical fact, but an assertion of individuality which provides an opportunity to voice subjective fears about illness and pain – an assertion of subjective feeling which certainly exceeds the model of relatively pure clinical descriptions evident in the first third of the century.

While Huxham voices tender and empathetic feelings for his wife's suffering, this new subjective voice remains juxtaposed, within the same missive, with the unmistakable rhetoric of the new science physician. Huxham's medicine-by-post continues:

> She never had her Catamenia regularly either as to Time, or Quantity – her whole Family had weak nerves, tho' naturally cheerful & brisk Spirits – Several of them have fallen into, & even of, dropsical Disorders.

> About 12 months since, driving Home very hard for 5, or 6, miles in a Chariot, not too easie. She found about 2 or 3 Hours after her Legs were very much swol'n, almost as high as her Knees – She never had any thing of a like nature before....

> At ye beginning of March last She was seized wth a bilious hysteric Cholick... wth great Costiveness and very high colour'd Urine wch was soon carried off by common Methods – but an obtuse Pain or Soreness remained in ye left Hypochondrium, just under ye Spleen, but wth out Swelling or any considerable Induration.

Despite all treatments and moderation in diet:

> [H]er Swellings have been rather kept from encreasing than carried off; nay I fear they rather advance.... her Discharge by Stool is now free & easie, often times wth much yellow & black bile – but her Urine is in very small quantity, very thick & high colour'd, & deposits a vast Deal of red brick colour'd Sediment.

> She takes daily & constant Exercise by Riding, walking, &c & bears it well, & hath been a considerable Time in ye Country in a very fine pure air. (MS 6141)

The history thus concludes with a consideration of four of the six non-naturals: diet, evacuations, exercise, and air. Jurin's prescription (penned onto Huxham's letter) is his very own *lixivium lithontripticum!*

It is instructive to compare the medicine-by-post rhetoric of Huxham to that of Jurin. John Huxham was a regular correspondent of Jurin. He collaborated with Jurin in collecting cases which demonstrated the safety and efficacy of smallpox inoculation, and they frequently compared notes on the relationship of meteorology and health. However, Huxham, as physician, betrays a humanity in his letters that anticipates the greater subjectivity that is emerging with the medicine of sensibility, and even a turn for the dramatic that also becomes more prominent in subsequent decades. In the case of Dr Seymour, a patient with advanced liver disease, we have the rare occasion to compare the rhetoric of Dr Jurin directly with that of Dr Huxham in response to the same complicated private-practice patient.

Dr Huxham is first sees Dr Seymour, but on 7 January 1729/30, he seeks advice from Jurin: 'The affairs given are so uncertain and lacking in stability that we are in quite a slipping way: even the helper is sometimes forced to ask for help and the doctor for a doctor.' Huxham describes the patient as 'a man of fifty, a doctor of this famous Province, [who] has for one or two months now been suffering from serious madness'. Huxham ventures that 'The patient had lived too richly and luxuriously, perhaps drinking to excess....' He explains, with emphatic drama and metaphor, that he was 'called to this patient, with an excellent doctor who is a friend of mine, and I flew to the rescue stretching out helping hands'. Huxham then resorts to a most objective account of his classic treatment of Dr Seymour, consisting of 'generous' bleeding, 'preparations of Antimony, which I greatly approve of in madness',[66] and 'Wilson's cure-alls' which tend either to 'cause violent vomiting, or stimulate the bowels, frequently and very gently'.[67] As in the letter regarding his wife, Huxham juxtaposes new science objectivity with eruptions of feeling.

A subsequent letter from Dr Huxham to Jurin, dated 29 March, 1730, explains that 'For some considerable Time after I wrote you poor Doct^r Seymour' had become 'more calm & rationale, his furious Exacerbations Shorter and Seldomer'. But following this remission, 'he grew again very outrageous & mad, his urine was exceeding bilious & very Small in Quantity'. Huxham continues with a very precise clinical description of a man suffering from the effects of end-stage alcoholic cirrhosis: 'his whole Skin was tinged of a yellow icterick colour, his Belly became very tense & his Legs swelled at ye anckles.... He now continues, sometimes falling into a violent Fit of weeping & yet in ye midst of it artfully contriving mischief.' Huxham lists numerous medicines that he has been using, and advises Jurin that 'we keep him chiefly on a vegetable diet'. He wonders also, putting in scientific observation, that the 'moon seems to have little or no Effect on him, wch I have frequently observ'd in other maniacks; 'tho for ye Reason they are term'd Lunaticks'. After a long list of questions for Jurin, Huxham says, deferentially, that 'Till I have ye Honour of your Answer, I shall not give him any more medicines with out ye most evident necessity.' He concludes that 'I am the first in ye name of unhappy Doct^r Seymour & his Family to return you their sincere and hearty Thanks for your generous and kind Advice for Him and his deplorable circumstances. – And then for my own for ye many Favours I have received from You....'[68]

In one of the rare autographs penned by Jurin concerned with a private practice consultation, Jurin shows concern for Dr Seymour's tolerance for treatment, but his tone remains mostly objective and removed from the patient's suffering – friendly but much more impersonal (rhetorically) than Huxham:

I was yesterday favour'd with your Second account of Dr Seymour's case, in answer to which I have little to say to ye Symptom's he lately labourd [*sic*] under, they being so judiciously & happily remov'd by your Prescriptions. I would only infer from them, that we must be cautious of using great evacuations, & rather allow length of time for ye cure, than be too hasty in attempting it: but in this you & I are intirely of ye same sentiment. (MS 6141)

After some detailed discussion of medications, including a 'rougher vomit... once in a fortnight,' but the withholding of 'Evacuations' should the patient 'incline to ye low, mopish way', Jurin considers the meteorological effects raised by Huxham, responding that, 'As to ye Moon, I am of your mind, having never seen any of those cases, that I had any dependence on it'.[69] Jurin's adherence to, and trust in, empirical observation remains firm, and he demonstrates, in his measured medicine-by-post reply to Huxham, that he is more distinctly fixed in the mould of the new science physician than his esteemed colleague. Huxham's medicine-by-post is a rhetoric in transition, located between the doctor of new science and the doctor of sensibility whose voice will predominate over the next decades.

The assertion that the medicine-by-post of the first decades of the eighteenth century were predominantly influenced by the prescriptions of new science rhetoric is challenged by the rather dramatic medicine-by-post correspondence of Mary Ferrers – the aristocratic wife of Washington Shirley, second Earl Ferrers – to the famous Dr Hans Sloane (1660–1753).[70] This correspondence is from the same period as the Jurin letters (Jurin served as Secretary to the Royal Society within a decade after Sloane). However, the letters from Lady Mary, unlike those of Bishop Cary to Jurin, are penned directly by the female patient. The rhetoric is much freer than the other letters we have examined so far, much more descriptive about the emotional distress of her situation. This said, however, the difference between this medical correspondence and the others in this chapter is, finally, more apparent than real.

The example of Lady Mary's letters is very instructive in clarifying that it was not drama alone which distinguished the rhetoric of sensibility from the rhetoric of new science but, rather, a whole new medical consciousness. The Ferrers-Sloane letters are also valuable in showing that a woman patient in the early-eighteenth century was able to be completely open with her physician about so sensitive a subject as venereal disease contracted from her husband – and that she might expect a very sympathetic and supportive male physician to listen to her narrative, even among the established physicians of a patriarchal British society.[71]

Mary Ferrers (d. 1740) was the granddaughter of Sir Gawen Corbyn, and was married to Washington Shirley (1677–1729) in 1704. It was a union that Lady Mary was to regret.[72] Indeed, she had good reason to apply urgently to her physician regarding a 'deplorable situation,' for not only had she contracted venereal disease from her husband, but the Earl now refused her funds to travel to Italy for treatment. She had intended to seek medical advice from the Montpellier physician, Antoine Diedier, to whom she had been personally referred by none less than Dr Hermann Boerhaave.[73] She implores Sloane, 'Indeed all you have seen me suffer falls so short of what I now endure... and if you judge it worthy y^r pity, I will take the freedom to entreat you that you will go to my cruel Lord and beg before him this sad circumstance.'[74]

It is clear that Dr Sloane has acted on his patient's behalf, as evidenced in this response from Lady Mary posted from Brussels (dated 29 November, year uncertain):

> I had sooner spoke my gratitude for the generous concern you express'd with respect to my compliance with Dr Boerhaaves opinion of my going into Italy and which my Lord intimated when he gave me his permission to make the experiment, which tho he says your sentiments were not the same, yet however you thought it reasonable I should for my own satisfaction make the tryal since so many had been already ineffectual. (BL MS 4058)

Sloane has intervened in the sensitive domestic conflicts of this aristocratic couple, and has sided squarely with Lady Mary, even though he is not convinced of the benefits of travelling to Italy for cure. He acknowledges her emotional and physical needs in the face of failed therapy and does not take personal or professional offence that English medicine has failed to relieve his patient's illness.

Lord Ferrers had proposed meeting the countess in Lisle, from where she was to proceed to Naples. However, the Earl changed his mind and demanded that his wife return to England, threatening, by the patient's account, that he 'will protest my [medical] Bills if I do not Instantly comply'. This great disappointment came, writes Lady Mary to her doctor:

> att a time when I am confin'd to my Bed with such a convulsion upon the orifice of my stomach that I can hardly swallow even liquid sustenance for my support[.]... [I]f you judge it worthy yr pity I will take the freedom to entreat you that you will go to my cruell Lord and beg him this sad circumstance, say that my last request is only his leave to preserve the wretched remnant of my life a little longer[,] at least that he will suffer me to endeavour it by makeing [*sic*] this immediate tryal for which I have a strong inclination.... [75]

Once again the countess finds a sympathetic ear and an effective intermediary in Sloane, for in a subsequent letter from Brussels she is able to thank her physician for his 'interposition'.[76]

A year later she writes to Sloane from Montpellier to report on her medical progress under Diedier's direction. In this letter, the patient frankly discusses her venereal infection and holds her husband fully responsible. She is exhausted by illness and treatment alike, and voices typical eighteenth-century patient scepticism towards her doctors:

> After having past [*sic*] five months in this country in an increase of all my complaints which together with the excessive heat hath reduced me to a state of Desperation and oblig'd me to comply with the proposal of passing once more through a course of mercury and the rather because as he [Diedier] is persuad'd that the whole of my illness proceeds from an Injury from my Lord so that he promises himself that by managing that remedy with great caution and continuing it 6 or 7 months it is yet capable to perfect my cure, and tho I am very far from that opinion, yet having no other resource so I am reduc'd to make the experiment and must say in justice to Monsr. Diedier that having been seven weeks in his method I have suffered no sort of inconvenience from it.... (BL MS 4058)

These letters from Mary Ferrers to Haas Sloane offer vivid proof of how completely eighteenth-century women were at the mercy of the patriarchal system in which they lived. Yet, these letters also reveal a less obvious and more benign (if still paternalistic) corner of this same patriarchal world. Mary Ferrers was apparently confident in approaching Sloane for help in this situation of domestic abuse, and she was uninhibited in telling Sloane about her venereal infection – a situation that might have produced great mortification. Sloane, for his part, is ready to assist her, and he does not dismiss the countess's medical complaints nor the urgency of her desire for treatment. Monsieur Diedier, for his part, showed complete frankness with his female patient about her venereal illness and allows her to be an informed participant in her therapy. There is no suggestion of male complicity, and both Sloane and Diedier were quite willing to implicate the Earl as the cause of his wife's unfortunate malady, not disguising the nature of the disease from the patient or pretending cure was achieved when, in fact, it was not.

Does the dramatic rhetoric of the Ferrers-Sloane correspondence force us to reconsider the presumption that medicine-by-post rhetoric in the early decades of the eighteenth-century was primarily objective in character? Certainly, there is a openness and sympathy evident in this correspondence that looks more towards Huxham than Jurin. Yet, the drama in Lady Mary's letters derive as much out of the domestic as the medical crisis. It is true that she despairs of her health: 'I am confin'd to my Bed with such a convulsion upon the orifice of my stomach that I can hardly swallow even liquid sustenance for my support.' She also complains that heat and symptoms have 'reduced me to a state of Desperation and oblig'd me to comply with the proposal of passing once more through a course of mercury'. Still, these are rather straightforward, if urgent, declarations of discomfort and medical necessity. The rhetoric here may anticipate, as with Dr Huxham, the opening up of subjective experience, but it is not a rhetoric that registerspain as arising from an exquisite delicacy of constitution. That was yet to come.

As speculation on the role of the nervous system in health and disease supplanted iatromechanical principles in medical thinking, so the rhetoric of new science lost favour with the patient. The transition in medical concern from hydraulics to nervous sensibility liberated the epistolary voice of the patient dramatically; subjective feeling was encouraged and, by the second half of the century, dominated medicine-by-post communication. Paradoxically, as the narrative of personal experience in disease revealed more that was private, one's illness became, increasingly, an acceptable topic for social 'conversation' – a narrative to share with others. The champion of this new rhetoric was a physician who first had to free himself from iatromechanical medicine and Newtonianism, a doctor who for a time had been as fully 'in the shadow of the *Principia*' as Jurin – the Bath physician, George Cheyne.

Notes

1. Garlick Hill, England, 7 August 1727, Wellcome MS. 6146. All letters to and from James Jurin cited in this paper are from The Wellcome Library for the History and Understanding of Medicine in London. (I am grateful for a Brandeis University Sachar Fund grant for supporting my research at the Wellcome Trust.) *The Correspondence of James Jurin (1684-1750): Physician and Secretary to the Royal Society*, A. Rusnock (ed.), (Amsterdam: Rodopi, 1996) contains many of the letters cited in this chapter. The Jurin medical correspondence presented in this chapter was examined and transcribed by me just prior to Rusnock's book coming to press, but I am most grateful to Rusnock for her extreme generosity in sharing her transcriptions with me (some not included in her final edition) before the actual publication of her exemplary edition of Jurin's letters. Citations for Jurin's correspondence in this chapter reference the Wellcome manuscript numbers and also pages in Rusnock (where applicable): for example, Wellcome MS no.; Rusnock, *op. cit.* (note 1), page numbers.

2. The Royal College of Physicians of London (chartered in 1518) had great difficulty in establishing its authority over medical practice. The College tried to limit the practice of medicine within a seven mile radius of the

centre of the London to Fellows and Licentiates of the College. Fellows were elected to the college and were exclusively Oxford or Cambridge graduates; other medical practitioners might be granted a licence after passing an examination and the payment of 'a stiff fee', but such licentiates had no voting rights. Disregard of the College's authority was reflected not only by limited membership but also by a decline in the number of Fellows and Licentiates from 136 to 78 over the twenty years following the close of the seventeenth century. Furthermore, a physician's standing with the College of Physicians seems to have weighed little with patients, even from the aristocratic classes; Queen Anne's personal physician, for example, was not a member of the College. Outside of London, the need for doctors in the provinces provided an opportunity for surgeons, apothecaries, and for the hybrid surgeon–apothecary, to practice without restrictions from the Royal College. The demand for doctors in the towns and rural areas outside of London was recognised by the right of bishops to grant an Episcopal licence bestowing the official title of 'Medici' on local medical practitioners. See G. Holmes, *Augustan England: Professions, State and Society, 1680-1730* (Boston: George Allen & Unwin, 1982), Chapter 6, especially 169–73.

3. See T.M. Brown, 'Medicine in the Shadow of the *Principia*', *Journal of the History of Ideas* 48, 1 (1987), 629–48. Also see A. Guerrini, 'James Keill, George Cheyne, and Newtonian Physiology, 1690-1740', *Journal of the History of Biology* 18, 2 (1985), 247–66; and Guerrini, 'Isaac Newton, George Cheyne and the Principia Medicinae', in *The Medical Revolution of the Seventeenth Century*, R. French and A. Wear (eds), (Cambridge: Cambridge University Press, 1989), 222–45. J. Wiltshire, in *Samuel Johnson in the Medical World: The Doctor and the Patient* (New York: Cambridge, 1991), provides an especially lucid description of the basics of iatromechanical principles as set out by the famous Leiden physician-professor, Herman Boerhaave (1668–1738), the influential founder of the iatromechanical system, see 76–82. H.J. Cook has further refined our understanding of Boerhaave's personality and medical philosophy in 'Boerhaave and the Flight from Reason in Medicine', in *Bulletin of the History of Medicine* 74, 3 (2000), 221–40.

4. The following biographical material comes from the introduction on James Jurin by A. Rusnock in her edition of *The Correspondence of James Jurin, op. cit.* (note 1), 8–61.

5. Although many English and Scottish students did return with the MD degree from Leyden, it was not uncommon simply to attend lectures of one's choosing without the intention of securing a medical degree. Some students 'were already in unqualified medical practice and were content to go back to it with their added experience, while others... used their Leyden training as a passport to a bishop's licence on their return to England and practised as

medici in the provinces'; see Holmes, *op. cit.* (note 2), 177. The Edinburgh
Medical School programme, established in 1726, was a response to the drain
of Scottish medical students to Holland (see Chapter 4 for details), but both
Edinburgh and Leyden served to provide access into the medical profession
for those who would have been denied the opportunity of attending Oxford
or Cambridge on religious grounds. Furthermore, the tuition at both
Edinburgh and Leyden was far more affordable than at the English
universities, partly because students could pick and choose which lectures to
attend and pay a fee only for those classes.

6. Rusnock, *op. cit.* (note 1),10.
7. Jurin may have been considered not sufficiently Jacobite in political leanings
   for some of Newcastle's citizens.
8. Rusnock, *op. cit.* (note 1), 11.
9. This pamphlet war is discussed more fully, below, to illustrate a particular
   brand of medical rhetoric during this period.
10. F.N. Smith, *Scientific Discourse: Gulliver's Travels and The Philosophical
    Transactions, The Genres of Gulliver's Travels* (Newark: University of Delaware
    Press, 1990), 152.
11. Vellication is the 'action of or process of pulling or twitching; irritation or
    stimulation by means of small sharp points; titillation and tickling', *Oxford
    English Dictionary.*
12. Wellcome MS 6146.
13. T. Sprat, *The History of the Royal Society of London (1667),* J. Cope and H.
    Whitmore Jones (eds), (St. Louis: Washington University Studies, 1958).
14. B. Vickers, 'The Royal Society and English Prose: A Reassessment', in
    *Rhetoric and the Pursuit of Truth: Language: Language Change in the
    Seventeenth and Eighteenth Centuries* (Los Angeles: University of California
    Press, 1985), 3.
15. Smith, *op. cit.* (note 10), 139.
16. R. Porter, 'Laymen, Doctors and Medical Knowledge in the Eighteenth
    Century: The Evidence of the *Gentleman's Magazine*', in R. Porter (ed.),
    Patients and Practitioners: Lay Perceptions of Medicine in Pre-Industrial Society
    (New York: Cambridge University Press, 185), 283–313.
17. Sprat, *op. cit.* (note 13), 111–13. The call for a 'primitive purity' of language,
    in which there is an equivalency of 'things' for 'words' was satirised by
    Jonathan Swift in *Gulliver's Travels.* During Gulliver's visit to the grand
    Academy of Lagado, at the School of Languages, the professors enlarge upon
    a 'Scheme for abolishing all Words whatsoever', words being deleterious to
    one's health through exhausting the lungs. In the opinion of the Projectors:

> Words are only Names for *Things*, it would be more convenient for
> all Men to carry about them, such *Things* as were necessary to

express the particular Business they are to discourse on... which only
hath this Inconvenience attending it; that if a Man's Business be very
great, and of various Kinds, he must be obliged in Proportion to
carry a greater Bundle of *Things* upon his Back, unless he can afford
one or two strong Servants to attend him. I have often beheld two
of those Sages almost sinking under the Weight of their Packs....

In a related Academy project, Swift alludes to the Royal Society's suspicion of
Latinisms. The 'Professors' at the School of Languages in Lagado aim 'to
shorten Discourse by cutting Polysyllables into one, and leaving out Verbs
and Participles; because in reality all things imaginable are but Nouns'.
Gulliver's Travels (1726), in *The Prose Works of Jonathan Swift*, H. Davis *et al.*
(eds), (Oxford: Basil Blackwell, 1939–68), 11:185.

18. See Brown, *op. cit.* (note 3).
19. These were all aspects of environment that the doctor could influence by
    advice on such matters as diet, travel, activity, alteration of habits, and
    avoidance of certain strong emotions. Galen distinguished between 'naturals',
    which comprised the body and its workings, and 'contra-naturals', which
    comprised disease. 'Non-naturals' were, therefore, a third category, neither
    intrinsic to body nor disease, yet affecting the state of health. The
    classification into six non-naturals is medieval, and physician–authors might
    subsume these non-naturals into fewer categories. (I am indebted to
    Christopher Lawrence for this helpful definition of the non-naturals.)
20. For the place of iatromechanical medical philosophy within Enlightenment
    medicine, and for a description of the limited components of physical
    examination available to physicians in this period, see R. Porter, *The Greatest
    Benefit to Mankind: A Medical History of Humanity* (New York: W.W.
    Norton & Co., 1997), ch. x, 'Enlightenment', 245–303.
21. Smith, *op. cit.* (note 10), 149.
22. *Ibid.*, 145. It was the editorial policy of *The Philosophical Transactions* in the
    first decades of the eighteenth century to leave it to readers to come to their
    own judgment on the worth of observations reported in the journal. See
    T.C. Bond, 'Keeping up with the Latest *Transactions*: The Literary Critique
    of Scientific Writing in the Hans Sloane Years', *Eighteenth-Century Life*, 22,
    2 (May 1998), 1–17; see also C. Bazerman, 'Reporting the Experiment: The
    Changing Account of Scientific Doings in the Philosophical Transactions of
    the Royal Society, 1665–1800', in *Shaping Written Knowledge: The Genre and
    Activity of the Experimental Article in Science* (Madison: University of
    Wisconsin Press, 1988), ch. 3, 59–79.
    A letter from 7 August 1727 from James Jurin to Thomas Dereham, an
    expatriate English Roman Catholic, is of interest in respect to the laissez faire
    attitude of the Royal Society. Jurin corresponded often with Dereham, who

associated with many Italian natural philosophers, in the hopes of encouraging scientific interchange of ideas between England and Italy. Jurin responds to Dereham's frustration at the long wait for responses from Jurin in his role as Secretary to the Royal Society:

> The Italian Virtuosi, I find, always expect, & you seem to require, that I should send you ye Opinion of ye Society upon ye several Papers you transmit to me. But this is what ye Royal Society never gives. They pronounce no Judgement upon what comes before them, but only return their thanks to ye Authors. (Rusnock, 365)

23. John Horsley to James Jurin, 1 July 1723, Widdrington; Wellcome MS 6146; Rusnock, *op. cit.* (note 1), 188–9.
24. Jurin to Horsley, 19 October 1723, Laur, Pountney Lane; Wellcome MS 6146, Rusnock, *op. cit.* (note 1), 202–3.
25. Jacob Johnson to James Jurin, 10 December 1727, Newcastle; Wellcome MS 6139. All subsequent letters of Henry Shafto and Jacob Johnson are found under this same Wellcome MS number.
26. 'Cephalicks... are all those Medicines which are good for Distempers of the Head', J. Quincy, *Lexicon Physico-Medicum* (London, 1726). See bibliography for the complete, very extended, title to this reference work.
27. From the letters of Dr William Cullen at the Royal College of Physicians in Edinburgh. This is from the collection desigated the 'Consultation Letters', the volumes of which are organised by date. See Chapter 4 on Dr William Cullen, for more specifics on this collection and its organisation. (The fuller text of this particular letter is also given in that chapter.)
28. J. Schneid Lewis, *In the Family Way: Childbearing in the British Aristocracy, 1760–1860* (New Jersey: Rutgers, 1986), 93.
29. However, there were exceptions. A delightful anecdote regarding physician fees is found in the Wellcome manuscript collection of letters of Catherine Hutton (1756-1846), a miscellaneous writer who collected autograph letters from girlhood. Hutton remarks in an annotation on a note of Sir Walter Farquhar (1738-1829), a successful Scottish apothecary turned physician:

> Sir Walter Farquhar was a fashionable physician, with a smooth insinuating manner. A certain Duchess put twenty guineas into his hand and said, 'the duke drinks too much: I wish you could cure him of this disorder'. He visited the duke, asked a multitude of questions, assured him he was in a very dangerous way, and concluded by limiting his wine. The prescription took effect, and the Doctor received a double fee. (Wellcome MS 5270, no. 26)

Regarding Henry Alexander, 'the celebrated Occulist', who performed cataract removal with a needle ['couching'], Hutton comments (on a paper, in her collection, with the signature of Alexander) that:

> his fee for operating on one eye is a hundred guineas; but if the patient is so fortunate as to have two eyes which want the operation (of couching) at once, he may have it performed on both for a hundred and fifty guineas. The fee, however, is not limited to these sums.; Lord Lowther gave Alexander a thousand pounds for two eyes; and was, moreover, so delighted that he could see to shoot partridges, that he sent him two brace out of the first six he killed. (Wellcome MS 5270, no. 55)

These anecdotes also bear witness that once a doctor was established the system of not discussing fees directly could work to the great advantage of the physician. See Schneid Lewis, *ibid.*, 93.

30. Vickers, *op. cit.* (note 14), 32–7.
31. Vickers, *ibid.*, 3.
32. Sprat, *op. cit.* (note 13), 112.
33. For a discussion on the battle of rhetoric between established physicians and irregulars, or empirics, see A. Guerrini, '"A Club of Little Villains": Rhetoric, Professional Identity and Medical Pamphlet Wars', in M. Mulvey Roberts and R. Porter (eds), *Literature and Medicine during the Eighteenth Century* (New York: Routledge, 1993), 226–44. See also R. Porter, *Health for Sale: Quackery in England 1660–1850* (New York: Manchester University Press, 1989), and Porter, '"I Think Ye Both Quacks": The Controversy between Theodore Myersbach and Dr John Coakley Lettsom', in W.F. Bynum and R. Porter (eds), *Medical Fringe and Medical Orthodoxy 1750–1850* (New Hampshire: Croom Helm, 1987), 56–78. A brief overview can be found in P.W. Child, *Discourse and Practice in Eighteenth-Century Medical Literature: The Case of George Cheyne* (PhD thesis, Notre Dame, Indiana, 1992), 122–4.
34. Rusnock, 'Introduction', *op. cit.* (note 1), 45; A.J. Viseltear, 'The Last Illnesses of Robert and Horace Walpole.' *Yale Journal of Medicine*, 56 (1983), 131–52: 132.
35. John Ranby, *A Narrative of the Last Illness of the Right Honourable the Earl of Orford: From May 1744, to the Day of his Decease March the Eighteenth following* [published with his *Treatise on Gun-Shot Wounds*] (London, 1745).
36. London: M. Cooper, 1745. In the Wellcome Library collection entitled 'Medical Tracts', Old Series, Vol. 1, No. 52, 32. Fielding praises Ranby several times in *The History of Tom Jones, A Foundling*; see Book VIII, Chapter 12, and Book XVI, Chapter 9.

Accusing Jurin of practicing quack medicine was all too apt under the circumstances. Jurin's stone-dissolving recipe was remarkably similar to the nostrum concocted by the notorious woman lay healer, Mrs Joanna Stephens. She had produced a mixture of powdered calcined shells (egg shells combined with oyster and snail shells) and soap, for which secret recipe Parliament paid her £5,000 in 1739. The ingredients contain lime which, in fact, might have helped dissolve certain types of stones. Jurin's concoction was several times more powerful, but the fact that he refused to divulge the contents of his *lixivium lithontripticum* – claiming that he did so for the public good – added to negative speculation surrounding the prescription and the death of Walpole.

37. James Jurin, *Expostulatory Address to John Ranby, Esq; Principal Serjeant Surgeon to His Majesty, and F.R.S., Occasioned by his Treatise on Gunshot-Wounds, and his Narrative of the Earl of Orford's Last Illness. By a Physician* (London: M. Cooper, 1745). This tract is available at the Wellcome Library, in Tracts, Early Printed Books, MSL tracts. Page numbers for this are included in text.

38. A. Guerrini, *op. cit.* (note 33), 230.

39. Holmes, *op. cit.* (note 2), 167.

40. C. McIntosh, *The Evolution of English Prose, 1700–1800: Style, Politeness, and Print Culture* (New York: Cambridge University Press, 1998), 15–19.

41. Jurin to Paul Dudley, 7 August 1727; Wellcome MS. 6146. Paul Dudley (1675–1751) was a natural historian as well as Governor of Massachusetts.

42. Thomas Worsley to James Jurin, 25 November 1746, Hovingham; Wellcome MS 6139, Rusnock, *op. cit.* (note 1), 488. 'Thomas Worsley (1710–1778), Amateur Architect and Surveyor-General for HM works Hovingham Hall, Yorkshire, North Reading' (footnote in Rusnock, *idem.*, 488).

43. Mordecai Cary to James Jurin, 1 August 1733, Clonfert; Wellcome MS 6140.

44. Cary to Jurin, 28 July 1733, Clonfert; Wellcome MS 6140, Rusnock *op. cit.* (note 1), 404. Tom Bentley, classicist, was the nephew of Richard Bentley.

45. June 1733, Clonfert; Wellcome MS 6140, Rusnock, *op. cit.* (note 1), 396–7. All the correspondence between Mordecai Cary and James Jurin cited here is found in Wellcome MS 6140. Only the first four of the extant eight letters in this correspondence are included in Rusnock.

46. F.N. Smith notes that the 'contemporary scientific prose' of new science often used analogy. 'Although comparison employed for the sake of elaboration was verboten to the Royal Society reporter, comparison for the sake of better explaining the subject at hand seems to have been acceptable, or at least unavoidable'. Smith, *op. cit.* (note 10), 146.

47. Chalybeate water contains iron salts.

48. It is only in a letter dated 28 July that the bishop acknowledges a response from Jurin for letters received on 12, 19, and 21 June (all missing autographs). Jurin jotted down prescriptions on the back of the letters he received from Cary, starting with the first letter of this correspondence. Nonetheless, Cary's 28 July note clearly states that Mrs Cary has been 'taking the course of Physick prescribed by Yours of 12th ult. [ultimo]' and nothing about prescriptions prior to this date.

49. Millepededa consisted of dried and powdered woodlice, used as a diuretic or deobstruent (a drug which removes obstructions to any bodily fluids or evacuation); see J. Worth Estes, *Dictionary of Protopharmacology: Therapeutic Practices, 1700–1850* (Canton, MA: Science History Publications, 1990). I do not see millepededa prescribed by Jurin in his prescription notes scribbled on the backs of Cary's letters prior to this date, but chalybeate waters are included. It is possible, therefore, that some instructions reached the bishop and his wife prior to Jurin's first full response on 12 June. More likely, this was recommended by a local practitioner of medicine, or the apothecary, and simply continued by Jurin.

50. 'Astrut' signifies 'protruding'.

51. 'Salivation ('ptyalism'), accompanied by a metallic taste, was a predictable side effect of all mercurial drugs, and was, therefore, often monitored as a guide to dose adjustment' from 'Hydrargyrus' in Estes, *op. cit.* (note 49).

52. Robert Burton, *The Anatomy of Melancholy* (1621), N.K. Kiessling, T.C. Faulkner, R.L. Blair (eds), (Oxford: Clarendon Press, 1990), Vol. 2: 3.

53. This prescription was appended by Jurin to back of 12 June letter from Cary.

54. 'Emmenagogue: A drug that promotes menstrual discharge by stimulating uterine vessels, or by virtue of its antihysteric properties' (Estes, 75).

55. Omoplatae – 'or *Homoplata*, from *Humerus*, the Shoulder and *Latus*, the Side; is the same *Scapula*, the Shoulder-Blade'. See Quincy, *op. cit.* (note 26).

56. In Quincy, *op. cit.* (note 26), 'Lentor hath been used by some antient Writers to Purposes now in neglect, and at present is chiefly retained from the Example of Bellini to express that sizy, viscid, coagulated Part of Blood, which in malignant Fevers obstructs the capillary Vessels, and is the chief Instrument of all those Mischiefs which then happen; see Bellini de Febribus.'

57. 15 January 1733/4, Dublin.

58. A 'scurfy spot' would be a scaling or encrusted skin lesion.

59. 8 February 1734/5, 'Clonfert or rather Eyrecour'.

60. Phthsical: wasting, or consumptive, symptoms.

61. Shallett Turner to James Jurin, 29 May 1726, Cambridge; Wellcome MS 6139. The blister referred to here is called a 'perpetual blister'. Cantharis (or cantharidis) was a blistering agent made from powdered Spanish flies (Cantharis vesicatoria). When applied externally, as blistering plaster, 'it first

operates as a general stimulant to 'artificially' remove fluid directly from the
body into the blister fluid, and indirectly into urine or phlegm, and then to
'relieve torpor' by diverting 'the impetus of the blood from the part affected
to the part of application'. The blister sometimes acts as an antispasmodic or
'counter-irritant' that reflexly reduces irritability, especially of the blood
vessels, thereby altering the circulation in patients with severe fevers, but
sometimes to stimulate the vascular and nervous tissues in adjacent
anatomical areas by 'counter-irritation'. For full effect, and when 'the object
is to produce a permanent effect, the application should be continued for
twelve hours, and on the scalp for twenty-four hours'. Estes, *op. cit.* (note
49).

62. On the mind–body relationship during the Enlightenment, see G.S.
    Rousseau (ed.), *The Languages of Psyche: Mind and Body in Enlightenment
    Thought* (Berkeley: University of California Press, 1990).
63. Turner to Jurin, 28 April 1726, Cambridge; Wellcome MS 6139.
64. Thomas Worsley to James Jurin, 25 November 1746, Hovingham; Wellcome
    MS. 6139, Rusnock, *op. cit.* (note 1), 488–9. Rusnock describes Worsley as
    an 'amateur architect and surveyor-general for HM works at Hovingham
    Hall, Yorkshire, North Riding'; see footnote in Rusnock, *idem.*, 488.
65. John Huxham to James Jurin, 8 June 1742, Plymouth; Wellcome MS 6141,
    Rusnock, *op. cit.* (note 1), 435–6.
66. Antimony: 'Tartar emetic, or antimony potassium tartrate, the most
    frequently prescribed of all antimony compounds.... Sedates the circulation,
    while it excites the secretions. Diaphoretic, cathartic, and expectorant at low
    doses, and emetic at high doses'. Estes, *op. cit.* (note 49).
67. Huxham to Jurin, 7 January 1729/30, Plymouth; Wellcome MS 6141,
    Rusnock, *op. cit.* (note 1), 380–1.
68. Huxham to Jurin, 29 March 1730; Wellcome MS 6131, Rusnock, *op. cit.*
    (note 1), 382–3. Seymour's 'madness', associated with 'weeping' and
    'mischief', so well-described by Huxham, corresponds to the modern
    medical diagnosis of hepatic encephalopathy, a confusion associated with
    high blood ammonia levels in cirrhotic patients. Of note is that we still treat
    this particular problem by altering diet and with medicines which produce
    diarrhoea since intestinal bacteria are thought responsible for the ammonia
    production and producing other metabolic products which affect mental
    function in liver patients. Modern treatment avoids protein, as in meat,
    which is broken down into ammonia in the gut; so Huxham's use of a
    vegetable diet (for whatever logic) is consistent with present day dietary
    advice. Diuretics also remain a staple of treating the ascites and oedema
    which collect in cirrhotic patients, and now, as in the eighteenth century,
    physicians resort to tapping the abdomen to remove ascitic fluid directly. In
    short, the medical treatment for the complications of cirrhosis have not

changed all that greatly since Huxham and Jurin, only the rationale behind the treatment and the form of the medications. It is not surprising to read that Huxham had some success with his therapeutic regimen in this case. However, surgical advances have certainly occurred since the eighteenth century, and in this day and age Dr Seymour would undoubtedly be a candidate for a liver transplant – but only if he were able to remain abstinent for six months to a year!

See Chapter 5, in which I discuss excerpts of Henry Fielding's remarkably objective and precise account of his own end-stage cirrhosis in *The Journal of a Voyage to Lisbon*.

69. Jurin to Huxham, 4 April 1730, Garlick Hill [London]; Wellcome MS 6141, Rusnock, *op. cit.* (note 1), 384–5.

70. Hans Sloane had a very successful private medical practice in Bloomsbury Square. He became Secretary to the Royal Society in 1693, a post he held to 1712. During his tenure he revived publication of *The Philosophical Transactions,* which had been suspended in 1687. Sloane became President of the Royal Society in 1727 (the same year he was appointed first physician to King George II), and his tenure lasted until 1741. Queen Anne was one of his patients, among many luminaries of English society. However, Sloane was known for his generosity, a benefactor to various hospitals and leaving his whole salary to Christ's Hospital where he was the physician-in-charge, and never turning away a patient who could not pay his fee.

71. This subject is discussed more fully in Chapter 4. But I have found in the letters I have examined from all periods of the century that women patients were generally quite free in discussing their medical conditions in medicine-by-post, and that the male physicians were immensely sensitive and responsive to the physical, psychological, and social problems of their women patient correspondents.

72. Mental instability, and more than a streak of cruelty, seem to have run in the Shirley family – most famously, Laurence Shirley, the fourth Earl Ferrers, whose wife (also Mary) was able to convince the House of Lords to grant her a Parliamentary Separation on the grounds of extreme cruelty in 1758. Laurence Earl Ferrers was hung at Tyburn two years later for shooting, execution style, his land steward who had become receiver of rents after the separation.

73. Antoine Deidier (d. 1746) was a physician and professor of chemistry at Montpellier. Dr Richard Mead, in the 'Preface' to his expanded, eighth edition, of his *Discourse on the Plague* (1722) prominently, but critically, mentions Deidier's experimental methods to prove that bile is the most contagious body fluid of plague patients. Deidier had injected dogs with the bile from persons who had died of the plague, and these animals uniformly developed classical signs and symptoms of the disease. Since dogs did not

seem to contract infection by scavenging on the dead bodies of plague victims, Deidier argued for an alimentary aetiology of the disease. Mead, however, found Deidier's experimental method faulty by Royal Society standards.

74. The letters of Mary Washington Ferrers in the Sloane collection at the British Library, MS 4058, ff. 327–33, are undated as to year, and the various catalogues of this collection are unhelpful. The dates of neighbouring letters in the folio cannot be relied upon to provide even an approximately correct year. However, the letters to Sloane cannot have been written later than 1729, the year of the Earl's death. Hermann Boerhaave, the famous Leyden professor of medicine consulted by Lady Mary, died in 1738.

75. Lady Mary received an annual allowance (probably 'pin money') of £800. She was only requesting additional funds 'to fix me with necessarys for the journey'.

76. This letter, dated February, is no. 332 in folio MS 4058 but must come before letter no. 330 as the countess is still in Brussels and thanking Sloane for a successful resolution of her conflict with the Earl, allowing her to make the journey to Italy. The venereal therapy is described in letter no. 330 and would have been written to Sloane the following November.

3

George Cheyne: A Very Public Private Doctor

> Perhaps I may pick out among my many Letters received from Time to Time
> some others that either describe their Cases or record their Cure, which may
> be a Consolation or Encouragement for you, and might be of Service to
> others in like Cases when I am dead and gone, for my Letters and
> Correspondence are not the meanest Part of my Works and Experience.
>
> George Cheyne to Samuel Richardson[1]

George Cheyne (1671–1743), the prominent Bath physician and medical
celebrity, was enormous. To begin with physical appearance, at one point in
his life Cheyne claimed to have weighed thirty-four stone, nearly five
hundred pounds. His personality was as extravagant and distinctive as his
person, and he figured largely in the public eye. He authored over twelve
books on medical subjects, but from the 1720s, when he turned to writing
specifically for the lay public, he became 'perhaps the most popular English
writer of practical medical works targeted at the "general reader"'.[2] These *ad
populum* works spawned multiple editions, including foreign language
translations, and secured his reputation right up to the close of the century.
His most popular work, *Essay of Health and Long Life* (London, 1724) had
eleven English language editions, the last in 1827, a Latin version in 1725,
as well as foreign editions published in Paris, Brussels, Frankfurt, Dresden,
Leipzig, and a New York edition appearing in 1813.

Cheyne was a prolific correspondent, and he incorporated letters from
his successful medicine-by-post practice into works such as *The English
Malady* (1733).[3] The highly successful *Observations concerning the Nature
and due Method of treating the Gout, for the use of my Worthy Friend, Richard
Tennison, Esq.: Together with an Account of the Nature and Qualities of the
Bath Waters* (1720) was an expanded prescription-by-post for his patient.[4]
Cheyne believed firmly in the therapeutic value of the letter:

> [M]y way to my Friends and Advice to them is to lay it down as a Law that
> I and they write always in such a Compass of Time and sit down accordingly,
> and let the Pen write on to fill up what Nature, Affection, or Providence
> suggests; and it very rarely happens but you are diverted yourself in the Time
> and amuse your Friend if he is not otherwise strongly engaged, for all forced,
> laboured Writing in familiar Letters is generally irksome to both.[5]

He was physician and friend to Samuel Richardson, Alexander Pope, Samuel Johnson, and David Hume, and to society figures such as 'Beau' Nash, master of ceremonies for Bath, and George Grenville, politician and future Prime Minister. His medico–religious writings recommended him to the Countesses of Huntingdon, 'one of Methodism's first aristocratic patrons', and influenced the religious philosophies of both John Wesley and William Bentley.[6] It is little wonder that medical historians have been fascinated by Cheyne in recent years.[7]

However, my particular interest in this chapter is to show that Cheyne was certainly among the most crucial transitional figures in altering the eighteenth-century doctor–patient relationship through the influence of a highly personal and original blend of rhetorical devices found in his medicine-by-post. Roy Porter has said of Cheyne that 'his writings on chronic disorders proved particularly pivotal, encapsulating past wisdom, while formulating new philosophies for the future.'[8] Most true; but equally important, it was Cheyne who set the example in rejecting the restrictive objectivity of new science rhetoric and encouraged his patients to be expansive and subjective in describing the experience of personal illness.

Cheyne's ultimate medical authority, as in the case of Jurin, resided largely in his being a prominent and visible representative of the fashionable medical beliefs held by his patients – consistent with Jewson's model of medical patronage, discussed previously. However, Cheyne played a much greater role than Jurin in actually shaping what was fashionable. In making his own transition from iatromechanical medicine to embracing a human physiology centred on the nerves, Cheyne became the icon for a complex melding of medical, social, and intellectual trends. He masterfully used his own personal history as valetudinarian to reify those trends and to create a unique bond with his patients and the public. As Steven Shapin has noted, Cheyne's public claim to expertise was his micromechanical knowledge of the 'invisible world' of the body, yet what contributed most to his private practice success was that 'Cheyne was a virtuoso in using the informal channel' of letter, personal communication, and word-of-mouth to promote his authority and the confidence that his knowledge – and personal experience as both doctor and invalid – was fully dedicated to the welfare of his patients, who were uppermost in his thoughts at all times.[9]

Reformulated by Cheyne, the experience of malaise became, for both the individual and society at large, not only appropriate subject matter for medicine-by-post but its central theme. The correspondence of personal illness became a social commodity whose rhetoric was defined by the emerging medical discourse on nervous disorders and nerve sensibility so effectively popularised by Cheyne.[10] As such, the epistolary language of medicine-by-post shared the same rhetorical origins as the novel of

114

Figure 3.1

*George Cheyne (1671–1743). Line engraving by J. Tookey, 1787,
after J. van Diest. Courtesy: Wellcome Library, London.*

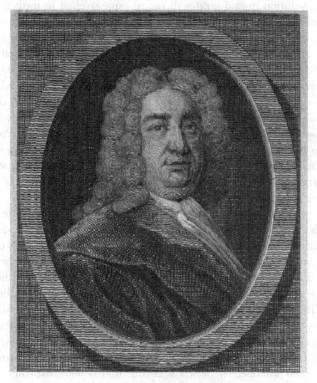

*Signature of George Cheyne.
Courtesy: Huntingdon Library, California.*

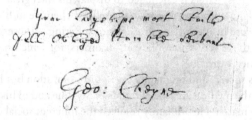

sensibility. It seems inevitable that George Cheyne and Samuel Richardson
should have become friends, avid correspondents and followers of each
other's work. It is also not surprising that the personal letter should have

represented to both men the most reliable repository of experience and index of true feeling. Cheyne exhorted his patient, Richardson, '[B]e frank with me and all honest Men, else you will be to blame, for we cannot know one another's Hearts but by our Tongues or Pens.'[11]

The evolution toward greater rhetorical expressiveness in medicine-by-post, fuelled so effectively by Cheyne's example, had its origins in a major change in speculative medical thought in Britain during the third and fourth decades of the century. This was a move away from the iatromechanical–hydraulic interpretation of the body to a view which favoured the centrality of the nervous system as the determinant of health and disease. But whereas the iatromechanical model of the body had been a leveller of social class – describing the body in terms of pumps, tubes, and fluids – the new nerve physiology re-established a biological hierarchy in which sensibility replaced blood as the measure of worth. A heightened susceptibility to fashionable disease states, such as 'the spleen', became associated with people from the upper strata of society who showed great social refinement as well as those who were absorbed in artistic or intellectual endeavours.

It is evident how such a medical theory might appeal to an aristocratic class whose members felt encroached upon by an increasingly prosperous and vocal middle-class that aspired to the accoutrements and titles of the gentry while rejecting the aristocratic ideology of 'birth makes worth'. Paradoxically, the new medical system facilitated social mobility by making 'gentility' attainable to the middling class through the emulation of the new 'sensibility'. As Paul Langford explains: 'The emphasis on feeling provided... flexibility and removed the sense of repressive social exclusiveness which marked a more aristocratic view of the world.'[12] Such upward mobility was especially available to the well-educated, middle-class professional man; and doctors who attended upper-class clients understood that they 'were expected to conduct themselves as gentlemen and knew the commercial importance of doing so.'[13] The rhetoric employed by Cheyne in his medicine-by-post letters is calculated to display his own great sensibility and thereby to claim authority to advise the refined clientele in his practice. His credentials were his own years of exquisite suffering – those years in which he endured those very same 'Nervous disorders' for which he was now the self-proclaimed expert.

Cheyne's success and originality lay not in innovation but in his masterly synthesis of the medical and social trends of his time and in his ability to find a rhetoric to match. He brilliantly resolved the inherent social contradictions and tensions of the new nerve physiology so as to give it national appeal to both upper and middle classes alike. In his popular medical tracts, Cheyne glamorised the class of patients who were most susceptible to 'nervous Distempers' by redefining vulnerability as a mark of privilege associated with the upper ranks of society – those with refinement, material success, or with remarkable intellectual or artistic gifts. However, Cheyne equally dramatised the intense 'Miseries' associated with the privilege of having delicate nerves, and he did not make it either desirable or fashionable to remain ill.[14] Hypochondriacal states were the consequence of nerves debilitated by 'high living', from overindulgence in diet and drink, and from physical inactivity. The 'English malady' was the price to be paid for living in a richly civilised and commercially successful society.[15] The cure was to renounce the excesses that harmed the physical body – and, in turn, the spirits – and to strive for the more healthy habits exemplified by the middle-class: sensible diet, a regimen of moderate exercise, and a devout heart to keep the passions in check.

Cheyne, himself of middle-class origins, was thus able to flatter his upper-class patients by addressing their singular constitutions while acknowledging, as subtext, the middle-class perception of the aristocracy as debilitated by a pervasive vitiation of moral character. His letters to patients are prescriptions for abstinence from overindulgence written in a rhetoric filled with religious metaphors and invoking Providence. The pain of Illness, and the deprivations required for cure become, alike, a form of penitence for the valetudinarian; the reward for the compliant patient is not only recuperation but great moral self-satisfaction. Cheyne advised Richardson: 'In a Word next to eternal Happiness... is bodily Health, and best worth giving up every Thing for it, and in Truth all true Religion consists in Self-denial and Resignation. God grant us both these two invaluable Means.'[16]

In letters – and his most successful books – Cheyne was able to construct a medical philosophy out of a blend of his own case history, disparate medical traditions (both classical and Christian), and contemporary medical theory. He forged a rhetoric that perfectly communicated his very original synthesis of medicine with religion and private illness with societal ills. The English malady was at once a personal and a public disease, and Cheyne's philosophical and rhetorical amalgam gave him prominence and authority not only in the treatment of individual patients but as doctor to British society as a whole.

I have divided this chapter into four parts to elucidate Cheyne's rise to the position of medical icon and to describe the origins and character of his strikingly individual and influential rhetorical style. His medicine-by-post communications figure prominently throughout. A biographical section considers his life up through 1720 – the year he began medical practice in Bath – early intellectual influences and the profound effect of protracted physical and mental ill health on his eventual medical philosophy and rhetorical strategies. This is followed by a discussion on the 'public' nature of 'private' medical correspondence, an eighteenth-century phenomenon that is critical in understanding how Cheyne's medicine-by-post might have had such a broad influence not only on the rhetoric of his own generation but also an ongoing effect on the character of doctor–patient correspondence well into the second half of the century. A third section describes Cheyne's controversial role as physician–celebrity in the context of the medical ethics of the period and suggests why Cheyne's private and public readership were so receptive to his moral and spiritual message. The last part of the chapter considers in detail Cheyne's rhetorical style and epistolary stratagems in his medicine-by-post practice as well as the influence of his style on the rhetoric of his patients. I have included abundant examples of Cheyne's urgent, quirky, deliberate, and individual epistolary style to support my arguments but also, I hope, simply to delight the reader with the character and language of this fascinating eighteenth-century, larger-than-life personality.

Foundations for becoming an icon

The career trajectory of Dr George Cheyne – medical celebrity, author of *The English Malady*, and committed medicine-by-post correspondent – would be inconceivable without the backdrop of his dramatic personal early history. Most importantly, Cheyne capitalised on his own medical history, his struggles with the 'the spleen', to form a bond with his patients on the basis of shared suffering, promoting himself as a doctor of great empathy and sensibility. His books and letters overflow with examples of a dissolute past life, of immoderate diet and drink, inattention to bodily exercise, and inevitable nervous collapse. As Anita Guerrini has observed, Cheyne was highly unusual for his time in that 'far from hiding behind the physician's persona, Cheyne laid himself bare, in all his unlovely bulk and tortured soul, to the reader's gaze.'[17] He wrote to Richardson: 'I have nothing to conceal, not my Faults and Frailties.'[18] Yet Cheyne's narrative account of his own vulnerability and recovery through a regimen of diet, exercise, and spirituality, the regimen he later marketed so effectively, served not only as a bridge to his patients but created a public persona of himself as icon of the recovered hypochondriac.

Cheyne was born in 1671 in Methlick, Aberdeenshire. As Roy Porter has lamented, 'in view of his later trials and traumas in managing his bodily appetites, it is especially frustrating that the formative years of Cheyne's life are veiled in obscurity.'[19] We do know that the Cheynes were an established Scottish Episcopalian family 'distantly related to Gilbert Burnet', the Bishop of Salisbury and Whig historian.[20] Nevertheless, Anita Guerrini informs us, Cheyne's 'social position was highly ambiguous' in that he was 'the son of a tenant farmer' and 'descended from a family who had once owned land but had lost it.'[21] He was provided with a classical education and was enrolled, in the late 1680s, at Marischal College in Aberdeen, presumably destined for a career in the Church. As mathematics tutor to John Ker, subsequent Duke of Roxburgh, he had his first important exposure to pietism. This religious movement, which was to have a profound influence on Cheyne's subsequent religious attitudes and medical philosophy, was an offshoot of late-seventeenth-century Lutherism. Pietism encouraged an intense personal spiritual devotion of the heart over the mind; and there is perhaps some irony that the definition of 'pietist' in Johnson's *Dictionary* is attributed to Cheyne's relation, Bishop Burnet: 'One of a sect professing great strictness and purity of life; despising learning and ecclesiastical polity; a kind of mystick.'[22] However, it would not be until after great personal trials and disappointments that Cheyne came to embrace pietism with earnest devotion.

At the close of the century, Cheyne found himself engaged in scholarly pursuits in mathematics and medicine under the influence of the Edinburgh physician Archibald Pitcairne, among the first and most energetic of the circle of iatromechanists who were attempting to apply Newtonian physics to medicine.[23] Cheyne became engrossed in this project, writing treatises that promulgated Pitcairne's medical philosophy and expanded upon it. At this time in his career, he was fully dedicated to the idea that Newtonian principles should be applied to medical physiology and practice. In this belief, he belonged to that group of physicians whom Theodore Brown has described as 'Newton-struck', those doctors who were reconceiving medicine 'in the shadow of the *Principia*'.[24] Pre-eminent in this group, and personally acquainted with Newton, were James Jurin, James Keill, Richard Mead, and Henry Pemberton. Among the devotees who were not part of Newton's immediate inner circle but who sought to win his favour and 'that of their Newton-admiring contemporaries' were the three Scottish physicians: Archibald Pitcairne, William Cockburn, and George Cheyne. For all of these 'Newton-struck' physicians, explains Brown:

> hydraulic iatromechanism was a positive alternative to the loose hypothetical speculations about peculiarly shaped particles and pores that in the 1680s and 1690s had very quickly become iatromechanical orthodoxy. Iatromechanism itself was a desperate attempt to make physicians *appear* modern and up-to-date while keeping traditional methods of diagnosis and therapy intact.... Hydraulic 'Newtonianism' gave physicians of the next generation a sense of methodological improvement, moral uplift, and optimism for the future as well as a *rhetoric* which might please a Newton-admiring and nationalistic British clientele. To a large extent this strategy seems to have worked in helping to build successful medical careers [italics mine].[25]

Under Pitcairne's sponsorship, and after obtaining his MD from King's College in Aberdeen, Cheyne moved to London in 1701 as mathematics tutor to William Ker, the younger brother of John. A dissolute life, which had begun in Edinburgh in the company of Pitcairne, escalated when Cheyne moved to London. Anita Guerrini informs us, 'Whereas he had been dismissed from his Edinburgh tutoring position for drunkenness, he fit in well with the Ker brothers... a life of parties, drink, and sex, punctuated by bouts of gonorrhea.'[26]

In trying to build his medical career and make connections with the right sort of people, Cheyne frequented the pub and coffeehouses, gormandising his way into morbid obesity. By 1705, his physical and mental health had spiralled out of control due to this dissipated way of life. In one of many narrations of that period in his life, Cheyne tells Richardson:

> I had been so exceedingly fat, unwieldy, and overgrown beyond any one I believe in Europe, that I weighed 34 Stone, this had so stretched my Skin and Belly that when my Fat and Belly was shrunk to common Size by many repeated Vomits (at first once or twice a Week), want of Sleep, a perpetual Lowness, Loss of Appetite, and an Inability to Digest any Thing but Milk and Bread, my Guts fell out through the Cawl where the Spermatic Vessels perforate it and made a Kind of Wind Rupture which was some Years a Breeding unheeded.[27]

Cheyne fell into deep despondency over his failure to establish himself as a significant iatromechanist author and successful private physician in London. Of the 'Newton-struck' group, Cheyne appears to have produced the least convincing mathematical models of hydraulic iatromechanical physiology, and by the early 1720s Cheyne was apologising in print for his early authorial efforts which he now regarded as the 'unripe Fruit' of youthful enthusiasm.[28]

In later writings, both letters and popular medical tracts, Cheyne would describe himself at this stage of his life as displaying the protean symptoms of hypochondria. In the eighteenth century, the meaning of this diagnosis differed from our twentieth-century idea of an imaginary invalid. Rather, explains medical historian Michael Barfoot, it was a condition 'uniformly interpreted as one in which a particular state or quality of the imagination, however caused, exerted a morbid effect on the body'; that is, the patient experienced real physical sequellae as a consequence of a particular mental state, which itself might have arisen from the disordered sensory input of damaged peripheral nerves (as described more fully below). Patients with 'the hyp' had multiple symptoms, among which gastrointestinal complaints were especially predictable.[29] It was this morbid condition that Cheyne reconceived for British society in 1733 under the rubric of *The English Malady*. In a chapter of that work entitled 'The Author's Case', Cheyne reiterated his own trials to show the depths to which one could 'plunge' by immoderate living but offered his own example to illustrate the possibility of recovery through sobriety, attention to diet, exercise, and spiritual wholeness.

Cheyne's recuperation from 'the hyp', however, took many years. From 1705, when he returned to Scotland, until 1732, when he felt he was fully restored to health, Cheyne suffered multiple relapses of 'the spleen' which he ascribed to self-indulgence in diet and laxity of good habits. At age seventy, looking back at this period in his life, Cheyne willingly confessed to Samuel Richardson:

> [M]y Case was at first worse I think than any One's I think I ever read or saw
> – a putrified [sic] overgrown Body from Luxury and perpetual Laziness,
> scorbutical all over, a regular St Anthony's Fire every two months, regularly
> the Gout all over Six Months of the Year, perpetual Reaching [*sic*], Anxiety,
> Giddiness, Fitts, and Startings.[30]

After another exacerbation of his condition in 1710, Cheyne consulted Dr Taylor of Croydon, a clergyman known for his enthusiastic endorsement of an all-milk diet for various ills. The beneficial effect of this diet made a lasting impression on Cheyne. He subsequently translated this personal experience into medical advice for his own patients, advocating a predominantly milk, seed, and vegetable diet for the treatment of gout and hypochondria. Cheyne had also been impressed with the medicinal effects of the spa waters at Bath. His first major success in writing for the public addressed treatment for gout and the beneficial properties of Bath waters. This was published in 1720, the same year Cheyne set up permanent residence in Bath and started what was to become a flourishing medical practice. Cheyne's personal history suggests how naturally he came to embody, both literally and symbolically, the preoccupying health issue of his day, hypochondria, or as Cheyne lists its other appellations: 'nervous Distempers, Spleen, Vapours, Lowness of Spirits', and which 'by Foreigners, and all our Neighbours of the Continent', explains Cheyne, 'are In Derision called the ENGLISH MALADY.'[31]

Medicine-by-post: a public private endeavour

For a reputable physician such as Cheyne to display such candour about his own trials and derelictions was no doubt a great selling point with both the public and his patients. But to claim that Cheyne's private practice letters influenced a transformation in the rhetoric of eighteenth-century doctor–patient correspondence implies that his private consultation letters were, in fact, public. This was the case; for not only were medicine-by-post letters shared, but news concerning personal illness circulated freely in social circles. Add to this, however, that Cheyne – like his acquaintance and sometime patient Alexander Pope – was expert in using the vagaries of the eighteenth-century book trade to place his 'private' letters in the public sphere as a means of self-advertisement. What was remarkable in Cheyne's public performance, however, was the extreme of unembarrassed self-revelation, passion, exuberance, and sensitivity that he brought to centre stage in the doctor-patient relationship and its language. His was truly a fresh voice in a stale and predictable medical theatre.

Cheyne diligently set the example in being frank about his own private illness in order to encourage his patients to be equally forthright. Such trust was necessary for a satisfactory therapeutic outcome; withholding information, for modesty or other reasons, could only obfuscate diagnosis and delay proper treatment. Cheyne exhorted Samuel Richardson to keep him fully informed about his medical state:

> I have not written to you of late because I really had not Materials, having suggested to you all I knew about mending or preserving your Health in my several former Letters, and not hearing of any new Symptoms or the old ones exasperating else. I hope you know me too well and my Manner... to be any longer shy with me but to use me with that Freedom that becomes Persons designing the same Ends.[32]

A young Countess of Huntingdon, in her mid-twenties, might be excused her hesitation in speaking plainly about the haemorrhoids associated with her recent pregnancy, but Cheyne tactfully expresses impatience with such reticence:

> You have suffered a great deal for want of sufficient explication. Now when I, considering the case as entirely conquered, find the cure as yet imperfect, I must advise your ladyship to still more care and caution, least you irritate that tender part.... I fear you have suffered by taking so many [medicines] without a full notion of your case.[33]

Incomplete clinical information to formulate an effective medical regime was always a potential problem in medicine-by-post, but for Cheyne it was not only the factual details that mattered. For him, a consultation letter was a matter of attitude, the uninhibited willingness of the patient to confide all to one's doctor. As he counsels Richardson: '[B]e frank with me... else you will be to blame.'[34] A 'frank' medical history was not, in and of itself, therapeutic in the manner of a religious confession, but it served as evidence of trust in one's physician, and as such it was an acknowledgment of the doctor's authority and a sign that the patient was morally committed to follow whatever regimen was prescribed for cure.[35]

Unfortunately, in the imperfect world of eighteenth-century private practice, as in the case of the Countess of Huntingdon, it was not unusual for Cheyne to hear news of his patient's condition through gossip: 'I am most heartily sorry that you have been so extremely ill as Mrs Cotter informs'; or, 'Mrs Coles made me believe the physicians had called your complaint a gravel colic, which made me write as I did.'[36] It is the very public nature of private illness that requires Cheyne so often to write to the Countess in defence of his regimen:

> As to your diet I am loathe to bring you to an entire milk and vegetable diet if I could help it. I know it would cure entirely, in time, of all your complaints and make you look beautiful, healthy, and gay, as you should. But it is particular and inconvenient in the world, and all man and womankind will be up in arms against me, and your ladyship will often be told you are killing yourself by Dr Cheyne's whims.[37]

News of satisfaction or displeasure with a doctor circulated quickly by way of letter or word-of-mouth, and Cheyne laboured ceaselessly in his own letters to rectify any misreading of his character or therapeutic intentions that arose in the busybody public scrutiny that was a fact of eighteenth-century medical life.

Medical correspondence, like other eighteenth-century letters, was 'private' only in the sense that a letter was addressed to an individual. Even in matters of personal health, correspondence was becoming what Habermas has described for the eighteenth-century letter in general, a vehicle of personal communication that was composed with the possibility, even likelihood, of being shared with an 'audience' beyond the individual to whom it was addressed.[38] Lawrence Klein, in his work on gender, has further refined the distinctions between the meaning of 'public' and 'private' in eighteenth-century Britain. Klein asserts that the most common application of the word 'public' referred to a state of 'sociability', whereas 'private' meant 'solitary'. Any matter, no matter how personal, that invited 'perception' or even 'participation' by others, outside the home, was considered 'public'.[39] Klein's purpose is to show that eighteenth-century women were not excluded from public life but active participants in a 'public' life that was a continuum of the home. If we allow that illness was an experience which was centred in the home for both men and women, then illness should be considered 'public' very much along the lines described by Klein. Roy and Dorothy Porter write that 'eighteenth-century letters, and no doubt even more so, its tea-table chit-chat, teemed with talk of courses of physic, operations and the "fortunes of physicians".'[40] Judith Schneid Lewis observes of the relationship between man-midwives (accoucheurs) and their aristocratic patients that the 'ability [of the doctor] to appear both honest and reassuring, in letters as well as in person', was 'essential to his good standing with the entire aristocratic circle surrounding the patient.'[41] The intense interest of the public, and the uninvited commentary by outside doctors in the medical conditions of such figures as Robert Walpole, Queen Caroline, or King George III, should be recognised as typical of the 'public' nature of personal illness rather than exceptional breaches of patient confidentiality occasioned by the celebrity status of these patients.

That middle-class patients also partook in this circulation of personal medical information can be inferred from the work of Habermas about the general character and purpose of eighteenth-century bourgeoisie correspondence. However, we have more direct evidence of this in the correspondence of Samuel Johnson (see Chapter 1) who was not exceptional in this respect. Cheyne both invites and facilitates in the circulation of the medical histories of his middle-class patients, doctors such as Dr Cranstoun (see below) and numerous others as we shall see. Richardson's troubles were not private matter. When the publisher questioned the efficacy of Cheyne's recipe after only two weeks, Cheyne responds to Richardson's impatience by snapping back, 'Did you think it was a supernatural Cure of Distempers, Witchcraft or Enchantment?' But Cheyne is especially annoyed that his patient should listen to ignorant if well-meaning advisors who impute any 'Difficulties and Puzzles' to Cheyne's regimen instead of the lingering effects of illness: 'I thought it might satisfy you they [Richardson's symptoms] were not exasperated by it [Cheyne's regimen] as all your wise Counsellors, Friends, and Familiars made you dread.'[42] If there was more open 'public' interest in aristocratic or celebrity patients, there was certainly ample medical gossip among the rising middle class as well, concerning each other's state of health, and ready opinion on a doctor's qualifications.

This social network by which patients pooled their common experience with illness, doctors, and competing therapies, ensured that they were making some kind of informed decision and protecting themselves from truly harmful charlatans. In an age that did not legislate medical ethics, communication among patients was the most substantial safeguard against bad medicine. Although an Oxford or Cambridge degree might suffice the Royal College of Physicians that a colleague was of good standing, patients held their own kangaroo court on a physician's character and ethics through informal conversation and the circulating private letter. What is remarkable is that this very same court, so prompt to discredit a doctor's character and prescriptions, betrays so little concern about matters of confidentiality other than in cases of venereal disease and madness.[43] Cheyne, for all his keen sensitivity to public and private opinion, shows no compunction in his letters about sharing medical news. Indeed, in his letters to the Countess of Huntingdon and to Samuel Richardson, Cheyne never reassures them of an obligation to privacy even as he is revealing the details of other patient histories to them!

This is not to suggest that private-practice patients did not expect their physicians to be discreet, but any idea of patient confidentiality was subsumed within the tradition of a code of gentlemanly conduct rather than any specific code of medical ethic or claims to privacy.[44] It was in his role as 'gentleman' that Cheyne feels compelled to make the following disclaimer in the 'Advertisement' preceding part three of *The English Malady*, that portion of the book in which he has provided actual case histories from among his own patients to illustrate various forms of the malaise:

> [I]t was by no means convenient or proper to publish their Names without
> Leave; and I was unwilling to put my friends and Patients to the Pain, either
> of a Consent or Refusal, and resolved even to bear the slur of Forgery, and
> let the Whole rest on my own Credit, rather than contend with Difficulties.
> I have therefore mentioned their Names, only in those Cases where I was
> absolutely at Liberty; but solemnly declare, that the others were such in the
> main, as I have represented them.

But this said, Cheyne is quick to qualify his statement by assuring interested readers that:

> [I]n any particular Case, if called upon, I am ready to assign the Person,
> under proper Conditions, and have always describ'd the Case from the Name
> and Character of the Patient, and the History of the Distemper placed before
> my Eyes.[45]

Whenever it served Cheyne's purpose to recommend his medical practice, or his particular dietetic regimen, he discovered acceptable, if somewhat disingenuous, ways to reveal more about the eminent patients in his practice.

In *The English Malady*, for example, the 'anonymous' cases are introduced in a manner that surely tantalised his readers to engage in a guessing game of who's who: 'A Tender *young Gentleman*, of great Worth and Ingenuity, here in our *Neighbourhood*', 'A Lady of *great Fortune* in this Town, eminent for her great *Charity*, *Piety*, and *fine Breeding*', 'A *Gentleman* well known, and as much belov'd by all that know him for his *fine Parts*, *Great Probity*, and the distinguish'd Figure he has constantly made in the *Senate*', 'A *Knight Baronet* of an *Ancient Family*, by keeping bad Hours, in attending

125

upon the Business of the *Parliament*, and living freely about Town', and so on. The italics are all Cheyne's, and serve conveniently to announce the quality of his clients and the scope of his practice.[46]

That the patients were fully cooperative and even encouraged such public display of their medical conditions is evidenced in a letter to Cheyne from his patient Dr Cranstoun, which forms one of the case histories in *The English Malady*.[47] While Cranstoun's letter, dated 20 September 1732, takes the form of a personal doctor–patient interchange, it is candidly composed with eventual publication in mind, to be included in Cheyne's forthcoming medical opus. Cranstoun is enthusiastic about Cheyne's book project, and writes:

> What you are pleased to communicate, of a *Treatise* you design for the Press, gives me great Pleasure.... And tho', at best, I'm always at a vast Loss for Language and Expression, I must beg you'll forgive my careless Freedom in this: While I write with Ease and Openness to a Friend: if you can but take the Meaning, I hope whatever Use you please to make of it, you'll be so kind as to treat me and it as your own.[48]

Cheyne takes Cranstoun at his word, and makes certain to include Dr Cranstoun's effusive encomium to Cheyne as well as the basic case history:

> The clear distinct Knowledge, from small imperfect *Hints*, you had at first of my Distemper, was equally surprizing, with the positive Assurance of Success, with which you pressed to persuade and encourage my following your *Method of Care*; nothing but mature Experience and well-taken Observations, upon certain Principles of *Science*, cou'd have warranted, or supported a Prediction more like *prophetick Security* than *physical Prognostick*, which hitherto has answer'd; as I have faithfully the Condition [ie. the English malady].[49]

Medicine-by-post, then, was an entirely respectable and effective way to promote one's practice within a particular segment of society.

Indeed, Cheyne thoroughly exploited the self-promotional possibilities of medicine-by-post. When the Countess of Huntingdon has moved to the countryside for reasons of health, Cheyne alerts her of neighbours who are also his patients: 'one you already know, Lord Bateman... gay as a bird'; the others include 'Mr Reynolds, a counsellor [*sic*] and a gentleman of estate, of wretched nerves and a high scorbutic disorder. He lives entirely on milk and vegetables with seeds, and drinks milk and water.... The third is a merchant of the city, who only summers in Hertfordshire.' This short list serves a similar purpose to that in *The English Malady*, calling attention to the distinguished clientele who follow Cheyne's medical advice. He concludes the letter, 'I beg my humble duty to my Lady Gower.... Desire her to be careful, for I fear she is but a tender and delicate constitution, even more so than your ladyship.... I sent Sir William Stanhope away better. Two of his brothers are here my patients now, all nervous and low.'[50]

Cheyne is quite prepared to forward letters from one patient to another in order to promote patient confidence. To convince the Countess to continue her regimen: 'I send you enclosed a copy of a letter I lately had from a vegetable [eater] of 72 years, who was in mortal agonies here last summer. He is a considerable person in the House of Commons – but this only to yourself, for your encouragement and to persevere and to hope all.'[51] Cheyne's warning, 'but this only to yourself', should be read not as concern about patient confidentiality but solely as urging discretion in the use of news about another patient. If patient confidentiality had been at issue, then the impropriety would have been in sharing any information at all. But Cheyne's purpose in letting the Countess of Huntingdon see the letter from a prominent society figure is not simply to exhort her, by example of other therapeutic successes, but to encourage her trust by the fact that other important and worthy people depend on Cheyne's good character. In a system of patronage, the doctor depended entirely on such word of mouth and of pen.

Another shared letter, from one William Moore of Salisbury, dated 26 October 1742, was preserved by Richardson in his volume of Cheyne's correspondence. This letter served Cheyne admirably as a testament to both his medical skill and character as a physician of refined feelings. He hastened to forward it to Richardson within a week of receipt, describing the writer of the letter as 'One who was vapoured, low Spirited, weak, feeble, and quite miserable, who by Vomits, his low Diet, and some other Helps mentioned to you, is as you will see.' Between the lines of Moore's letter we can appreciate how completely the patient adopted Cheyne's persona as a doctor of sensibility – supremely empathetic with both physical distress and human frailties:

> When you first assisted me in my Extremity you pleasantly intimated what was the common Practice of Patients – 'God and the Doctor we alike adore, just in the Nick of Danger, not before' etc. But I hope I have convinced you (though in a very Troublesome Manner) that I am not unmindful of you. No, so long as I am conscious of my Existence I shall have a quick Sense of the Instrument of my Happiness. And whereas I formerly troubled you with doleful Complaints I could now gladly tire you with Accounts of a more pleasing Nature, but I know my Distance. However, I thought your frequent and kind Inquiries after me demanded a thankful Acknowledgement.... [D]id I pay a due Regard unto those two Directions, viz't. Daily Walking and

abstaining from Butter, I believe I should not have the least Allay to my Health – the former is not always in my Power and therefore cannot blame myself on that Account.... As to my indulging in Butter, which really is a Transgression, I submit to the Penalty of a Vomit.... In all other Things I am punctual and persevering....

That God may preserve you valuable Life and continue to bless your Labour for the Good of Mankind is the Prayer of Sir.[52]

The letter is part confession; Moore acknowledges that he was not the most compliant of patients, inclined to share 'doleful Complaints' in a 'Troublesome Manner' and reluctant in following Cheyne's advice. But the unspoken drama of his recovery is evident in the phrases he uses to describe his physician as the 'Instrument of my Happiness' who 'assisted me in my Extremity.' Moore has also adopted Cheyne's medico–religious language of illness and regimen as forms of penitence.[53] The patient describes his dietary slips as 'Transgression' and his vomits as the 'Penalty' he must pay for restoration of 'Health and Tranquillity.' Surely Richardson, of all people, must have appreciated Moore's epistolary skill at turning a simple thank-you note into a form of narrative punctuated by expressive feeling and moral reflection. That Cheyne should have shown Moore's letter to Richardson is evidence that all three men shared a common vocabulary of sensibility to describe illness. Moreover, these correspondents must have shared a common belief in the efficacy of letter-writing as a spiritual reinforcement of therapy as well as an obligation to spread the good word of Cheyne's regimen.

Medicine-by-post was thus an ideal place for Cheyne to trumpet his own sensibility. For example, with the Countess of Huntingdon he shared his concerns and joys about other patients. It is the message of his own sensibility that should be read into Cheyne's report to the Countess that 'Lady Gore's case (*for which I am heartily concerned*) I fear it is obstruction from a lung case' [italics mine].[54] Cheyne instantly conveys to the Countess his heartfelt pleasure in the felicitous news that, 'I have just now received a letter from Lady Fr. Hastings at Ladstone, who acquaints me that all her disorders and complaints, and particularly those at her stomach and at her months [menstrual periods], are entirely gone, and she says all her friends tell her she looks fresh, clear, and plump by her milk and vegetable diet.'[55] But perhaps nowhere is Cheyne more transparent in his effort to portray himself as the physician of sensibility than in this reflection he shares with Richardson:

You need not question that I am sufficiently apprized of and have felt the Grief, Anguish, and Anxiety such a Distemper must have on a Mind of any

128

Degree of Sensibility and so fine and lively an Imagination as yours, and it is
happy for Mankind that they cannot feel but by Compassion and Consent
of Parts (as One Member feels the Pain of Another) the Misery of their
Fellow Creatures of their Acquaintance; else Life would be Intolerable.[56]

In an age where the code of the gentleman was the sum and substance of
medical ethics, portraying oneself as a doctor of exquisite sensibility was an
announcement of one's professional morality, and was meant to inspire
confidence in one's therapeutic decisions regardless of actual outcome. For
practical purposes, this system of medical ethics was generally acceptable,
though the age was far too sceptical for any physician to think he might gain
absolute and unquestioned trust from his patient. Nonetheless, to prove
oneself morally superior to one's professional competitors was part of
everyday life in the eighteenth-century medical marketplace, and medicine-
by-post was an effective means to propagate information about one's
professional character.

From the start, Cheyne clearly appreciated that he could best circulate
his ideas and enhance his reputation – and his practice – through print.
Though bordering dangerously close to the methods of advertisement of
quack physicians, Cheyne found a reputable way to publish testimonials to
the efficacy of his regimen, and to proclaim the quality of his practice, by
making public selected correspondence from his private practice. Some
patients who normally anticipated having their letters circulated selectively
among segments of their acquaintances, and who were great advocates of
Cheyne's regimen, might have *volunteered* their letters for publication, as in
the case of Dr Cranstoun. Cheyne, like Richardson, recognised the
verisimilitude implied by the personal letter:

> I chose to give the *Case* in the *doctor's* own Words, thinking it would be more
> satisfactory in its *native Dress*; for tho' He modestly thinks it might want a
> little of the modern polishing, yet the strong good Sense, the nice
> Observations, and the unaffected Simplicity, is infinitely preferable to all
> *Varnish*, and shows *him* equally an excellent *Physician*, and a Man of *Probity*.
> Other Cases of the same Kind under my Care, I have from several *Gentlemen*
> of the *Faculty*, which shall be produced (if necessary) in due Time, after
> obtaining their Permission.'[57]

The rhetoric of correspondence allows the patient to speak directly to
other patients, without the interference of the medical author, and the effect
is one of sincerity and taste which helps to overcome reader suspicion of self-
promotion associated so entirely with the bills of mountebanks and
charlatans. This approach seems to have been very successful with the public

Cheyne intended to reach, though his medical colleagues remained more than sceptical.

However, not all patients would be anxious to reveal their private medical histories to the public at large. So, to enlarge the pool of letters that he could publish, especially those from high-society clientele, required the savvy of someone who was familiar with the intricacies of the eighteenth-century book trade – and Cheyne was fully equipped to meet the challenge. By 1720, Cheyne was establishing himself in private medical practice in Bath, and he had just published his first medical tract designed for public consumption, *Observations concerning the Nature and due Method of treating the Gout, for the use of my worthy friend, Richard Tennison, Esq.: together with an account of the Nature and Qualities of the Bath Waters.*[58] The title suggests the origin of the work, a prescription-by-post intended for private use by Tennison. However, Cheyne claimed he decided to enlarge and publish his instructions to Tennison, fearing 'its being pyrated' once he discovered copies of the original letter circulating among other sufferers of the gout.[59] The possibility that unscrupulous booksellers might pirate his letter for their own profit was not an idle concern in a print world harbouring such notorious characters as the 'unspeakable' Edmund Curll. On the other hand, writers themselves were quite prepared to seize the opportunities provided by the perilous uncertainties of the book trade. They could plead the necessity to publish 'leaked' private communications with public figures, insisting that only an authorised publication would respect the intentions and propriety of the correspondents. Cheyne had a low threshold when it came to circulating or publishing what had begun as private communication. If the serendipity of piracy had not in fact occurred in a particular instance, Cheyne would readily imagine the possibility in order to convince himself and his patients of the need to go public with their medical histories for the sake of accuracy and for the universal benefit of other sufferers like themselves. Publishing the contents of previously private medical correspondence served Cheyne by simultaneously advertising his practice and his regimen while boosting book sales.

As the eighteenth-century book trade made the transition from a patronage system to a commercial enterprise, authors quickly realised they must elbow their way into the territory of the bookseller if they were not to be swindled out of profits due to them, and they would have to fight for their rights with any means available. Cheyne was among those authors who fully appreciated the challenge. He adapted readily to the rapidly emerging world of the print marketplace. As with his advice on gout written for Tennison, Cheyne took the same tack a few years later on some 'Rules of Health' he had posted to Sir Joseph Jeckyll (1663–1738), Master of Rolls –

using the occasion of a possibly 'miscarried' document to argue for some urgency in turning private advice into public domain:

> I should be extremely sory [*sic*] for such a Mischance. Least it should fall into the Hands of the pyrating Booksellers without the corrections of my Friends and the additions (which are Large) and some few alterations and amendments I have since made in it to make it of more use. Upon the Intimation you made me in your first I have entertained some thoughts of making it more Universal and publishing it. But shou'd be glad to know your opinion and that of any friends you have communicated it with if it has come to your hands. I have now finish'd it as compleat [*sic*] as I can make it and add to it a preface[.] [A]mong many other matters[,] I have mentioned that it was design'd first intirely [*sic*] for your use but made more universal and published that others might reap benefit by it if it cou'd afford any. I shall continue or ommitt [*sic*] this or let it continue in its privacy as you shall approve.[60]

In using the abuses of the 'pyrating' booksellers as an excuse to recycle private letters into published works, Cheyne was in good company. When Edmund Curll released an unauthorised collection of some 'youthful' letters Alexander Pope had penned to Henry Cromwell (first cousin once removed of Oliver Cromwell), Pope used the occasion as reason to have published his own edition of these letters in 1735. Cheyne identified with Pope's experience with the book trade: 'He is certainly an honest, ingenious Man, extremely easy in his Circumstances, but has suffered much from the Book-sellers', said Cheyne to Richardson. In the same letter, Cheyne offers his own observations on the booksellers: 'specious Curls was the gentlest Expression I had of them all, who have got so plentifully by me.'[61] But Cheyne, like Pope, was clearly no fool when it came to knowing how to profit from his prolific epistolary output. Through the circulation of private letters and by taking advantage of the book trade, Cheyne was able to advance his medical career and make a great impression on a large public outside of his own practice.

But the degree of Cheyne's popularity and influence depended on yet another crucial factor, and that was Cheyne's skill at stitching together a seamless new kind of medical rhetoric from the diverse fabrics of apparently contradictory medical traditions and contemporary trends: joining classical and Christian medical traditions; pairing the newest and most fashionable medical speculation with elements of pietism and middle-class Puritanism; attaching personal autobiography to national malaise; and, finally, combining the language of natural philosophy with the language of sensibility. Cheyne's capacious eclecticism and gift for synthesis inspired him to invent a rhetoric that could contain all these diverse elements and which must have appealed to a public itself so inclined to eclecticism in medicine, a public which held the hand of established medicine while eagerly dabbling in self-medication and empiric cure-alls.

In searching for an authorial voice and an epistolary style that would encompass his broad medical view, Cheyne fashioned a highly individual medical rhetoric, distinct from the prescriptive language of new science, and which asserted the importance of individual subjectivity. This made a profound impression on his patients and the public. Cheyne engendered a new fashion in medicine-by-post rhetoric, not only by example but by enjoining patients to respond in kind, as part of a spiritual communion, a republic of valetudinarian letter-writers.

The next section will examine in some detail the substance and appeal of Cheyne's individual medical philosophy and regimen (with all its contradictory elements) and considers why the public was so ready to embrace his message.

Cheyne's particular rhetoric, and hence the rhetoric he encouraged his patients to use in narrating their own medical conditions, must be understood as an amalgam of the contradictory elements he pulled together to form his own epistolary style. Most important among these qualities – and the ones with which his patients and the public could most readily identify – were spirituality and sensibility.

Spirituality: a new medical regimen and a new medical ethic

Cheyne's lively private practice at Bath attests to his personal appeal, and Selina Hastings (the Countess of Huntingdon), Dr W. Cranstoun, and William Moore approved greatly of his character in letters to acquaintances or to the doctor himself. The Countess of Huntingdon remarked in a letter to her husband from Bath in 1741, 'Dr Cheyne has been with me and has been talking like an old apostle. He really has the most refined notions of the true spiritual religion I almost ever met with.... I receive much light and comfort from his conversation.'[62] The impressive popularity of his books, running into multiple editions throughout the century, suggests that the public found both his message and his rhetorical style compelling. But the public's eager reception of the man and his writings must be explained, in part, by Cheyne's acumen in tapping into several major developments taking place in the medico–public sphere in the first third of the century. What Cheyne offered the public – and what his admirers must have recognised (consciously or subliminally) in his writing and person – was a prismatic representation of themselves, of British society, transformed by 'new' trends in medical speculation which actually had their roots in the late-seventeenth century but were only now coming fully into public consciousness.[63] Cheyne performed the function of ambassador between the world of medical theory and society, much as David Hume was to assign himself the role of ambassador between 'the Dominions of Learning [and] those of Conversation'.[64]

Two major intellectual legacies of the late-seventeenth century were especially responsible for creating the intellectual environment in which Cheyne's medical philosophy could flourish and liberate doctor–patient communication from the manacles of new science rhetoric with its proscriptions against subjectivity. The first of these was Thomas Willis's meticulous anatomical dissections and reinterpretation of the function of the nervous system which prepared the way for a physiology based on nerve sensibility. The other was John Locke's redefinition of the meaning of 'personal identity' – of 'individuality' based on human consciousness and sense perception in place of the traditional religious view of identity limited to an immortal and unchanging substantial soul.

Willis's magnum opus, the *Cerebri anatome* (London, 1664), in which he established the brain's dominant role in the function of the nervous system and, importantly, concluded that the soul is restricted within the body to the brain, was the basis for the eventual displacement of iatromechanical physiology by a physiology centered on the nervous system and which was the foundation for the concept of 'sensibility'. As G.S. Rousseau explains, once 'the soul is limited to the brain, as Willis and his followers in the 1660s contended, then nerves alone can be held responsible for sensory impressions, and consequently for knowledge.[65] Although Cheyne's more sophisticated patients might have been familiar with the works of physicians Richard Blackmore and Nicholas Robinson who, in the 1720s, had abandoned humoral-based theory in favour of a mind–body interrelationship based on the nerves, Cheyne was unquestionably the most effective populariser of a 'new' physiology of the nerves based on Willis's work.

John Locke had been a medical student under Willis. While a direct or specific influence of Willis's work on Locke has been impossible to document, it seems most likely that the new speculation concerning the centrality of the nervous system contributed significantly to Locke's interpretation of knowledge as based on perception and sensation. He expanded on this in the second edition of his *Essay on Human Understanding* in 1694, proposing that 'personal identity' is the product of a human consciousness which itself was formed by sensory perceptions and impressions. Locke argued that 'identity' could not be proven to reside in some immortal, indivisible, and unchanging 'substance' answerable to God, which was the eschatological view of 'individuality' offered by established religion. Instead, he postulated – expanding on Descartes – that all we can know with certainty is our own conscious state, and therefore it must be consciousness *assisted by memory* which produces our idea of a personal identity that exists *over time*. This idea spawned heated theological and philosophical public debate in the first decades of the eighteenth century, especially over the question of where to place moral responsibility if there were no constant, substantial soul but rather an ever-changing self formed and influenced by sensory input. Locke was satisfied that moral accountability resided in the fact that a function of consciousness involved 'concern' about one's behaviour, and that there was, ultimately, a consistency in how one's 'consciousness' judged one's own character and actions. Alexander Pope, in his poem 'Epistle to Cobham', called this overriding principle of consciousness the 'ruling passion'. Although this moral question remained a thorny issue in intellectual circles, by 1740, Locke's conception of the individual was popularly acknowledged and many medical writers had begun to use 'consciousness' synonymously with 'soul'. [66]

Cheyne's audience would have had ample opportunity to be indoctrinated to Locke's notion of the self either directly, through pamphlet wars on the subject (satirised by the Scriblerus Club), or indirectly through the works of contemporary authors who promulgated Locke's ideas of personal identity in their art. Among these authors were Cheyne's friends and patients, Alexander Pope and Samuel Richardson.[67] It is inconceivable that Cheyne was not familiar with Locke's reformulation of individuality and that he would not have found it compatible with his own therapeutic agenda which placed such a premium on individual experience and taking personal responsibility for one's habits to preserve, or else restore, bodily and mental (spiritual) health. Indeed, Cheyne was to complement and reinforce Locke's concept of 'consciousness' and personal responsibility with pietism – another seventeenth-century legacy which was being reinterpreted by the eighteenth century – to produce his own particular mix of medicine and morality.

Cheyne brilliantly codified and vitalised the paradigmatic shifts in scientific speculative thought inspired by the work of Willis and Locke to meet the needs of the British public of the 1720's and 1730's.[68] He took the medical and philosophical conjecture of Willis and Locke and transcribed it into a practical model of nervous disorders experienced through individual sensibility and tempered by individual passions and moral responsibility. As the most successful ambassador between a medical world now on the cusp of replacing iatromechanical principles with a physiology founded on the nervous system, Cheyne became a medical celebrity. This fact, naturally, galled many British physicians. They were not only suspicious and jealous of Cheyne's popularity but resented that his influence with the public interfered with their own medical practices. By addressing the public at large through his books, Cheyne was going over the heads of his physician colleagues. An anecdotal story in this regard concerns the famous Dr Richard Meade who, out of frustration and by way of retribution, is said to have departed from his usual practice of waiving his fee for the clergy when a man of the cloth insisted on following dietary advice taken from one of Cheyne's books even after Meade had strongly discouraged the cleric from such a course.[69] Such reactions to Cheyne, however, only confirm his popularity with the public as an able interpreter of medical theory and a bellwether of medical fashion.

Anita Guerrini has described the important role Cheyne played in the social history of medicine as not so much defining a new biology but rather in making 'explicit the links between biology and spirituality.'[70] Much of Cheyne's great appeal to patients lay in how he seamlessly incorporated Christian medical traditions and classical medicine. His medical practice and writings were the product of a classical education tempered by personal, physical, and psychological trials and by the sincere belief that his own medical recovery was realised through the force of spiritual renewal. The result was a unique and attractive medical amalgam which, I believe, allowed Cheyne to accomplish that great 'coup', as Roy Porter describes it, of 'reorienting the notion of an English malady', from an undesirable mental and physical state:

> [T]o a sociology of success, abundance, and (over)consumption; to a physiological site – the nerves – which being internal and hidden from the eye, sidestepped the physically disgusting features scorbutic, glandular or venereal disease; and to a cluster of symptoms – the state of the spirits – which were intrinsically fascinating to the sufferers themselves.[71]

'Spirits', here, should be understood to encompass both the physiological state of the nerves and the psychological state of the patient. For Cheyne, in somewhat circular reasoning, spiritual strength supplied the will to persist in whatever regimen was required to restore physical integrity to the nerves and, from thence, relieve the patient of his hypochondriacal state and disordered 'spirits'.

When Cheyne advised a mode of life consisting of reasonable exercise and proper diet, he was convinced by his own personal experience that such habits would maintain the unobstructed flow of 'animal spirits' in the nerves, preserving healthy tone and restoring damaged nerves to their ideal function.[72] His regimens attended to the management of the classic non-naturals of Galen, and he also applied iatromechanical principles to ensure the 'unobstructed flow' of blood and other body fluids – but all this to the end of maintaining the vigour and tone of the 'solids' and, in consequence, the 'spirits.' When Richardson developed some swelling in his legs, Cheyne accordingly reassured his patient:

> Your Head, Spirits, and Strength will be the better; they are not dropsical nor even can be: they are only the Laxity of the Solids and the Thickness of the Curd of the Blood whereby the Heart is not able to force the Blood upwards so quickly in the Veins as its own Weight carries it downwards in the Arteries. We call it anasarcous. You will see its Cure in my last Book, which is only by Water Drinking.[73]

While Cheyne, at this time, still adhered to the basic principles of iatromechanical medicine, he had dispensed with complicated mathematical details and concerned himself with more general therapeutic manoeuvres to prevent stasis. The goal of Cheyne's regimen was primarily to stall, or reverse, the deleterious effects on the nerves and other solids caused by immoderate diet, alcohol, uncontrolled passions, and the sloth of luxurious living.[74]

The teaching in the established medical schools (as Cambridge and Oxford) was that an improper lifestyle upset the proper balance of the non-naturals and would bring on an illness 'unique to the sufferer', a situation that 'was essentially a disturbance of fluid equilibrium to be managed by a personal attendant.'[75] Cheyne did not disagree with this fundamental concept of disease, but he also had his own very distinctive philosophy about treatment that made his approach seem radical and which was an anathema to his conservative professional colleagues. To begin with, Cheyne was unusually emphatic about the role of the 'passions' (one of the non-naturals) in affecting individual health and recovery from illness, in the power of the patient's mental state to aid or else sabotage therapy – an issue that would have been of much less concern to his iatromechanical colleagues who counted primarily on the good effects of vomits and cathartics. Cheyne also was adamant about the virtues of a 'low diet' that was an all milk and vegetable diet and, with some individual variation, prescribed this to all his patients – a uniformity of treatment that weakened the indispensable authority over the patient desired by most physicians. The suggestion that patients might adopt a regimen of diet and exercise to maintain a healthy state without requiring the regular interference of a medical 'personal attendant' was an obvious threat to business of medicine as usual. The idea of patient autonomy flew directly in the face of established medicine and would inevitably expose the unwary patient to the perils of self-help regimens in the vacuum of professional experience. For established physicians there were clear moral implications attached to what they saw as Cheyne's fostering of medical irresponsibility. It was a matter of medical ethics.

Cheyne was enough of an iatromechanist in his early days, and trained in the mainstream of British medicine, to shun Paracelsian-type therapeutics. He was entirely sceptical about the value of 'Chemical nostrums and the wild Dreams of pyrotechnical Enthusiasts as *Helmont*', and he vigorously discouraged Richardson from experimenting with this form of treatment:

> I have studied Chemistry and read most of all the Rational and Philosophical Chemists, but never could make any Thing of them that I could rely on, and even despise Boerhaave for his Brags of some of his chemical Medicines which I have ever found false on frequent Trial.

> ...It were very strange if the Almighty had not offered to us a less intricate Cure of Diseases than these laborious and difficult Trifles; and I never saw a chemical Medicine of any Kind that I could not *over-match* with a natural and simple one.[76]

However, he did share with the Paracelsian tradition a strong 'Christian philosophy' of medical therapy – a tendency to simpler and less traumatic cures than were used by his classically-trained colleagues.[77]

If he was radical in certain respects, Cheyne was also perfectly in keeping with developing medical trends in accepting the nervous system as having a predominant role in the mediation of bodily functions and modulating the impressions received by the mind. In seeing the nerves as the core system affecting health and disease, he was aligning himself with distinguished physicians such as Richard Blackmore and Nicholas Robinson. 'Nervous disorders' were now seen as the consequence of a loss of tone and a general laxity of the nerves which could eventuate in associated mental disturbance as well as bodily ailments. It was first and foremost an unhealthy physical state, through diet and lack of exercise, which predisposed to damaged nerves which, in turn, influenced the function of the brain through sensory input. To manage one's 'passions' was to ensure habits that maintained the body's physical fitness and prevented the development of serious nervous disorders such as hypochondria ('the hyp') or the yet more worrisome and refractory condition of melancholia.

Excessive intellectual effort also created a condition which predisposed to upset of the nerves, brain, and stomach, all of which were physiologically connected through the web of the nervous system. Scholars, literati, and all those with artistic inclination were, along with persons of social refinement, considered to have especially vulnerable and delicate nerves and, thereby, were especially susceptible to falling victim to the symptoms of the English malady. Cheyne warned:

Now, since this present Age has made Efforts to go beyond former Times, in all Arts of *Ingenuity, Invention, Study, Learning,* and all the contemplative and sedentary Professions... the Organs of these Faculties being worn and spoil'd, must affect and deaden the whole *System,* and lay a Foundation for the Diseases of Lowness and Weakness.... *Great Wits* are great *Epicures,* at least men of *Taste.*[78]

The nexus of nerves, mind, and stomach, was considered especially prone to illness in the man of sensibility who could, however, claim the burden of his valetudinarian condition as a mark of distinction. So it is not surprising that Samuel Richardson – as much the embodiment of the writer of sensibility as Cheyne was the embodiment of the English malady – readily accepted that he was a victim of the English malady and sought Cheyne's medical advice for his nervous ailments. Cheyne fully commiserated with the author:

Now as to yourself, I never wrote a Book in my Life but I had a Fit of Illness after. Hanging down you Head and want of Exercise must increase your Giddiness. The Body I added will get the better of the Spirit.... Your Friend and Mine, Mr Bertrand, tells me you look full puffed, short necked, and Head and Face bursting with Blood, as if by your Application and sedentary Life the whole System was spouted into your Head.[79]

A bridge was created between the therapeutic concerns of medicine with the moral intentions of the authors of the novels of sensibility. Both described the trials of the sensitive individual. For both Cheyne and Richardson, spiritual and moral strength were important to one's well-being, and literature might play a vital role in physical and mental wholeness.

David Shuttleton, in *'Pamela's Library': Samuel Richardson and Dr Cheyne's 'Universal Cure',* illustrates how the friendship and literary association of Cheyne and Richardson confirms the reciprocal influence of medicine and art in this period. 'Nervous sensibility' provided a reservoir of interpretive possibility for the artist (such as Richardson) to describe not only the font of moral sensitivity in his protagonists but in himself as inspired artist. Cheyne hoped to engage Richardson in a joint project to create and publish a list of medical and morally sound literary readings that were appropriate for an imagined (expanded) library of Richardson's popular fictional heroine, Pamela. Although Cheyne was unable to entice Richardson to complete such a project, his own eagerness for it illustrates Cheyne's conviction that well-chosen medical and moral reading material would benefit the public health in both body and mind. Indeed, Cheyne hoped to divert the mind from the, ultimately, harmful physical effects of melancholy by applying, to use David Shuttleton's words, 'Christian reform as collective cure'.[80]

Cheyne's medical programme to relieve patients of symptoms of the English malady was attractive in that it was tempered by moderation in all its aspects but still demanded just enough personal sacrifice and effort to make his patients feel a moral satisfaction in having earned the restitution of their health. His predominantly milk and vegetable diet only infrequently required complete abstinence from meat and alcohol, and his prescription for exercise consisted of walking, riding in a coach, use of a swing, and even being brushed by one's servants. The most vigorous form of healthy exercise was horse riding. However, an indoor, do-it-yourself, substitute for horse riding was available in the form of the 'chamber-horse', an exercise machine which Cheyne recommended highly to Richardson: 'I wonder you get not an Amanuensis and dictate to him riding on the new Chamber Horse so well known in London. It is certainly an excellent Contrivance for the Sedentary, Studious, and Thinking Part of Mankind, as I have tried by Experience.'[81] This exercise, wrote Cheyne, was 'admirable and has all the good and beneficial Effects of a hard Trotting Horse except the fresh Air.' Cheyne himself used this device an hour every day in fair weather and promised to 'do more when the Weather will not permit me to walk in the Garden or ride my Coach.'[82]

Cheyne studiously set the example for his patients, trotting out his own experience at every opportunity in his letters, thereby ensuring his credibility and authority as physician while contributing immensely to his own appeal as a public figure:

> I have been often under that Terror and Anxiety you mention and always suffered to Extremity if the Chariot was accidentally stopped.

> Drilling along I found to be the best Day Time Opiate to my Anguish, and I could have wished I could have lived, eat, drunk, and slept in a Vehicle.[83]

While exercise played a vital role in maintaining the tone of the nerves and the solid elements of the body, it also served to divert the mind from an inclination to melancholy induced by sedentary occupations and deep study.

Cheyne's rhetorical energy and dramatic effect is a hallmark of his style, as in this advice to his author friend:

> I am gay, lively, and debonaire, and free from every Ail but the Infirmities of Age; yet under all this Difficulty I walk in my Garden or in my Hall 3 Hours every Day without which I fear I could not go on so well. If ever you are hurt it will be by Sitting and Plodding, and therefore for God's Sake and your Family's Sake give it over and become a perpetuum Mobile.[84]

While the symptoms of disease, and dis-ease, ought to be cured with measures such as these, the spiritual life remained a critical adjunctive therapy to diet and exercise – to fortify the patient with the will to persevere in the dietary regime and to maintain a regular physical exercise programme to restore physical robustness and psychological peace. Ultimately, the mutual dependence of mind and body was weighted more towards the influence of the body. Nonetheless, virtuous living and the contemplation of spiritual matters were seen to hold the passions in check and thereby forestall mental disequilibrium. Once disequilibrium occurred, vomits and pills were to be employed only as supplemental therapy when other measures to restore a healthy physiological state had failed.

The spiritual dimension of Cheyne's medical project – including his own spiritual transformation – contributed immensely to his success as author of popular medical tracts and to his personal appeal for individual patients. Cheyne was writing at a time when the medical profession lacked any codified system of ethics, yet Cheyne seemed to fill this void by substituting the classical ideal of physician character with a newer trustworthy goodness founded on sensibility, spirituality, and the virtues of moderation. What the medical profession had inherited from its seventeenth-century predecessors was what Andrew Wear calls an 'assertive rather than deliberative' ethics in which 'ethics were put to work in the struggles of a medical market-place largely unregulated by law.' Established physicians in London proclaimed that their privileged Oxford, or Cambridge, education had conferred on them the Aristotelian ideal of the virtuous man whose character must be 'acquired by habit over time by a process of learning that is not innate.'[85] It was apodictic in the Hippocratic corpus and the writings of Galen that proper professional conduct was inseparable from character and that long years of study were necessary to forge the character of the ideal physician. An Oxford or Cambridge medical education was presumed, by the elitist medical circles, to imbue its students with 'right reason', that is, 'a particular kind of reason central to the moderate Anglican outlook, derived from scholastic ideas about the connections between virtue and the knowledge of God and nature.'[86] Without more specific standards for professional conduct, the charge of unethical behaviour could be levelled conveniently at any rival physician or competitive group of practitioners, or anyone offering a new surgical procedure. But established physicians were equally the target of irregular doctors who accused them of unethical behaviour evidenced by greed and exclusivity, by arrogance and pretension. 'Rhetoric, advertising, and denigration became mixed with medical ethics' and 'the imputation of danger and harm could be placed on any medical practice.'[87] Cheyne could not avoid the medical marketplace rhetoric, and his novel medical ideas and self-promotion through publication were roundly condemned by many of his fellow physicians. Yet Cheyne brought a new voice to the medical marketplace that seems to have impressed his patients, and much of the public, as more genuine, more moral, and less self-serving than that of many of his medical competitors.

Such medical–celebrity status as Cheyne's went hand-in-hand with vulnerability to public attacks on one's moral principles and medical ethics. Cheyne's dietary regimen, no less than Jurin's bladder-stone concoction, *lixivium lithontripticum* (see Chapter 2), was regularly criticised by the established physician community. In addition to defending himself in print against the slurs of competitors, Cheyne needed to reassure his patients that they were getting the best possible medical care. Insinuations by a rival physician that a regimen was unsound, or even unsafe, and malicious gossip, were incessantly eroding the doctor's hard-earned reputation.[88] Cheyne exposed himself to accusation of quackery by established physicians who identified empirics by the blatant advertising of their practices to the public through bills or *ad populum* medical tracts. Cheyne was obliged to defend his reputation in print. He claims in the 'Advertisement' to Part Three of *The English Malady*, that 'the obvious Sneer of its being a Quack's Bill has been the least Part of the Difficulty; for when I set about finishing this Work, for the Benefit of the Sedentary, Tender and Decay'd, I made a Sacrifice of some part of my Vanity and Interest.'[89]

Cheyne upset the medical *status quo* by transforming medicine from the exclusive property of the trained physician to a personal endeavour which required a more active role and responsibility on the part of the patient, giving the patient a greater power over his or her own body. He was redefining medicine as a common-sense knowledge supported by Christian principles. Such a threat to the established profession raised personal attacks by physicians upon Cheyne's character as well as on his regimen. Cheyne was forced to find a rhetoric that refuted such frequent personal slander while maintaining his moral high ground as medical ambassador to the public.

In a letter to the Countess of Huntingdon, dated 15 April, 1734, he writes, 'I durst not have adventured to advise you a total milk and vegetable diet, for I have heard your hysteric colic (for which London physicians were sent for) was charged to my account.'[90] Similar concerns are evident in Cheyne's letters to Richardson:

> If I knew, believed, or were not convinced beyond the Possibility of a Doubt, that only the Continuance in your Diet believing, as the Mystics say, in Opposition to reason, and hoping, as Scripture says, against Hope, can only at last cure you, you cannot think I could so obstinately persist to oppose the Opinion of your Physician, you Surgeon, your Wife, and your Religious Friends. What Interest can I have in being thus bigoted? I know if you die I

shall bear the blame; it will be my Regimen and Method that has killed you, and you know I have not the Power of Life and Death. God forbid; but this I can say in the Presence of my Maker, that if Providence designs to save you, I know no other Means than those I have advised you.... If you must die and Heaven has said so, your death will be much gentler, and if He has ordained you to recover I have shown you the only Way known to me, or, I think, knowable.... I will willingly bear the Blame of all to have a Chance to save and restore you.[91]

With both the Countess and Richardson, Cheyne readily invokes Providence and often imagines himself martyr to the cause of his patients' medical recovery. His appropriation of religious imagery to serve his particular and individual metaphorical use would seem egregious if it were not for our knowledge of Cheyne's serious conversion and the approbation he received from very devout patients and religious leaders. Among the most devout was the Countess of Huntingdon, who received this note from her doctor:

[T]ho I have been pelted to death on your ladyship's account I so truly honour and esteem your ladyship, and I think I know the honesty of your heart, that I suffer with pleasure, since in my conscience I am persuaded I have put you the only way possible to secure so valuable a life, and preserve you at present from greater sufferings during the cure than you could be under any other method known to men....[92]

Cheyne shared, to a certain extent, with his more conservative medical colleagues a tendency to blame failed therapy on patient non-compliance with medical orders, and to see this as a moral failing on the part of the patient. Christopher Lawrence, in 'Ornate Physicians and Learned Artisans', explains that the philosophy taught at the Edinburgh Medical School during the years 1726–46 was 'based on the non-naturals and stressed the importance of personal responsibility in the maintenance of health and cited moral failure as a cause of disease.'[93] Women patients were regarded as especially prone to heed the advice of friends over that of their physician, mistaking sympathy for qualified judgment. Cheyne betrays this stereotypical attitude when he questions the Countess's resolve to remain on his diet: 'I only feared that the number of persons those of your rank must see and hear might frighten or sneer you out of your purpose.'[94] Of course, Cheyne equally chided Richardson also for being distracted from his medical regimen by well-intentioned intruders. Any patient who invited treatment from any but a regular medical man was culpable of encouraging the spread of quackery and unethical practices.[95]

However, Cheyne was able to incorporate a tradition of Christian ethic into his attitude toward patient treatment that made the often necessary admonishments to patients seem less censorious. In contrast to classical medicine's focus on the individual patient, the alternative Christian tradition of healing was associated with gentler cures which were more holistic and homeopathic in nature than the harsh purging and bleeding treatments of classical medical practice. Cheyne was certainly prepared to employ the same timeworn methods of his medical colleagues, but he tempered his treatments with sensitivity for the patient's toleration of therapy.

Furthermore, the Christian tradition of health care encouraged a philosophy of self-help and looked favourably on the self-administration of herbal and other gentle remedies.[96] While Cheyne gave his patients very precise regimens to follow (not always so gentle), he paid respect to the personal judgment of his patients regarding their own physical needs. He writes to the the Countess of Huntingdon:

> I am extremely rejoiced you continue so well; I was always for your ladyship's giving into a little white meat, after that by vomits, powderous medicines, exercise, and a low diet you had sufficiently sweetened your blood, opened the obstructions in the glands, and taken off that inflammation.... I advised continuing so long in a low diet of vegetable food and unfermented liquors, for fear of bringing back these acute pains and inflammation to any degree. After that was sufficiently obviated and removed, I was always for your returning to a white meat diet, by slow degrees and slight trials.[97]

Cheyne's diffidence to his patroness-patient is very much in character for the eighteenth-century physician as described by Jewson; he puts on the best face possible given the *fait accompli* of the Countess's decision to resume a diet with meat.[98] But Cheyne also seems genuinely willing, more than most doctors of the period would be, to relax professional authority in the face of patient self-determination. His manner recalls Samuel Richardson's ideal of the sensitive physician, Dr H. in *Clarissa*, whose humanity stands in such contrast to the affected and imperious manner of doctors satirised in Restoration and eighteenth-century plays and novels.[99] In another letter to the Countess, Cheyne voices a confidence in his patient's judgment so consistent with his own religious beliefs that one is convinced of his sincerity even if tinctured by the flattery expected from a middle-class physician in addressing an aristocratic patron:

> You must ever follow the directions of nature and your own observations, for nobody can inform you so well as your own feelings what and when such or any evacuations is to be made, for nature and your feeling will point it out. Providence and its sovereign has got you in his power, and you must only

attend to him, and he will bring you by such feelings to the condition he wants you to be in.[100]

Cheyne, however, cannot always maintain this epistolary high ground, especially when he feels threatened by a rival physician. In this letter of 25 February, 1736/7, from Bath, Cheyne does not hesitate to invoke Providence to trounce the competition:

Madam

Your ladyship does me but justice when you think I have been as anxious about your health as if my own life depended on it, and it was that made so frank in telling you my mind, when you made that great jump in your medicines and diet by other advice, which I own both frightened and hurt me, solely on your account, for tho I have no great opinion of the professor's skill in practice, especially on British constitutions, yet sure I am had I drawn up the case, as I think I know it best from long observation and much enquiry, I am positive he could not have advised such a method, and I think it is because good Providence intended to save you, that you so soon and so slightly felt the inconvenience of it, for all the cases I have recovered I never go before the calls of nature, and it is very happy for your ladyship that you have so quickly returned to the simplicity of the dietetical Ghospel [*sic*] under which in due time I doubt not you will acquire a firm a stable state of health.[101]

Cheyne's rhetoric, here, belies his implied objectivity, the claim that this letter is 'solely on your account', as he writes to the Countess. This is a very carefully crafted letter in which Cheyne suggests that Providence is his particular medical colleague in watching over the health of the Countess. He feigns personal disinterest as regards the consultant called in to attend the Countess of Huntingdon, and avers that the only object of his anxiety is the patient's safety. Yet Cheyne makes a point of raising questions about the consultant's reputation and offers the view that this physician – obviously foreign – betrays an unfamiliarity with the constitution of English patients in general and, worse, has been dismissive of the particular constitutional needs of the Countess. Cheyne sets up his rival as typical of the presumptuous and authoritative, classically-trained, physician who would rather summarily prescribe a difficult regimen of harsh cathartics and emetics than devote 'long observation and much enquiry' to become truly intimate with the particular constitutional needs of the patient. In place of the classical medical approach imposed on the Countess by his rival, Cheyne invokes Christian ideals of healing by emphasising his own very personal concern with his patient's well-being and his sincere happiness that the

Countess has 'returned to the *simplicity* of the dietetical Ghospel' [italics mine].

As Anita Guerrini explains in 'The Hungry Soul, George Cheyne and the Construction of Femininity', Cheyne popularised the mystical notion that there was 'an inverse relationship between weight and spirituality: the less matter, the more spirit.'[102] In 1705, when he sought help for his own spiritual recovery, Cheyne found inspiration in George Garden, an old friend and Episcopalian clergyman. Garden believed in a personal mystical religion which he had adopted from seventeenth-century Scottish academics and churchmen, and from the writings of Antoinette Bourignon, a Flemish mystic. A more contemporary influence on the pietist circle was Jeanne Guyon (1648–1717) who inspired her followers, which included Garden and Cheyne, with her 'radical passive quietism' and an 'anti-Cartesian discourse which replaced reason with emotion.'[103]

Cheyne's mix of diet and spirituality, Guerrini claims, was especially attractive to women patients in the upper ranks of society. His milk-centered diet was associated with the maternal and with the domestic, while the male-associated diet of beef, large quantities of poultry, and alcoholic beverages, was frowned upon. Cheyne invited the upper classes of the British society to recognise in themselves an extreme susceptibility to the debilitating effects of excessive passions because of their natural and inherent tendency, as a class, to nervous sensibility. In women, this malaise of the privileged classes was readily identified with 'hysteria'; men with identical symptoms were said to be hypochondriacal and assumed to have very sensitive, effeminate constitutions. In prescribing to both sexes a cure that called attention to good diet and spirituality, Cheyne was honouring those attributes most associated with the feminine role in society. Paradoxically, this gendered cure was meant to restore vigour to nerves which had been weakened and thought to be effeminised.[104]

This said, Cheyne did not necessarily have an easy time convincing women patients to stick with his demanding diet. As he put it to Richardson, 'I have been preaching this Doctrine these 30 Years and ever found it hardest to persuade Women and Parsons.' Cheyne claims that:

> [T]hose that know me and my late Book will say I am... one of [women's] stoutest Panegyrists and... have found 50 Women for one Man at Church and Sacrament, but their Sufferings not being so intense as Men's, and their being more used to Sickness they are rarely brought into the greatest Abstinence.'[105]

This is an extraordinary statement, indeed, from a physician so attentive to his women patients and so popular with them. If Guerrini is not overstating the appeal of Cheyne's brand of medicine with women patients – and the evidence strongly supports her assertion – then we must assume that women patients largely accepted the image of themselves as experienced valetudinarians of frequent but inconsequential ailments as compared to men.[106]

Richardson's fictional heroines certainly do not support Cheyne's view of women. Fearing that Richardson's wife might be interfering with a regimen he prescribed for her husband, Cheyne writes to his patient:

> I hope Mrs Richardson is not like the rest of her Sex or Kindred known to
> me who I fear would rather renounce Life than Luxury.... But I have always
> found it the most difficult Thing I ever undertook to get a Wife's Consent to
> confine her Husband to a low Diet, much more to bring themselves to it.[107]

Such criticism could hardly be levelled at Clarissa or Pamela – but perhaps they are the exception that prove the rule? In any case, Cheyne qualified his remarks on Mrs Richardson by acknowledging (in a previous letter) that 'what I said of Women applied to Mrs Richardson, was from her Relation to one of the staunch Epicures [*sic*] I ever knew, Husband and Wife.'[108]

Cheyne, who in his early years had himself been the staunchest of epicures, avoided extremism in his religious beliefs and was moderate in religion as he was in his medical prescriptions. For all his interest in pietism and Methodism, there is no evidence that he ever left the Anglican church.[109] He was resolved to remain faithful to the moderate ideal of Anglicanism. Guerrini comments that 'Cheyne's modification of both the physical and religious extremes of asceticism and enthusiasm proved greatly appealing to the classes who frequented Bath, enabling them to ameliorate both their bodies and their consciences under the rubric of a fashionable sensitivity.'[110] Cheyne's medical philosophy, however, based on the relationship of the physical to the spiritual, had a major influence in shaping both the religious and medical beliefs of John Wesley and George Whitefield, the founders of Methodism, both of whom read Cheyne's work and corresponded with him. It was Cheyne's particular concern with the connection of spiritual and physical health that made him so desirable as a personal physician for Selina Hastings, the Countess of Huntingdon.[111]

The moral themes in Cheyne's popular medical books, and perhaps even more strikingly in his consultations-by-post, cannot help but spill over into a discussion of class – for he presumes to recommend to his aristocratic and upper-class patients a change in style of life to a pattern of habits and spiritual values which most closely approximate the middle class. His medical advice, directed as it is to the most materially successful members of

British society was, in effect, a directive, for health's sake, to emulate the model of moderation offered by the middling orders of society.[112] In this recommendation, Cheyne was self serving, insinuating himself, a physician of the middling rank, as the indispensable herald to the upper classes of that wholesome lifestyle they ought to assume.[113] Cheyne at once dramatised the differences between classes (in terms of excessive consumption versus moderation in diet, inactivity versus activity, etc.) while blurring the boundaries between them: making heightened sensibility a distinctive mark of social work for the upwardly mobile middle class. At the same time he invited genteel, titled patients to relieve the medical consequences of disordered nerves, due to an opulent lifestyle, by imitating the sensible habits and example of moderation exemplified by middle-class restraint in consumption. Cheyne, as a professional medical man, and reigning arbiter on 'nervous sensibility', was particularly well situated to play role of ambassador between the classes – a role he vigorously cultivated. His rhetoric was subtly crafted for the purpose of dissolving the barriers between himself and the upper-class patients he served.

Cheyne was engaged in a carefully constructed project of self-fashioning which permeates both his life and his rhetoric. He literally and symbolically embodied the transitional changes occurring in medicine after the heyday of iatromechanical medicine, appropriating to himself the themes of sensibility, of individual experience, and of deep personal spiritual fervour, as part of medical cure. His prescription of a moderate lifestyle tapped into the socio–economic changes of the period in which the middle class saw themselves as achieving the refined sensibility of the aristocratic class but without succumbing to the moral laxity caused by excess. Cheyne, whether by instinct or by calculation, successfully put himself forth as the representative of these changes, and as intermediary between the classes as well as between the domains of science and society.

Most important to his project, and to his self-fashioning, was to find a rhetoric that was direct, deliberate without risking offence, simultaneously authoritative and congenial – a rhetoric which would allow him to insinuate himself into the private lives of the aristocracy while maintaining his integrity as a physician with a strong middle-class message. He also had a survivor story to tell, a type of spiritual biography, of physical wholeness enabled through spiritual strength. A tall order, but one filled brilliantly by Cheyne.

Dr Cheyne's medicine-by-post: inventing a rhetoric

I have argued that Cheyne was the most public representative, even an icon, of a series of transitional moves occurring in the second quarter of the eighteenth century. For this role, he discovered a particularly effective rhetoric that bridged classical and Christian medical traditions, brought iatromechanistic principles under the umbrella of nervous sensibility, and which sought to authorise with his upper-rank British patrons those middle-class values of moderation and ascetic diligence in matters of personal health. This rhetoric both reflected and effectively contributed to the blurring of class and gender lines, in message and, as we shall see, through a mix of genteel and common prose. Whether blue blood or middle class, man or woman, all were invited by Cheyne to a slice of the sensibility pie.

Cheyne's persona in his books and medicine-by-post served as literary type for the English malady that he was professing to cure; his rhetoric extended this persona and contributed to creating that persona. It is not surprising that the rhetoric which informs his popular medical tracts equally characterises his private correspondence with patients. As Paul Child informs us, in his dissertation on the rhetoric of Cheyne's published medical tracts, Cheyne acknowledged that his published works were largely an outgrowth of his consultation-by-post practice.[114] And this acknowledgment invites us to look for the same artifice and rhetorical tactics which mark Cheyne's published medical works in his medicine-by-post practice – a voice designed to be distinctly audible in the eighteenth-century medical marketplace.

That Cheyne sought a distinctive voice, and achieved it, is quite evident from a letter he sent to Richardson in 1740:

> Mr Leake[115] told me in his dark confused Manner that a good Friend of mine had desired I would give him some Account of the Cheltenham Waters to be inserted in a new intended Edition of the Journey through England.... I guessed you at least to be concerned in it through you did not care to be known.... [B]ut you must mind to dilute my strong Terms and Metaphors, and to expunge my Shibboleths else I shall be found out which I would not be upon any Account whatsoever.[116]

Carey McIntosh, in *The Evolution of English Prose, 1700-1800*, explains that while eighteenth-century schools perpetuated the classical skills of oratory, a New Rhetoric was developing mid-century which re-oriented classical rhetoric to a growing print culture and was 'uniquely poised to speak to the needs of the emerging middle class'.[117] The contributors to this movement were largely Scottish intellectuals who had 'common roots in the new aesthetics and psychology of the middle third of the century' and who incorporated the philosophy from the 1730s and 1740s on 'ideas of sympathy, imagination, perception, taste, beauty, and evidence.'[118] Indeed, 'politeness and refinement played a leading role in the New Rhetoric... yoked with the ideal of civilization.'[119] Cheyne's own prose style was not New Rhetoric, but rather a mix of genteel and common prose; yet his popularisation of 'nervous sensibility' anticipates a culture of refined, 'feminised' rhetoric.

Cheyne's prose combines a deliberate genteel refinement with the colourful informality of early-eighteenth-century common speech – signalled by use of colloquialisms, solecisms, and archaic words.[120] While the general public may not have developed, as of yet, particular sensitivity to the use of 'correct' grammar and qualities of genteel prose style which distinguished the efforts of many of the newer orators and literati, there was a palpable ground swell within intellectual circles to establish an English worthy of national pride, a language which could restore a lost 'literary self-esteem' and cultural self-confidence.[121] Cheyne knew that his readers included literati, not only Richardson and Pope, but also Johnson, Hume, Berkeley, and Chesterfield.[122] One would expect, therefore, that Cheyne would wish to emulate the prose of these writers. However, McIntosh places Cheyne among those 'strong-willed middle-class writers' who 'seem to have decided to ignore more genteel standards and be informal as they pleased', writing 'coarse, vigorous, colloquial English', much like the prose of Matthew Bramble in his letters to Dr Lewis in Smollett's *The Expedition of Humphry Clinker*.[123] But Paul Child, in his dissertation on Cheyne's rhetorical style in the popular medical tracts, appreciates a dichotomy between Cheyne's impulse to please the general public with an 'unaffected style' while impressing his more educated audience with stylistic elegance.[124] Charles Mullett has commented on the shift in epistolary prose style between the formality of Cheyne's letters to Selina Hastings, and the 'absolute informality' of his letters to Richardson.[125]

My reading of Cheyne's prose style in his correspondence with patients is consistent with Child's interpretation of the published works – that there is an ever-present back-and-forth between the common and the genteel. However, I find this ongoing opposition of styles particularly intricate in Cheyne's medicine-by-post. Although it is hard to prove whether Cheyne's prose style is simply the product of a natural admixture of prose forms or the product of a felicitous and deliberate rhetorical compromise, I would argue that the consistency of Cheyne's writing strongly favours the latter interpretation.

The case studies in *The English Malady*, represent a clientele largely in the upper ranks of society, as one would expect from a successful practice in Bath. This fact must have required Cheyne, a physician of the middle class, to acknowledge the superior social status of his patients by using what McIntosh has designated 'courtly-genteel' prose – a linguistic heritage based on 'a small number of abstract, almost technical terms derived from the social environment of the court. It is a vocabulary which acknowledges the power of the monarch to "will" actions, and to grant "favour", and infers obligation, duty, and dependency on the part of those who attend the powerful.'[126] Outside the court, such language was meant to signal refinement and sensibility and, as such, was becoming increasingly the language of written prose.

Cheyne often employs the courtly-genteel style in his correspondence, for example in the opening of a letter addressed to the Countess of Huntingdon, 28 August 1732:

> Madam,
>
> I have the honour of your ladyship's today, and am more and more confirmed in what I knew before – that you will not suffer your well-wishers to be without any kind of expression of goodness and generosity. I have nothing I can say to purpose, nor anything that is not far below your ladyship's merit and benificence [*sic*], and must remit you to a superior court, where I hope your good works may be rewarded with their hunderfold [*sic*] here, as well as eternal felicity hereafter.[127]

But it is most characteristic of Cheyne's letters that he combines the 'common' language with the genteel style; one form may follow on the heels of the other, or else common vocabulary or coarse syntax may be incorporated into a deliberate and complex sentence structure. In the letter quoted above, Cheyne mentions that,

> I blame my own stupidity extremely in not putting you in mind that water, blood warm, is preferable to cold water or indeed in your case to wine itself. I know a person of great tenderness and delicacy who by that alone preserved a weak constitution many years and is now at 70 one of the most robust persons in England, and can bear wine now very well, but does not want it.
>
> I extremely approve and rejoice at your ladyship's courage in your diet, not to make you a hugeous compliment. (28 August 1732)

The sentence order is strained in the writer's effort to achieve a seemingly unaffected elegance of style. Cheyne cannot resist throwing in asides, characteristic of his epistolary manner, that interrupt the flow and even the tone of his letter. Instead of ending the sentence with 'and can bear wine now very well', he adds parenthetically 'but does not want it', superfluous fluff except that it introduces a kind of chattiness that must have appealed to his patients. The following paragraph opens in the genteel manner only to make use of the word 'hugeous', a usage described in Johnson's dictionary as 'a low word for vast', but which Cheyne must have employed for its friendly, colloquial effect. In this mix of prose styles, Cheyne seems to have aimed for a happy rhetorical compromise between studied politeness and simple directness.[128]

This effort to express warm familiarity within a framework intended to demonstrate gentility – with due respect for the patient–patron – is evident in essentially all those letters sent by Cheyne to the Countess of Huntingdon. For example, in this early letter from Bath, 3 June 1732:

> Madam,
>
> I have the honour of your ladyship's [letter], and one of the greatest pleasures I can possibly receive is having been the instrument in the hands of Providence of restoring so useful and valuable a health in some degree, which I hope by the same influence to be enabled to perfect without flattery or compliment. Tho I see many, there are few I honour more or wish better to than your ladyship. It would look like the first, if I should tell you all the good things were said of you after you were gone (and we at Bath are not much used to flattery behind our backs).[129]

Cheyne's desire to display both respect and familiarity creates a fractured style. The rhetoric is strained as Cheyne insists on his servile position yet concludes by teasing the Countess, in a parenthetical aside, that flirts with impropriety. His effusive praise of the 25-year-old Countess in August (cited previously) praises 'your ladyship's courage in your diet', but in doing so Cheyne rather boldly assumes the right to comment on the character of his patient despite the wide gap in their social station. The paragraph begins with that disingenuous disclaimer that the doctor does not intend to pay the Countess a 'hugeous compliment', but continues with Cheyne doing precisely that in the form of an elaborate, flattering, rhetorical inquiry:

> Do you know many ladies of your rank, quality, youth, and necessary high living that has sense, virtue, or indeed faculties capable of conviction, resolution, and courage to enter upon such a course of self denial for these poor disregarded low things (such as they are commonly reckoned), of good spirits, cheerfulness, health, and long life; and pray what is all the grandeur and glory in the world without them? (28 August 1732)

Perhaps the difference in age, Cheyne is 61 at the time of this letter, encourages this familiarity, but it is still remarkable that Cheyne should so openly denigrate 'grandeur' in conversing with aristocracy. Cheyne brings his religious convictions to bear on his sentiments in this letter, and one might conjecture that Cheyne intends to erase the social status difference between himself and the patient by insisting on their common religious inclinations. The effect, however, is disconcerting. Cheyne's message is that what makes the Countess so extraordinary is her maturity in valuing those things not usually appreciated by members of a privileged class. Cheyne's rhetorical style only exaggerates the contradictions inherent in the content of the letter. While he aims for a deliberate elegance of prose in the use of a series of words balanced against another series: 'rank, quality, youth, and necessary high living' with 'sense, virtue, or indeed faculties capable of conviction', he throws in asides and informal phrases such as 'hugeous compliment' or 'high living' that deflate pretensions to formality. Finally, the noticeable fault in agreement between 'ladies' and 'has' creates yet another contrast of respectable old-fashioned usage that calls attention to itself, partly because it feels as if this more properly belongs to colloquial speech than to written prose. Such solecisms, couched as they are among so many epistolary niceties, seem deliberate, and could betray an intention, conscious or not, to dispel the class difference between the doctor and his patron–patient.

By comparison, two letters from Dr John Burton (1710–71) to the Countess of Huntingdon, written in the early 1740s, show a much more usual doctor–patient epistolary style.[130] Burton's style shows a far more consistent use of courtly/genteel prose than is to be found in Cheyne. An accoucheur and an antiquary, Burton was the son of a London merchant. He studied at Leiden and received his MD at Rheims. He was known to have Jacobite leanings, and eventually became the satirical target of Lawrence Sterne in the shape of Dr Slop in *Tristram Shandy*. Nonetheless, Burton had a considerable reputation as an accoucheur. His epistolary tone with the Countess is never familiar, though Burton clearly wants to communicate his sensibility and personal involvement in the Countess's health as well as in that of a young lady who has been referred to him by the Countess:

Yr Ladyship will do me the great Honour if you will please to inform me how the Method I lately recommended to you with Dr Douglass succeeds. I have great Dependance on the Opening Pills[131] which you take every 4th Night; as a very efficacious, tho a gentle Remedy....

I shall be further oblig'd to Yr Ladyship if you would do me ye Favour at the same Time to acquaint me how yr young Lady finds herself that I prescrib'd for the beginning of August. Her Case was complicated; Short cough, Hectick Fever, Loss of Flesh, with Obstruction of ye Viscera in General. These Symptoms appear'd to me not very favourable. I consider'd them with ye greatest attention and shall be glad to know ye Event of ye Directions I sent to Yr Ladyship. I cannot but have a particular Concern for any One that Yr Ladyship thinks fit to recommend to me; and shall be always with ye highest Regard

Madam
Yr Ladyship's most faithful
& most Obedient Servant[132]

Mullett has commented that the letters from Cheyne to Richardson 'contrast pleasantly with the Cheyne-Huntingdon correspondence in their absolute informality', but this is not entirely true.[133] In one of Cheyne's early letters to Richardson, before the success of *Pamela* had turned Richardson into the famous author, Cheyne addresses his printer in a letter that strongly recalls the 'Hugeous Compliment' letter to the Countess:

Dear Sir,

I truly think myself much obliged to your Civility and Friendship. I have a sincere Regard for you and am convinced you are a Man of Probity and Worth beyond what I have met among Tradesmen. There is no Doubt there are many worthy Persons of that Class, but it has been my Misfortune to meet with but a few that had Parts and Probity both, and you may be assured if I be an honest Man myself I must value such.[134]

The force of the compliment rests, as it does in the case of the Countess, by pointing to the exceptional qualities that the correspondent displays in contrast to others of the same class (or professional) origin. In both the letters to the Countess and to Richardson, the compliments are constructed in a formal style that declares its syntactical and verbal intentionality. To place this in Carey McIntosh's prose scheme, there is a 'written' quality in many of Cheyne's letters which calls attention to itself and demands to be distinguished from spoken language. Nonetheless, Cheyne's polite style often becomes forced, as in this note to Richardson in January 1739/40:

I hope you know me too well and my Manner of acting with the Lovers of Virtue and its Source, whom I profess to love and serve with my Power, to be any longer shy with me but to use me with that Freedom that becomes Persons designing the same ends.[135]

Ironically, this attempt at formal prose includes a solecism, 'but to use' – for 'but that you will use' – and the sentence is rambling, failing at any attempt at balance or periodicity.[136]

Paul Child has claimed that Cheyne, in his published works, 'cultivated all the best stylistic features of eighteenth-century prose elegance: parallelism, balance and caesura, antithesis, epigram, periodic sentence structure.'[137] More precisely, however, while Cheyne was certainly aware of such prose refinements, he did not always employ them with consistent finesse in his correspondence, and this may well have been intentional on his

part. This said, there can be little doubt that Cheyne often strove for a type
of 'literary' prose form in his letters. For example, in the following
communication to the Countess, Cheyne makes extensive use of anaphora –
here, the repetition of the phrase 'I am afraid' – to dramatise his concern
that he has not received a response to his last letter:

> I am afraid your ladyship's [letter] or mine has miscarried; I am afraid you
> have been out of order in such a manner as not to admit any delay. I am
> afraid I have fallen in disgrace with your ladyship, contrary to my most
> earnest intention. I am afraid something of great concern has happened to
> the valuable and honourable family – in short madam, I am afraid of a
> thousand contrary things.[138]

The effect works well to communicate to the Countess Cheyne's
intensifying anxiety, that his state of mind has as much to do with his
concern that he has displeased his patron, as it does with the state of her
health. Cheyne makes abundant use of metaphor and similes for pure
literary effect, ignoring the proscriptive limits of new science rhetoric, which
studiously restricted the use of conceits to occasional illustrations drawn
from nature. Cheyne gladly indulges in rhetorical play and dramatic effects,
and even dietary advice is often accompanied by startling images. In a letter
of 3 August 1734 to the Countess, Cheyne insists that for a physician to
advise anyone who suffers from only a moderate condition to depart from a
moderate diet would be as if 'I should advise a man to snuff a candle with a
bullet shot out of a cannon.'[139] Or, encouraging Richardson to stay away
from fermented liquors which impede digestion: 'A Man that would drink
Nothing but Tepid Toast and Water might throw the Bridle on the Neck of
the Animal and let him follow his own Instinct.'[140] Still, 'there may be Times
and Season when a little Indulgence in Chicken and a Glass or two of Wine
may not only be convenient but necessary, as a Person stops to take his
Breath in ascending a steep Hill.'[141] Cheyne exhorts Richardson to persist in
a low diet and not be discouraged: 'The Weaker you are, the higher will be
your Recovery, like the Recoil of a Tennis Ball.'[142] Furthermore, 'it cannot
become worse, more severe or dangerous that it was before he began it, no
more than a Conflagration can become worse on pouring on some Water or
removing some of the Fuel.'[143] This analogy is dramatically extended in a
subsequent letter:

> When I put you on the Regimen and Method all I scrupled about was it
> being late in your Life and, your Headwork having been extra-ordinary,
> whether it could come in Time enough to cure totally these Symptoms,
> which were Reasons for my Advising the Regimen and Method. I knew if a
> Fire was scattered or extinguished in some of its Materials, it could not

readily, if the same scattering and extinguishing Method was continued, rise to Conflagration, ie. a new or dangerous Distemper, but if warm Ashes or hot Coals might not be continued till it turned into Powder. I was not secure but now upon removing the dead Coals, pouring out Water gently, and opening the Bottom to give Air, I find the Appearance by Management that a gentle clear Fire is probably to be put together again.[144]

More succinctly, the Countess is instructed that she must increase her diet 'by slow degrees, as corn grows, and by insensible steps, and never till the juices are entirely sweetened and the glands pervious.'[145] In a light-hearted mood, Cheyne uses metonymy to introduce the Countess to other devotees of his diet: 'You have three neighbours – vegetable, milk, and low livers – patients of mine in your neighbourhood.'[146]

The letters to Richardson are filled with imagery that makes use of religious analogy, especially when Cheyne needs to encourage faith and persistence in treatments that may take up to three years for full noticeable effect: 'I am extremely concerned that you should have Reason still of Complaints and Suffering but that is the Fate of all honest Men in this Life, which is a State of Trial and Probation for another Mansion.' In such instances, Cheyne recalls his own medical trials in a rhetoric evocative of Protestant spiritual biography. Cheyne offers his personal experience as reason he is able to empathise so profoundly with his patients. He has trod the same path as those he treats and can vouch for the value of his system: 'But I must not flatter you that you will not have your Purgatory and Purification. They pass through Death who do at Heaven arrive, says the Poet; but I think I can lead you through the State having passed it, I hope.'[147] Or again, in this letter from several months later:

[H]aving suffered in my own Bacon to a higher Degree that I ever read or heard of in any other Person I can describe the Road better and advise in the dangerous Steps, personal Experience being infinitely more secure than the most learned and penetrating Speculation.[148]

Cheyne envisions the affliction of the English malady as a form of religious purification, a virtual *Pilgrim's Progress*. In a prolix passage, Cheyne describes the 'Disorder' plaguing Richardson as:

[O]ne of the most effectual Means infinite Goodness could contrive to beget true Humility, to show the Nothingness of Creature comforts and sensual Enjoyments.... a temporal Purgatory;... and I earnestly pray both you and me and all those who love the Lord Jesus in sincerity they may have this Effect, and that our Purification may be in this Life.[149]

Cheyne portrays himself as a physician of great sensibility, and he reassures the Countess of Huntingdon that should he encounter 'the least coldness or indifference' from her as a result of his actions, 'I have a faithful monitor in my breast that would punish me as I deserved.'[150]

Mullett, whose editions of the letters of Cheyne to Huntingdon and Richardson give him authority on Cheyne's style, singles out Cheyne's 'capacity for idiomatic, even epigrammatic, expression and his gift for sharp characterisation.'[151] It is not hard to find examples of this gift in the correspondence. Writing from Bath to the Countess of Huntingdon, Cheyne explained that he was being criticised for occasionally referring patients to other spas. He therefore requested that she stop at Bath for a few days before going on to the Bristol waters which he had recommended. He continues:

> [T]here is such a universal malice against me here for sending people abroad (as I did my Lady Walpole lately) and to Bristol that I have been threatened with being mobbed, and some interested people spread it that I was sending the P. of Orange there, so that I durst scarce walk the streets... for the lower people think it is better to let people die here than send them elsewhere for their recovery.[152]

However, Cheyne concludes this letter by assuring the Countess that threats shall not deter him from doing what he thinks proper, and that 'Providence will take care of the rest, though I wish I had a little more of the wisdom of the serpent, provided I had the innocence of the dove with it.' In this few lines, Cheyne is able to be witty, play the martyr for his patients, advertise his practice, place himself firmly within the upper echelon of society, and remind the Countess of their mutual spiritual concerns. It is a miniature rhetorical tour de force.

Cheyne delights in the possibility of the pen. He enjoys a turn of phrase whenever possible, as when he writes, 'Tho I see many, there are few I honour more or can wish better to than your ladyship.'[153] The gratuitous phrase 'Tho I see many' serves primarily to flatter the ear as well as the patient and, once again, reminds the Countess of the popularity of Cheyne's practice. Yet the rhythm of the sentence is unquestionably pleasing and more effective than if Cheyne had restricted himself to the more direct compliment that 'There are few I honour more', etc. As we have seen, balance and parallelism are features of Cheyne's self-conscious 'written' prose, and in speaking of a diet that is both beneficial in pregnancy and useful to relieve haemorrhoid itching he advises, 'This is excellent food for your child and a sovereign remedy for your complaint.'[154] In his more expansive moments, his prose is effusive, stringing words in series: 'All the poor abilities, long experience, and warmest zeal I possess shall ever be employed to do, write, or wish for the temporal and eternal felicity of your ladyship and all your concerns.'[155]

However, Cheyne could trip over his own elaborate constructions, as in this urgent communication of 6 September 1735:

> All you describe I have felt and gone through, even almost to distraction, but I persevered in spite of sneer, puzzle, fright, and terror, well knowing I should be less miserable under this method than any other higher or stronger, and if I was to die I should go off in less misery. I thank God I have been long perfectly well by perseverance, and for the dimior[156] of our system I would not go through the same misery willingly and knowingly by returning to the higher regimen. I found nothing relieve but evacuations of one kind or another when sick, sleepless, or much oppressed. A vomit in lesser degrees, a Scotch pill, I chewed tobacco when spittings came on,[157] never stopped any evacuation nature pointed, drank Bristol water, chewed a bark on an empty stomach, sometimes a bit rhubarb, rode much, walked often, kept good hours, amused with agreeable, friendly company or innocent pastime, and time and patience under God conquered all at last; and so I have an absolute certainty it will do with your ladyship.[158]

The syntax is hard to follow and the parallelism is awkward, but these flaws in style are compensated in other ways. There is the enormous energy here: what begins as stylised prose slips into a run of very terse phrases marked by a staccato rhythm – a list of symptoms and therapy that is compelling by its sheer fecundity. Furthermore, the segment teases the reader by imitating the flavour of common speech within a framework that is self-conscious in calling attention to its 'writtenness'.

This fecundity of expression, a characteristic of early-eighteenth-century poetry and prose, has been well-described by Margaret Ann Doody in *The Daring Muse*. 'Expansiveness', she writes, 'is a fact of this literature, both in form and style', and she attributes its attendant zest for life to the Augustan appetite whetted by the success of imperialism.[159] Married to this 'impulse' for satiety is an obsession for 'complexity' and 'inclusiveness' (a mark of the new science rhetoric, as was described in Chapter 1). This carried over into a fascination with dialectic and presenting both sides of an argument – as in John Dryden's *Absalom and Achitophel* (1681). Cheyne's letters to the Countess often lean towards the dialectic, in this case the compulsion to anticipate what his detractors would be likely to criticise in the regimen he prescribed for her.

Both Margaret Ann Doody and Carol Houlihan Flynn point to a prominent connection between the impulse to prolixity in prose and the subject of health and mortality for eighteenth-century writers. Verbal energy seemed the means by which authors hoped to fend off any valetudinarian state and even forestall death. 'Silence, stasis and death – these ideas are associated by Augustan poets with the idea of the ending of a poem', says Doody,[160] and in 'Running Out of Matter', Flynn remarks that 'medical theorists and early English novelists' alike 'were committed in their different ways to... cheat, if not conquer, death', employing intense modes of 'stimulation and diversion in their ironically fatal battles against closure':

> Early novelists, like medical writers against the spleen, were searching for ways to come to terms with a mortality becoming all too pressing in a secularised world. While the medical therapists warn against the dangers of solidification, for to allow one's juices to grow stiff and solid is to harden into death itself, the writers of fiction resist ending their narratives... with digressions, anachronistic disruptions, parodic tailpieces that turn upon themselves, and metaleptic misspellings.[161]

Cheyne's therapeutic regimen was as concerned with rhetoric as recipe, and his often pressured 'common' rhetorical style partakes of the same impulse as the styles of his literary counterparts in fiction – to resist closure and the enervation of the nerves, mind, and body. His prose recommends, by its example, a gusto for life meant to overwhelm the inertia of a replete, therefore sick, society. For example, in the following letter to Richardson, Cheyne overwhelms us with the profuseness and optimism of his instructions to Richardson:

> I think you are Right to give up your Cold Bathing at least for the Winter Season and revive it in the warm Weather when it will be more beneficial.

> [...] Walk much in your Room and use a Journeyman or an Amanuensis's Hand in your Writing if possible. Go to Bed by Times and do most of your Business in the Morning. Take a Scotch Pill or two once in Ten Days or a Week.[162] Your short Neck is rather an Argument for a Vomit now and then than against it, for no long necked Animal can vomit, and Vomits are the best Preservatives from Apoplexies after little Phlebotomies, but I hope you shall need no more till the Spring.[163] But when the Stomach is free from Phlegm and Choler as it seems your's is little gentle Bleedings once in a Quarter may be sufficient.... Trouble yourself with no more Cold Bathing in any shape this Winter. I think from yours you are in the best Way I know, and you need only go on and trust the rest to Providence to which Protection and Direction I commit you and yours.[164]

Cheyne's energy spills directly over into matters other than health in the paragraph that immediately follows: 'Be so good as by a Line on Receipt of this to acquaint me what you learn or hear among the Criticks and Conoisseurs [*sic*] about my Book, and how it takes and passes off in your Metropolis.'

Achieving moderation in habits requires diligence. The self-destructive tendencies of high livers is an energy that must be transformed into a verve for reforming the self. Diversion is the key to successful therapy. David Shuttleton, explaining the manner in which 'Cheyne endorse[d] the therapeutic value of literature, the importance of proper diversion', offers this observation by Cheyne from the *Essay on Regimen* (1740):

> It is much more entertaining to play with Ideas, Philosophic Conjecture and such Amusements, how weakly soever founded, as tend to make Virtue and its source amiable, justify the Conduct of Providence, and mend and rejoice the Heart without hurting the Head, than to dwell on the dark Side of Things, that leads to Pyrrhonism, fatalism, Infidelity and Despair.'[165]

Cheyne wrote to Richardson that he is much 'obliged' to him, and would be to any 'Friend or indeed any honest Man' who would send him 'amusing, interesting, and sober Books, Pamphlets, or such like' which would serve as 'agreeable Means to help me spend without Anxiety or Dejection between 6 and 8 the only Time lies heavy on my Hands....'[166]

Intellectual diversion, carefully judged so as not to become too deep and therefore perilous in its own right, can entertain the mind and counteract the inclination to spleen, just as various forms of exercise. Among the most effective diversions, however, is letter writing itself. As in the epigraph of this chapter, Cheyne exhorted Richardson that 'my Way to my Friends and Advice to them is to lay is down as a Law that I and they write' on a regular basis, 'always in such a Compass of Time and sit down accordingly, and let the Pen write on to fill up what Nature, Affection, or Providence suggests.'[167] 'Whatever else you do', Cheyne admonishes his patient, 'fail not once a Week to let me hear from you, for I will not fail to amuse you somewhat by my Letters.'[168] But Cheyne's urging should not be misread as an invitation to trivial employment. For Cheyne, the letter is, in the words of Alexander Pope, 'a window in the bosom'; and so Cheyne implores Richardson '[B]e frank with me, and all honest men else you will be to blame, for we cannot know one one another's Hearts but by our Tongues and Pens.'[169]

Cheyne's patients clearly learned to imitate Cheyne's rhetorical recipe of art and heart, of science and sensibility. Dr Cranstoun, in his letter to Cheyne shows the transitional rhetoric forces at play in medicine-by-post. He promises, that this is to be an '*Abstract*... wherein, without the least Reasoning, Conjecture or Term of *Art*, I shall confine it to simple Narration of most essential matters of *Fact*.'[170] That is, he is promising an account of personal illness that adheres to new science rhetorical strictures. But while Dr Cranstoun makes every effort to be meticulous and objective, he also readily introduces striking subjective exclamations about the severity of his condition:

> But the warm Season allow'd me to drag a feeble and distressed Body abroad, and that as far as *Tunbridge*; I made a Trial of the Waters there, you know, without any Success, returning to *London* in as great Distress as ever; I wanted much to be determin'd, doubtful if I should be carried towards *Bath* or Home....

> At this Time... when exhausted more than ever, the Purging, by a little Assistance of the *Opiats*, after a Day's Nausea and *Vomiting*, was abated, which preserved the remaining Life. I then began to be exact in *Diet*....

Cranstoun's analysis of his urine specimen, although precise, is more poetic than scientific:

> I was often fretted with *strangurious Symptoms*. I took Notice of one Phenomenon in the *Urine*, which I never remembered to have seen, or heard, or observ'd before, which was the *Pellicle*, which is commonly carry'd on the Top, was powdered with exceeding small *Shining Particles*, like *Golddust*; the Sides of the Glass beset with the same, and the *mucous* Cloud in the *Centre* wrought full of them: These glittering *Atoms*, when gathered on the Finger, had the Feeling of fine hard Dust, and the *Urine* saturate with these, at its first Evacuation, would sparkle and rise in the *Glass*; at such Time there was deep Disorder and the *Oeconomy* and *nervous System*.[171]

Compare this with Bishop Cary's restrained and 'useful' description of his wife's urine posted to Dr Jurin in the previous chapter. There is a whole poetic dimension to Cranstoun's letter that exceeds the 'natural' similes of the Bishop. But that Cranstoun indulges in such vivid expression should hardly be unexpected from someone who introduces his case history to his physician, 'And now Dr *Infandum*! – *Jubes renovare Dolorem*.'[172]

By the close of the first half of the eighteenth century, the subjective description of illness by the patient had become fully sanctioned by the medicine of sensibility. To subjectivity would be added a rhetoric of urgency and drama, an increasingly dominant feature of medicine-by-post over the ensuing decades of the eighteenth century. Cheyne shared in a letter to Richardson, 'I think Lowness of Spirits in its extremest Degrees the only Misery in Life. If any Thing is Purgatory of Hell be worse I would prefer annihilation to it if possible; and better Spirits are the only solid Evidence of the Mending of the Constitution.'[173] The dramatised representation of illness marched in step with the novel of sensibility. One need only look at the selected passages from Richardson's *Clarissa* to appreciate how accurately Richardson reflected the new ideals of the doctor–patient relationship and the inherent rhetorical drama of the sick bed and the doctor-patient conversation around that scene. Cheyne set the example for Richardson when he wrote to the author: 'I speak and think out. I have nothing to conceal, not my Faults and Frailties.'[174] Cheyne had opened the door to the expression of one's personal drama in medicine-by-post, and such expression would flourish even more in the second half of the eighteenth century.

Notes

1. 7 November 1742, Bath. *The Letters of Dr George Cheyne to Samuel Richardson (1733–1743)*, C. Mullett (ed.), (Columbia: University of Missouri, 1943), LXXIV, 115. The original letters of Cheyne to Richardson are not extant or else remain undiscovered. What is available to us is a version of the letters which Richardson had transcribed into a notebook by a copyist. These are quite readable, though the copyist often encountered difficulty interpreting Cheyne's handwriting and was forced to omit words. Richardson left clear instructions in the book that the material in it was not to be published or 'lent' out to persons who might pirate it for their own purposes. In this, he was following the instructions of Cheyne who urged Richardson to 'destroy all my Letters when perused... I would not be counted a mere Trifler, as these long Nothing-Letters, merely to amuse you, would show me.' This sentiment is less consistent with Cheyne's character than the quotation at the head of this chapter. See Mullett, 'Preface', *idem.*, 19–20. All letters are from Bath unless otherwise noted. Mullett has identified letters in this correspondence by Roman numerals in addition to dates of correspondence. All subsequent reference to the Cheyne-Richardson letters will be cited as follows: Cheyne/Richardson, date of letter; note reference, Roman numeral of letter in collection, and page number in Mullett, as in note 5, below. All letters are from Bath unless otherwise noted.
2. R. Porter, 'Introduction' to George Cheyne, *The English Malady (1733)*, R. Porter (ed.), (New York: Tavistock/Routledge, 1991), ix.
3. *The English Malady* was published in London, 1733, with six editions appearing by 1739.
4. London, 1720, with 10th edition appearing in 1753. A list of Cheyne's publications, with dates of subsequent editions, has been compiled by Charles Mullet, though he does not claim his bibliography is complete. See, Mullett, *op. cit.* (note 1), 12–13.
5. Cheyne to Richardson, 19 November 1742; Mullett, *op. cit.* (note 1), LXXV, 117.
6. D. Shuttleton, 'Methodism and Dr George Cheyne's 'More Enlightening Principles',' in R. Porter (ed.), *Medicine in the Enlightenment* (Amsterdam:

Rodopi, 1995), 316–35; quotation is from 323. That Cheyne was friend and doctor to Pope and Richardson is certain. Mullett says that Johnson 'approved' of Cheyne, but does not identify him as a patient (Mullet, 'Preface', *op. cit.* note 1, 7) though Allan Ingram includes both Johnson and Hume in a list of patients and friends of Cheyne in his *Patterns of Madness in the Eighteenth Century: A Reader* (Liverpool: Liverpool University Press, 1998), 83.

7. Most recently, A. Guerrini, *Obesity and Depression in the Enlightenment: The Life and Times of George Cheyne* (Oklahoma: University of Oklahoma Press, Norman, 2000); also, S. Shapin, 'Trusting George Cheyne: Scientific Expertise, Common Sense, and Moral Authority in Early Eighteenth-Century Dietetic Medicine, *Bulletin of the History of Medicine*, 77 (2003), 263–97.

8. R. Porter, 'Consumption: Disease of the Consumer Society?', in J. Brewer and R. Porter (eds), *Consumption and the World of Goods* (New York: Routledge, 1993), 63.

9. Shapin, *op. cit.* (note 7), 296–7.

10. For a seminal and provocative essay on the relationship of seventeenth-century anatomical studies on the nervous system and the novel of sensibility, see G.S. Rousseau, 'Nerves, Spirits and Fibres: Toward Defining the Origins of Sensiblity', in R.F. Brissenden and J.C. Eade (eds), *Studies in the Eighteenth Century III: Papers Presented at the Third David Nichol Smith Memorial Seminar, Canberra, 1973* (Buffalo: University of Toronto Press, 1976); reprinted with postscript by Rousseau in *The Blue Guitar* (Messina, Italy), 2 (1976), 125–53.

11. Cheyne/Richardson, 13 May, 1739; Mullett, *op. cit.* (note 1), XXIV, 49.

12. See P. Langford, *A Polite and Commercial People: England 1727-1783* (New York: Oxford University Press, 1989), 66–7 and 464. Also, Michael McKeon, 'Historicizing Patriarchy: The Emergence of Gender Difference in England, 1660–1760', *Eighteenth-Century Studies*, 28 (1995), 297.

13. *Ibid.*, 72–3. The most successful eighteenth-century doctors were known to command large fees and boasted enormous incomes that permitted them to enjoy a nearly aristocratic lifestyle and social status. The fact that such a degree of professional success was attained by only a few did not deter those tempted by such prominent examples.

14. Porter, 'Introduction', *op. cit.* (note 2), xxxiii.

15. This world of material luxuries is brilliantly captured in miniature in Alexander Pope's satirical *The Rape of the Lock* (1714), most especially in the description of Belinda's 'Toilet' where 'Unnumber'd Treasures ope at once, and here/The various Off'rings of the World appear' (Canto I, lines 129–30). As noted above, Pope was a friend and patient of Cheyne.

16. Cheyne/Richardson, 2 May 1742; Mullett, *op. cit.* (note 1), LXI, 96.

17. A. Guerrini, 'The Hungry Soul: George Cheyne and the Construction of Femininity', *Eighteenth-Century Studies* 32, (1999), 282.

18. Cheyne/Richardson, 13 May 1739; Mullett *op. cit.* (note 1), XXIV, 49.

19. Porter, 'Introduction', *op. cit.* (note 2), xiv. Porter indicates that there is some uncertainty as to Cheyne's birthdate, but 1671 is most likely. The biographical material I present here is taken largely from two sources: Porter's 'Introduction' to *The English Malady*, *idem.*, ix-li, and from A. Guerrini, 'Case History as Spiritual Autobiography: George Cheyne's "Case of the Author"', *Eighteenth-Century Life*, 19 (May, 1995), 18–27, as well as her recent biography of Cheyne, *op. cit.* (note 7). See also D. Shuttleton, '"My Own Crazy Carcass": The Life and Works of Dr George Cheyne (1672-1743)', (PhD thesis, Edinburgh University, 1992).

20. Porter, 'Introduction', *op. cit.* (note 2), xv.

21. A. Guerrini, *op. cit.* (note 17), 281.

22. Shuttleton, *op. cit.* (note 6), 316–35. Cheyne's religious beliefs are discussed more fully below.

23. Pitcairne had lectured at Leiden University. Among his students was Herman Boerhaave who later became one of Europe's most renowned professors of medicine and who strongly promoted the iatromechanical view of the body.

24. T. Brown, 'Medicine in the Shadow of the *Principia*', *Journal of the History of Ideas*, 48 (1987), 629–48. Also on this subject see A. Guerrini, 'James Keill, George Cheyne, and Newtonian Physiology, 1690–1740', *Journal of the History of Biology*, 18, (1985), 247–66.

25. Brown, *ibid.*, 646.

26. Guerrini, *op. cit.* (note 19), 19.

27. Cheyne to Samuel Richardson, 23 December 1741; Mullett, *op. cit.* (note 1), LI, 76–7. A stone is 14 pounds. Cheyne is describing, here, the development of a scrotal hernia with intestine (containing gas or 'wind') present in the scrotum.

28. G. Cheyne, *Essay of Health and Long Life* (London, 1724). Newton himself never overtly encouraged application of his physics to medicine though he seems to have respected the efforts of others who made this attempt. Nonetheless, with Newton's diminished presence at the Royal Society from 1722 onward because of declining health (he died in 1727), interest rapidly waned in advancing the cause of medicine based purely on mathematics and physics. Its proponents turned to other interests. Jurin devoted his energies to smallpox inoculation while others in the group turned to chemistry and other areas of scientific inquiry; many simply tended to their enlarging private medical practices.

29. M. Barfoot, 'Dr William Cullen and Mr Adam Smith: A Case of Hypochondriasis?', *Proceedings of the Royal College of Physicians of Edinburgh*,

21 (1991), 204–14. In fact, gastrointestinal symptoms of abdominal pain, gas, and irregular bowel movements, are so regularly described in letters by patients with the 'hyp' that I am entirely convinced the clinical picture corresponds most closely with what modern medical practice labels 'irritable bowel syndrome' or 'spastic colon.' Heartburn symptoms are often reported with great precision in letters by eighteenth-century 'hyp' patients to their doctors, though I have not seen these symptoms referred to other than descriptively.

30. Cheyne/Richardson, 23 December 1741; Mullett, *op. cit.* (note 1), LI, 77. 'Reaching' was a commonly used alternative spelling for 'retching' (see Johnson's *Dictionary*). 'Scorbutical' here refered not to the Vitamin C deficiency that plagued sailors but was a more inclusive term which indicated a state of general malaise with poor skin tone and ulcerations, and often wasting disease – see R. Porter, 'Introduction', in Cheyne, *op. cit.* (note 2), xxxi. However, the eighteenth-century usage of 'scurvy', outside the specific maritime disease, is hard to pin down. Quincy, in his *Lexicon Physico-Medicum* (1726) defines 'Scorbuticus, Scurvy' as: 'a Disease that some writers make various Distinctions about, tho not to any great purpose. It is a Condition wherein the Blood is unequally fluid, and is best remedied by *stimuli,* Exercise, and such means as assist in Sanguification [the production of blood from chyle].' 'St. Anthony's Fire' refers to erysipelas.

31. Cheyne, 'Preface', *op. cit.* (note 2), i.

32. Cheyne/Richardson, 12 January 1739/40; Mullett, *op. cit.* (note 1), XXXV, 58.

33. Cheyne/Huntingdon, 7 January 1733/4; in C. Mullett (ed.), *The Letters of Dr George Cheyne to the Countess of Huntingdon* (San Marino: Huntington Library, 1940), 33. The 'tender part', referred to again in other letters, suggests rectal pain from haemorrhoids, which would be associated with pregnancy and childbirth. In another letter Cheyne writes, 'I have been mortally afraid to give you anything to strengthen you, least it should inflame that tender part.' (December, 1733; Mullett, 30–1 *idem*). Astounding as it may seem to us, Cheyne also recommended horse riding to cure this condition – part of the accepted regimen to restore the balance of the 'non-naturals' (see Chapter 2).

All quotations from the Cheyne–Huntingdon correspondence, unless otherwise noted, are from Mullett. The Huntingdon Library was kind enough to provide me with a complete set of these letters on microfilm. Any important discrepancies, or questionable words, are noted in subsequent footnotes. But as Mullett explains in his introduction to the Cheyne–Huntingdon correspondence, Cheyne admitted to writing in great haste, and the autographs show frequent inconsistencies and eccentricities in contractions, spelling, capitalisation, and punctuation. I have therefore largely relied on Mullett's labours despite some unfortunate modernisation of the autographs (some of which I have reversed).

Mullett does not identify the letters from Cheyne to the Countess of Huntingdon by Roman numerals as he does in his edition of the Cheyne–Richardson letters; therefore, only dates of letters and page numbers are cited for this correspondence. All correspondence is from Bath unless noted otherwise.

34. Cheyne/Richardson, 13 May 1739, *ibid.*, XXIV, 49.
35. The adherence to a prescribed medical regimen was, in fact, considered by established physicians to be a moral obligation on the part of the patient. This is described more fully below.
36. First letter is circa 1730; Mullett, *op. cit.* (note 33), 2. The second letter is from 18 February 1733/4, *idem*, 37.
37. Cheyne/Huntingdon, 19 November 1733; *ibid.*, 28.
38. J. Habermas, *The Structural Transformation of the Public Sphere: An Inquiry into a Category of Bourgeois Society*, translated by T. Burger (Cambridge: MIT Press, 1989), 49.
39. L.E. Klein, 'Gender and the Public/Private Distinction in the Eighteenth Century: Some Questions about Evidence and Analytic Procedure', *Eighteenth-Century Studies*, 29, 1 (1995), 97–109
40. D. Porter and R. Porter, *Patient's Progress: Doctors and Doctoring in Eighteenth-century England* (Stanford: Stanford University Press, 1989), 28.
41. J. Schneid Lewis, *In the Family Way* (New Brunswick: Rutgers University Press, 1986), 109–10. For a related discussion of how 'private' and 'public' become melded in matters of medical care in the eighteenth century, see L.F. Cody, 'The Politics of Reproduction from Midwives' Alternative Public Sphere to the Public Spectacle of Man-Midwifery', in *Eighteenth-Century Studies*, 32, No.4 (1999), 477–95. Cody describes how the eighteenth-century man-midwife successfully promoted himself as the public sphere man of reason and science while portraying himself, equally, as private sphere 'confidante' to his patients and their husbands, the 'model of humanity' and sympathy.
42. Cheyne/Richardson, 2 February 1742, Mullett, *op. cit.* (note 1) LIV, 82.
43. Physician discretion in cases of venereal disease and mental illness is discussed in the following chapter; see letters of William Cullen and James Gregory.
44. See M. Fissell, 'Innocent and Honorable Bribes: Medical Manners in Eighteenth-Century Britain', in R. Baker, D. Porter, and R. Porter (eds), *The Codification of Medical Morality: Historical and Philosophical Studies of the Formalization of Western Medical* (2 volumes): *Volume 1, Medical Ethics and Etiquette in the Eighteenth Century* (Boston: Kluwer Academic Publishers, 1993),19–45. Patient confidentiality was not a legal question in the

eighteenth century and it was not until Gregory's *Lectures on the Duties and Qualifications of a Physician* (1772) that specific recommendations on patient confidentiality were spelled out in a code of modern medical ethics (also cited in chapter 1). Chapter 4 contains a discussion of Gregory's ethics in the context of Scottish Enlightenment medicine.

45. Cheyne, *op. cit.* (note 2), 263.
46. These descriptions can be found right at the beginning of each of the individual case histories in Part Three of *The English Malady, ibid.,* 267–97 *passim.*
47. 'The Case of the Learned and Ingenious Dr Cranstoun, in a Letter to the Author, at his Desire, in Dr Cranstoun's own Words', *ibid.,* 311–24.
48. *Ibid.,* 312–3. The letter from Cranstoun is dated 20 September 1732, from Jedburgh. The first edition of *The English Malady* was published in 1733.
49. *Ibid.,* 312.
50. Cheyne/Huntingdon, 19 November 1733; Mullett, *op. cit.* (note 33), 26–30.
51. Cheyne/Huntingdon, 15 April 1734; *ibid.,* 39.
52. Included in the Cheyne to Richardson letters; Mullett, *op. cit.* (note 1), LXXIV, 116–17.
53. See below for more detailed discussion of Cheyne's medic–religious rhetoric.
54. Cheyne/Huntingdon, 18 January 1733/4; Mullett, *op. cit.* (note 33), 36.
55. Cheyne/Huntingdon, 18 February 1733/4; *ibid.,* 37–8.
56. Cheyne/Richardson, 2 May 1742; Mullett, *op. cit.* (note 1), LXI, 94.
57. Cheyne, *op. cit.* (note 2), 324.
58. London, 1720. This book was extremely popular and went through ten editions by 1753.
59. P. Child, 'Discourse and Practice in Eighteenth-Century Medical Literature: The Case of George Cheyne' (PhD thesis, Notre Dame, Indiana, 1992), 227.
60. Cheyne to Sir Joseph Jeckyll, 9 March, 1724, Bath; University of Edinburgh Library, La.II.303.
61. Cheyne/Richardson, 12 February 1741; Mullett, *op. cit.* (note 1) XLI, 65. For more on the complexities of eighteenth-century book publishing, see the excellent discussion by Mullett in his 'Introduction' to the C/R correspondence, *op. cit.* (note 1), 20–5. The machinations of Alexander Pope to publish private letters is described by J.A. Winn in *A Window in the Bosom: The Letters of Alexander Pope* (Hampton: Archon Books, 1977); in particular, see the first chapter entitled 'Schemes of Epistolary Fame', 13–41. For more on Pope and the seamy underside of publishing, see R. Straus, *The Unspeakable Curll* (London: Chapman and Hall, 1928).
62. Quoted in Shuttleton, *op. cit.* (note 6), 325.
63. Rousseau, *op. cit.* (note 10), 145–6.

64. David Hume, 'Of Essay Writing', (1742) in E.F. Miller (ed.), *Essays Moral, Political, and Literary,* revised edition (Indianapolis: Liberty Classics, 1985), 535.

65. Rousseau, *op. cit.* (note 10), 136. For a very thorough analysis of Willis and his work, see R.G. Frank Jr, 'Thomas Willis and His Circle: Brain and Mind in Seventeenth-Century Medicine', in G.S. Rousseau (ed.), *The Languages of Psyche: Mind and Body in Enlightenment Thought* (Clark Library Lectures 1985–1986), (Berkeley: University of California Press, 1990), 107–46.

66. See C. Fox, *Locke and the Scriblerians: Identity and Consciousness in Early Eighteenth-Century Britain* (Los Angeles: University of California Press, 1988).

67. *Ibid.,* 127. The Scriblerus Club consisted of Swift, Pope, Gay, Arbuthnot, Thomas Parnell, and the Earl of Oxford. Along with Pope and Richardson, Fox specifically mentions the influence of Locke's concept of 'personal identity' on James Boswell and Lawrence Sterne. See also, R. Porter, *The Creation of the Modern World: The Untold Story of the British Enlightenment* (London: W.W. Norton & Co., 2000), 156–83.

68. Rousseau, *op. cit.* (note 10), identifies the work of Willis and Locke as causing a paradigmatic shifts in scientific thought in the Kuhnian sense.

69. See Porter, 'Introduction', *op. cit.* (note 2), ix–x.

70. Guerrini, *op. cit.* (note 17), 288.

71. Porter, 'Introduction', *op. cit.* (note 2), xxxii. Later in the 'Introduction', Porter further defines Cheyne's legacy: '*The English Malady's* originality lay in setting intemperance within a socio–historico–cultural overview, somatizing a familiar socio-moral critique of luxury within an iatro-mechanics of nervous disorders, in such a way as to normalise depressive disorders: sufferers, cheyne insisted, deserved sympathy not scathing satire,' *idem.,* xl.

72. See Porter, 'Barely Touching: A Social Perspective on Mind and Body', in Rousseau, *Languages of Psyche, op. cit.* (note 65), 45–80. Also, on 'animal spirits', see Frank, Jr, 'Thomas Willis and His Circle', *idem.,* 107-146. Willis separated the soul into the rational and animal soul; the animal soul was considered subservient to the rational (reasoning) soul and was present in both man and animals whereas the rational soul was to be found only in man. Furthermore, the animal soul (anima brutorum, or corporeal soul) had two parts, a 'vital soul' in blood, and the 'sensitive soul' which composed the circulatory elements of the brain and nerves.

73. Cheyne/Richardson, 27 January, 1742/3; Mullett, *op. cit.* (note 1), LXXIX, 122. Regarding the book mentioned in this letter, Cheyne adds, 'By the Way, Strahan has never had the Civility to Favour me with one Line since he had the Property of that Book. I will deal no more with Booksellers with God's Grace.'

74. For a particularly lucid explication of Cheyne's medical physiology, see the section in Porter's 'Introduction' to *The English Malady* entitled 'The animal economy', *op. cit.* (note 2), xix-xxvi.

    The term 'solids' in the eighteenth century was used by physicians to identify those parts of the body containing the fluid elements. Whether the nerves themselves were entirely solid or were, instead, tubules which transported 'spirits' back and forth to the brain remained a heated debate, of great theoretical significance, ever since the anatomical dissections of Thomas Willis in the second half of the seventeenth century. Electrical conduction through solid nerves was not yet conceived by anatomists, and some explanation of the mode of communication between body and brain through the peripheral nerves was critical for non-Cartesians. Willis could not identify a definitive lumen in the nerves through which corpuscular 'spirit' matter could travel, but as R.J. Frank, Jr explains, Willis postulated that these finer particles must 'flow through the liquid/solid matrix that was created by the grosser class of particles... as a stream of water flowing through a solid mass of gravel'; see Frank, *op. cit.* (note 65), 133.

    The philosophical significance of this anatomical question is explained most compellingly by G. S. Rousseau, *op. cit.* (note 10).

75. C. Lawrence, 'Ornate Physicians and Learned Artisans: Edinburgh Medical Men, 1726–1776', in *William Hunter and the Eighteenth-Century Medical World*, W.F. Bynum and R. Porter (eds), (New York: Cambridge University Press, 1985), 156.

76. Cheyne/Richardson, May 1742 [no day date, but placed by Mullett between letters dated 2 May and 'received' 17 May; Mullet, *op. cit.* (note 1), LXII, 96. Johannes Baptista van Helmont (1579–1644) was a major disciple of Paracelsian chemical medicine. Herman Boerhaave, although first and foremost a proponent of iatromechanical medicine (he had been a student of Pitcairne), was appointed professor of chemistry at Leiden in 1718, and he authored *The Elements of Chemistry* in 1731.

77. Cheyne's 'Christian philosophy' is discussed more fully below.

78. Cheyne, *op. cit.* (note 2), 54.

79. Cheyne/Richardson, 24 August, 1741; Mullett, *op. cit.* (note 1), XLIII, 69.

80. D. Shuttleton, "Pamela's Library': Samuel Richardson and Dr Cheyne's 'Universal Cure',' *Eighteenth-Century Life*, 23 (February 1999), 59–79.

81. Cheyne/Richardson, Spring 1740 (undated letter); Mullett, *op. cit.* (note 1), XXXVII, 61. The 'chamber-horse' consisted of a board (Cheyne insisted the board be 'as long as the Room will permit, 18 or 20 feet, 16 at least') supported at either end by a chair, and surmounted by a chair to sit upon. One could then bounce up and down on this apparatus as if riding a horse. Cheyne provided very specific instruction on how Richardson should construct the machine, including a method to raise and lower the board; see

letter XXXVI, 59–60. Also, on the role of exercise in medical therapy, see C. Houlihan Flynn, 'Running Out of Matter: The Body Exercised in Eighteenth-Century Fiction', in Rousseau, *The Languages of Psyche, op. cit.* (note 65), 147–85.

82. Cheyne/Richardson, 1740 (undated letter); Mullett, *op. cit.* (note 1), XXXVI, 59–60.

83. Cheyne/Richardson, 26 April 1742; Mullett *ibid.,* LX, 92.

84. Cheyne/Richardson, 27 January 1742/3; Mullett, *ibid.,* LXXIX, 123.

85. A. Wear, 'Medical Ethics in Early Modern England', in A. Wear, J. Geyer-Kordesch and R. French (eds), *Doctors and Ethics: The Earlier Historical Setting of Professional Ethics* (Amsterdam-Atlanta, GA: Rodopi, 1993), 98–130.

86. H. Cook, *Trials of an Ordinary Doctor: Joannes Groenevelt in Seventeenth-Century London* (Baltimore: Johns Hopkins University Press, 1994), 118. See also Cook's more extensive discussion of 'right reason' in 'Bernard Mandeville and the Therapy of "The Clever Politician"', in *Journal of the History of Ideas,* 60 (January 1999), 101–24. In regard to the passions, Cook explains that, 'Governing the passions by right reason was critical to the ability to live the good life in both body and spirit' (109). Cheyne's concern with the relation of the passions to physical health was, therefore, firmly based on classical tradition.

87. Wear, *op. cit.* (note 85), 104–5.

88. A case in point, which dramatically illustrates the great tenuousness of medical reputation, is that of Richard Croft. He had become accoucheur (man-midwife) to Princess Charlotte in 1817, based on his great popularity with the wives of the aristocracy. However, when Princess Charlotte died following a prolonged (fifty hour) labour and a stillbirth delivery, 'public outrage... could not be stemmed. Many of the reproductive casualties suffered by the aristocracy in the year following Charlotte's death were blamed on the shock of the event.' After Croft experienced a second ill-fated delivery that year, he committed suicide. See Schneid Lewis, *op. cit.* (note 41), 97–8.

89. Cheyne, *op. cit.* (note 2), 259.

90. Cheyne/Huntingdon, 15 April 1734; Mullet, *op. cit.* (note 33), 39.

91. Received by Richardson 17 May , 1742; Mullett, *op. cit.* (note 1), LXIII, 98.

92. Cheyne/Huntingdon, 9 August 1735; Mullett, *op. cit.* (note 33), 48.

93. Lawrence, *op. cit.* (note 75), 156.

94. Cheyne/Huntingdon, 3 August 1734; Mullett, *op. cit.* (note 33), 42.

95. Wear, *op. cit.* (note 85),106.

96. *Ibid.,* 110.

97. Cheyne/Huntingdon, 20 August 1737; Mullett, *op. cit.* (note 33), 59.

98. See Chapter 1 for a discussion of the client–patron relationship in private

practice as described by Jewson.

99. Compare with the example of Bishop Cary writing to Dr Jurin with concern about the severity of the regimens prescribed for ois wife, but with no apparent change in prescription made by Dr Jurin (in Chapter 1).

100. Cheyne/Huntingdon, 6 September 1735, Mullett, *op. cit.* (note 33), 50.

101. Cheyne/Huntingdon, *ibid.*, 58.

102. Guerrini, *op. cit.* (note 17), 280.

103. Cheyne/Huntingdon, 25 February 1736/7; Mullett, 283.

104. Guerrini, *op. cit.* (note 17), 284–6; also R. Porter, 'Introduction', *op. cit.* (note 2), xli.

105. Cheyne/Richardson, [?] February 1742; Mullett *op. cit.* (note 1), LV, 85.

106. Perhaps Cheyne was comparing, in particular, the hysterical diseases of women with the severe gouty attacks more frequent in men?

107. Cheyne/Richardson, 2 February, 1742; Mullett *op. cit.* (note 1), LIV, 82.

108. Cheyne/Richardson, [?] February, 1742; Mullett *ibid.*, LV, 85.

109. See the excellent discussion on this point by Shuttleton, *op. cit.* (note 6).

110. Guerrini, *op. cit.* (note 17), 288.

111. Shuttleton, *op. cit.* (note 6), 323. Lord and Lady Huntingdon became practioners of Methodism in 1739 and were known to sponsor preachers of the faith.

112. For a description of the British middle class, or 'middling orders' of society, see Langford, *op. cit.* (note 12), 61–8.

113. See Porter, *op. cit.* (note 2), xxxi; Cheyne 'held up for emulation the lifestyle of the "middling rank", whose activities and diet were best suited to the climate and condition of England.... Thus Cheyne hoped to civilize the aristocratic consumption habits, to become the Chesterfield of the table. The poor would be healthy through work; the rich would work at being healthy.'

114. Child, *op. cit.* (note 59), 227.

115. James Leak (or Leake) was Richardson's brother-in-law. He was a prominent Bath bookseller who got his start in 1724 by publishing Cheyne's *Essay on Health*. Leake, as representative of his trade, comes in for scathing *ad hominem* attacks by Cheyne in man of the letters to Richardson.

116. Cheyne/Richardson, 7 November, 1740; Mullett, *op. cit.* (note 1), XXXIX, 63.

117. C. McIntosh, *Evolution of English Prose 1700-1800: Style, Politeness, and Print Culture* (New York: Cambridge University Press, 1998), 10.

118. *Ibid.*, 157.

119. *Ibid.*, 166.

120. See C. McIntosh, *Common and Courtly Language: The Stylistics of Social Class in 18th-Century English Literature* (Philadelphia: University of Pennsylvania Press, 1986).

121. *Ibid.*, 12; also McIntosh, *Evolution, op. cit.* (note 117), 15–19,

122. See Child, *op. cit.* (note 59), 257.
123. McIntosh places Cheyne with Robert L'Estrange (publicist), Jeremy Collier (preacher) and Richard Bentley (scholar), as writers who resisted the refinement of English prose. The fictional Matthew Bramble would seem to be representative in his selective use of archaisms, colloquialisms, and solecisms, of many of the country squires of the period as portrayed in the eighteenth-century novel; McIntosh, *op. cit.* (note 120), 38, 132–3.
124. Child, *op. cit.* (note 59), 252–62.
125. Mullett, 'Introduction', *op. cit.* (note 1), 20.
126. McIntosh, *Common and Courtly, op. cit.* (note 120), 69–71,
127. Cheyne/Huntingdon, 28 August 1732; Mullett, *op. cit.* (note 33), 9–12.
128. See McIntosh, *op. cit.* (note 117), for a detailed discussion of the transition of eighteenth-century prose from an oral-influenced, informal, style, as used by Defoe, to a more refined, correct, and self-conscious 'writtenness', exemplified in the prose of Samuel Johnson. One important signpost of this evolution was the increased use of periodicity – that is, structuring a sentence so that the important word is saved for the very end. Samuel Johnson's prose style was especially influential in this respect.
129. Cheyne/Huntingdon, 3 June 1732; Mullett, *op. cit.* (note 33), 3–4.
130. On microfilm in library at Harvard University, HA 1143 and HA 1142.
131. I have been unable to confirm what this medication would have been, but in a personal communication with the late J. Worth Estes, author of the invaluable *Dictionary of Protopharmacology: Therapeutic Practices 1700–1850* (Canton: Science History Publications, 1990), he believed this was most likely some form of laxative to relieve severe constipation.
132. 7 November, 1741, Saville Street; *op. cit.* (note 130), HA 1143
133. Mullett, 'Introduction', *op. cit.* (note 1), 20.
134. Cheyne/Richardson, 10 February 1738; Mullett, *op. cit.* (note 1), VIII, 36.
135. Cheyne/Richardson, 12 January, 1739/40; *ibid.,* XXXV, 58.
136. Carey McIntosh, in personal communication, was most helpful in pointing out examples of grammatical flaws in some of Cheyne's attempts at more formal prose style.
137. Child, *op. cit.* (note 59), 257.
138. Cheyne/Huntingdon, 28 October 1732; Mullett, *op. cit.* (note 33), 13.
139. Cheyne/Huntingdon, 3 August 1734; *ibid.,* 41
140. Cheyne/Richardson, 12 September 1739; Mullett, *op. cit.* (note 1), XXXIII, 57.
141. Cheyne/Richardson, 10 January 1741/2; *ibid.,* LIV, 80.
142. Cheyne/Richardson, 26 April 1742; *ibid.,* LX, 91.
143. Cheyne/Richardson, 2 February 1742; *ibid.,* LIV, 83.
144. Cheyne/Richardson, 12 October 1742; *ibid.,* LXXIII, 113.
145. Cheyne/Huntingdon, 14 April 1736; Mullett, 55.

146. Cheyne/Huntingdon, 19 November 1733; Mullett, 26.
147. Cheyne/Richardson, 2 February 1742; Mullett, *op. cit.* (note 1), LIV, 83.
148. Cheyne/Richardson, 14 July 1742; *ibid.,* LXVI, 103.
149. Cheyne/Richardson, 22 June 1742; *ibid.,* LXIV, 100.
150. Cheyne/Huntingdon, 28 August 1732; Mullet, *op. cit.* (note 33), 12.
151. Mullett, 'Introduction', *op. cit.* (note 1), 7.
152. Cheyne/Huntingdon, 18 January 1733/4; Mullet, *op. cit.* (note 33), 35–36.
153. Cheyne/Huntingdon, 3 June 1732; *ibid.,* 3.
154. Cheyne/Huntingdon, 12 August 1732; *ibid.,* 7–9.
155. Cheyne/Huntingdon, 19 July 1732; *ibid.* , 6.
156. Mullett does not explain this word. It is not in the O.E.D., and I have struggled with the original manuscript (on microfilm) and have shown it to various scholars experienced in reading Cheyne's difficult scrawl. But anyone who has spent as much time transcribing Cheyne's handwriting, as Mullett, must have the letters right. So my translation of 'dimior' is 'demur', meaning a scruple or objection. This makes sense and my guess is Cheyne was spelling the word phonetically, not an unknown liberty in the eighteenth century.
157. Tobacco was actually thought to be beneficial in respiratory ailments!
158. Cheyne/Huntingdon, 6 September 1735; Mullet, *op. cit.* (note 33), 50.
159. M. Anne Doody, *The Daring Muse: Augustan Poetry Reconsidered* (Cambridge: Cambridge University Press, 1985). See especially the first chapter for a discussion on the influence of imperialism, and the 'impulse to expansion' on eighteenth-century literary content and style.
160. *Ibid.,* 189.
161. Flynn, *op. cit.* (note 81), 149–50.
162. Anderson's[Scots] Pills, first described by Patrick Anderson in 1635, was patented by Dr Thomas Weir of Edinburgh in 1687 and served as a 'cathartic panacea' consisting of aloes, jalap, gamboge and anisum. See Estes, *Dictionary of Ptotopharmacology., op. cit.* (note 131).
163. Cheyne is recommending that Richardson use Thumb Vomits. The method is described by Cheyne fully in a letter of October 24, 1741 (Mullett, *op. cit.* [note 1], XLV, 70–2.):

    I generally chew a Bit of Tobacco to open the Glands and make me spit, then I tickle the Uvula and lower, till I keck [start to heave], and then let the Spittle flow if it will; if not I am at it again, and thus 30 or 40 Times without Drink or any kind of Liquor, but perhaps after to wash my Mouth with cold Water.... As for myself and many of my Patients I always found when the Head was cloudy or the Spirits not flippant a good long Pumping in this Manner always brought them about.

Cheyne further explains that whether or not one brings up anything is inconsequential as it is:

> the Compression of the Muscles of the Breast, the Labour, that does the Work.... At least the Wind will be pumped up which has the same Effect with Choler and Phlegm. If you could get a Facility in it, it would be a great Relief, and is now a Diversion to me like riding the Wooden Horse with a Book and Candle.

164. Cheyne/Richardson, 26 October 1739; Mullett, *op. cit.* (note 1), XXXIV, 57-8.
165. Shuttleton, 'Pamela's Library', *op. cit.* (note 80), 68.
166. Cheyne/Richardson, 30 June 1742; Mullett, *op. cit.* (note 1), LXV, 102.
167. Cheyne/Richardson, 19 November 1742; *ibid.*, LXXV, 117.
168. Cheyne/Richardson, 29 August 1742; *ibid.*, LXIX, 108.
169. Cheyne/Richardson, 13 May 1739; *ibid.*, XXIV, 49. For Pope's letter containing the metaphor of 'a window in the bosom', see Winn, *op. cit.* (note 61), 200.
170. Cheyne, *op. cit.* (note 2), 313.
171. *Ibid.*, 320–1. 'Strangurious symptoms' indicates painful and difficult urination. the 'pellicle' refers to a film that forms at the top of certain liquids.
172. *Ibid.*, 313. 'Infandum, regina jubes renovare dolorem' is from Book II of Aeneid (1. 3): 'O Queen – too terrible for tongues the pain /you ask me to renew, the tale of how/the Danaans could destroy the wealth of Troy' – verse translation from Allen Mandelbaum of *The Aeneid of Virgil* (New York: Bantam Books, 1961).
173. Cheyne/Richardson, 2 April 1742. Mullett, *op. cit.* (note 1), LVIII, 89.
174. Cheyne/Richardson, 13 May 1739; *ibid.*, XXIV, 49.

4

The Correspondence of Dr William Cullen: Scottish Enlightenment and New Directions in Medicine-by-Post

Dr Johnson has been very ill for some time; in a letter of anxious apprehension he writes to me, 'Ask your physicians about my case.'

James Boswell, 7 March 1784,
to Drs Cullen, Hope, and Monro at Edinburgh[1]

In the second half of the eighteenth-century, the rhetoric of medicine-by-post took on a new character and purpose as speculation on the physiology of the nervous system was refined and elaborated by doctors of the Scottish Enlightenment, in particular Robert Whytt (1714–66) and William Cullen (1710–90).[2] The new physiology expanded the role of 'sensibility' in defining man as a reactive organism, especially sensitive to the influence of physical climate and social environment. Of equal importance, Scottish Enlightenment doctors now conceived of a total 'sympathetic' integration of body function – a communication between solid organs as regulated through the nervous system – with a sophistication unmatched in prior decades. 'Sympathy', explains John Mullan, was 'the principle of coherence of those signs which possess the body to reveal the effects of passion and feeling.'[3] In other words, sympathy was that principle which rendered sensibility visible and, therefore, capable of 'touching' other responsive human beings by arousing nervous vibrations within the spectator through the senses.[4] Sympathy was the common denominator of 'touch', of 'feeling', as physical sensation and as metaphor; it was the interface between private sensation and the social world.

Michael McKeon has suggested that in the earlier decades of the eighteenth century manly sensibility 'lent to the ungendered industrious virtue of Protestant descent a subtly feminine receptivity' that 'pointed ahead to the cult of sensibility at midcentury.'

One attraction, says McKeon, of 'aristocratic ideology had been its claim that inner virtue was visibly manifested in the external phenomena of rank, regalia, personal display, even complexion', but 'the cult of sensibility attempted to reinvent this notion of the body as a system of socioethical signification in terms of biological materialism that would evade the ideology of aristocratic privilege.' For Cheyne, the appropriation of the image of the 'Man of Feeling' – of 'nervous sensibility' – had served primarily to ingratiate him into the world of aristocratic patients and to validate his particular brand of moralism (as described in the previous chapter). However, Scottish Enlightenment doctors not only elaborated upon the ethical implications of sensibility in a far more sophisticated and deliberate manner to bolster their professional status, but specified a professional sensibility that was particularly male. If, as McKeon claims, 'the cult of sensibility was short-lived because masculinity was learning to elaborate its own, highly circumscribed mode of "public virtue", alternative but complementary to the private domestic virtue of women', then this process is especially clearly demonstrated in the medical profession of the late-eighteenth century in Scotland.[5]

Sympathy in the context of the Scottish Enlightenment was, as Christopher Lawrence advises, 'a special case of sensibility' responsible for the natural impulse of people to form social bonds with persons of like interests and to create civic institutions and select societies for the betterment of mankind.[6] In medicine, sympathy would translate into the new fields of institutional and public health, in establishing voluntary hospitals and clinics to serve the poor. A medical physiology based on sensibility and sympathy, as Lawrence has suggested, perfectly complemented, and supported, the goals of the Scottish Enlightenment intellectuals and the landed elite who saw their role as the 'custodians of civilisation', as the 'natural governors' of a yet 'backward society' needing 'improvement.'[7]

Although there was a general European move from the iatromechanical to a vitalistic conception of the body, only in Scotland did vitalism lead to such a unified speculative system in which the total integration of body function was dependent on the nervous system. In France, for example, vitalism was conceived as an independent force within each separate organ, and 'in London, John Hunter ascribed his "living principle" to the blood'; but 'the Edinburgh theory of the body and the Edinburgh theory of social order used a common concept, integration through feeling.'[8] Civilised man had developed into a finely tuned organism whose health rested upon the perfect harmony of his internal body environment which, in turn, must be fully integrated with his external physical and social surroundings. It was a delicate arrangement put easily into disequilibrium, into a palpable and visible disorder which called for the expertise of the physician. But, importantly, 'sensibility' – as enlarged by the physiological and metaphorical principle of 'sympathy' – was viewed not as a medical liability – as it had with Cheyne – but as a desirable constitutional trait which, even if predisposing to certain states of ill health, positively enhanced society, civilization, and self-worth.

Figure 4.1

William Cullen (1710–90), portrait by William Cochrane.
Courtesy: Royal College of Physicians, Edinburgh.

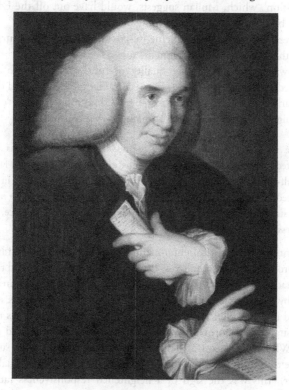

Signature of William Cullen.
Courtesy: Royal College of Physicians, Edinburgh.

John Mullan has taken issue with Lawrence's claim that Scottish Enlightenment leaders unreservedly adopted the model of sensibility and sympathy to describe the ideals of national improvement. The meaning of 'sensibility' in both literary and medical contexts, argues Mullan, always carried with it an aura of instability, the idea of a privileged state which inevitably teetered on the edge of self-absorption and a morbid isolation from society, as in melancholia. 'At the heart of such "theory" is disturbance and hesitation', which, Mullan suggests, would have put off the Edinburgh improvers by its potential to undermine 'ideological confidence'.[9]

However, my reading of medicine-by-post from the mid-century to later years of the Scottish Enlightenment suggests that 'sensibility', in large measure, was able to shed that quality of murky ambivalence that had confounded its meaning when, in the 1730s, George Cheyne had described a particularly 'English malady.' Barker-Benfield says that Cheyne 'embodied the campaign for the reformation of manners *and* consumerism':

> At one symbolic nerve center, where the culture's language was being generated, one finds a compressed combination of luxury and guilt, fashion and self-denial, sensuality and purgation; within such spirals, in fact, produced by them, was the elevation of the ambiguously susceptible nerves, whose state could be a sign of social superiority and Christian grace, or of weakness and nervous disorder.[10]

By contrast, Scottish Enlightenment medicine – as embodied by one of its most prominent representatives, Dr William Cullen – removed the moral stigma attached to disorders of sensibility. Instead of being a burden to be endured by susceptible (albeit privileged) persons whose nerves had been debilitated by imprudence of one kind or another, sensibility was redefined as the desirable and normal physiological state of highly civilised men and women. While the person of heightened sensibility was, to be sure, more vulnerable to certain types of illness than a less 'sensitive' individual (such as a labourer), this was the sign of a heightened responsiveness rather than simply highly irritable nerves.

Scottish Enlightenment physicians would not have argued with Cheyne's proposal that specific forms of malaise were the consequence of mankind's commercial and intellectual progress, but Enlightenment physicians also placed considerably more weight on sociability, with its commitment to consumerism, as a measure of physical well-being. Such a positive view of sensibility would be entirely consistent with Lawrence's thesis that medical speculation on human physiology was joined intimately with Enlightenment social ideology. Indeed, evidence for such a union can be discovered in the evolution of a new kind of doctor–patient rhetoric which routinely combines the medical with the metaphorical and the speculative with the practical.[11]

It is possible to define the ways in which the rhetoric of medicine-by-post of the Scottish Enlightenment reflected and disseminated the philosophy and concepts of speculative medicine of the period. The specific manner in which it did so is detailed in the course of this chapter, but certain critical elements of the new medical rhetoric can be enumerated here. To begin with, it reinvigorated a classical tradition of individualised medical care as an imperative of the doctor–patient relationship and assumed the professional authority implied in such a relationship. To that end, it largely rejected formulaic self-help programs – such as Cheyne's global approach to diet or the cure-alls of empirics – and asserted a complexity inherent in human physiology and responsiveness to environment that re-established the need for specialised professional knowledge and experience in times of illness. However, in true Enlightenment spirit, such knowledge was felt to be comprehensible to any person of intelligence, and patients were invited to understand and participate in their own treatment plans. Patient subjectivity in medical history became even more significant than it had been for Cheyne's patients; for now the patient's feelings were not merely the consequence of a 'nervous disorder' but intrinsic to diagnosis and treatment. The new rhetoric elevated sensibility to a quality of constitution not merely associated with privilege and abused nerves but with a natural and desirable evolution in mankind.

Such a positive view of sensibility gave licence to a richly emotive rhetoric in medicine-by-post; referential rhetoric was placed second to the drama of illness. In place of the rather confessional mode of Cheyne and his patients, personal stories now celebrated their hypersensitive constitutions. Dramatic rhetoric was, in fact, the counterpart – on the page – of sensibility made visible by theatrical (though genuine) somatic signs before an audience of intimates, the public, or one's doctor. Such patient language begged a particularly adept rhetorical response by the physician, displaying acute sensitivity without loss of that reassurance that attends unobtrusive authority.

However, interspersed among the predominantly hyperbolic medicine-by-post of this period, a different, more modest, utilitarian patient voice can be identified towards the close of the century. This voice may have been a reaction to the upper- and upper-middle-class cult of sensibility, a choice to emphasise the utilitarian aspects of Enlightenment medicine; or it may also have been the product of a larger and more diverse population of patients seeking medicine-by-post consultation. However, both the highly emotive, self-reflexive patient writer and the more self-effacing, referential patient writer are similar in how they translate the view of illness from a primarily internal disorder (such as a disequilibrium of fluids or a network of frayed fibres) into a view of malaise as the internal but visible response to things outside the body. It was a condition which called for the utmost skill of a physician, one with special intrinsic gifts of observation who had been schooled specifically in the interpretation of the complex semiotics of sensibility within the context of Enlightenment society.

While it is true that Scottish Enlightenment speculative medicine contained elements that were peculiar to that country – specific ideas promulgated by the university medical education curriculum and firmly integrated with Scottish Enlightenment philosophy – the example of Scottish medical practice is relevant to medical practice outside of Scotland. To begin with, actual therapeutic options were limited in the eighteenth century and 'regular' physicians throughout Europe and America did not vary greatly in their approach to treatment.[12] But furthermore, the influence of Scottish medicine beyond national borders was impressive.[13] Many Edinburgh-trained physicians set up practice outside of Scotland, either choosing to return to their native lands, or else simply unable to establish a medical practice within Scotland and forced to practise abroad. The other reason for the great influence of Scottish medicine on the Continent and in America was simply the prestige of the University and its star professors. The authority of Edinburgh physicians is evidenced by the many consultation letters received from patients and doctors well beyond the borders of Scotland, letters which attest to the far-reaching reputations of Cullen , James Gregory, and others.[14] As Christopher Lawrence has emphasised, 'there was no anomaly in Scottish medicine being a home-grown product appropriate for mass international consumption', albeit with modification in export.[15] In sum, there is reason to believe that the character and rhetoric of a major Scottish medicine-by-post practice, such as that of William Cullen, is relevant to medical practice outside of Scotland, though it remains necessary to recognise those traits that are specific to the medicine of the Scottish Enlightenment.

William Cullen

These elements of late-eighteenth-century medicine-by-post rhetoric that embodied the Enlightenment medical practice are well represented in the vast private practice correspondence of Dr William Cullen (1710–90). In the case of Dr William Cullen, we have a truly remarkable collection of medical correspondence from which to discover the character of late eighteenth-century medicine-by-post practice. Cullen was First Physician to the King in Scotland, President of the Royal College of Physicians of Edinburgh, and the pre-eminent lecturer at the University of Edinburgh's from 1755 till his death in 1790. In addition to his renown as authority on the relationship between illness and environment, Cullen was deeply committed to Scottish Enlightenment goals and counted among his close acquaintances David Hume and Adam Smith. He exemplified the spirit of 'improvement' and put speculative medicine into the service of practical patient care.

Cullen was born on 15 April 1710 in Hamilton, Scotland. He went to Glasgow University and, after a period as surgical apprentice to Dr John Paisley, he received his MD in 1740. However, after a few years spent in London, and serving as ship's surgeon, he returned to Edinburgh in his mid-twenties, for further medical training. He was a student founder member of the Medical Society of Edinburgh, a debating society which became the Royal Medical Society. Cullen set up practice in Hamilton in 1736, and William Hunter became his resident pupil and a partner in the practice for three years. Cullen then served as Doctor of Medicine from 1740, lecturing in chemistry, botany, materia medica (pharmacy) and the practice of physics. He was given a laboratory where he started his experiments in chemistry as it affected agriculture, a case of speculative science put to practical purpose in keeping with Enlightenment principles. It was at Glasgow that Cullen became close friends with Adam Smith and David Hume.[16]

Cullen accepted a position as professor of chemistry at Edinburgh in 1755. In addition to his famous lectures in chemistry. Cullen was always an immensely popular lecturer in whatever courses he taught, including botany, practice of medicine and institutes (theory) of medicine, materia medica, and clinical lectures at the Royal Infirmary. He published several academic medical texts which supplemented his student lectures, and soon after arrival in Edinburgh he became intimately involved in editing the authoritative *Edinburgh Pharmacopoeia*. With John Pringle, Cullen produced editions of the *Pharmacopoeia* in 1774, and again in 1783, that were notable for eliminating recipes of arcane complexity – Cullen distrusted polypharmacy – and those traditional ingredients which derived from long-standing superstition: 'the cobwebs, vipers, toads, snails, excrements, powdered skulls and the rest had gone'.[17] In addition to this impressive catalogue of academic appointments and activities, Cullen had an extraordinarily active private consultation practice.

Patient letters to Dr Cullen (from 1755) and copies of his own 'Consultation Letters', from 1768 to 1790 (the year of his death), are housed at the Royal College of Physicians of Edinburgh.[18] An overview of this collection by Guenter B. Risse identifies approximately 3000 letters from Cullen's private practice while he was professor of medicine at the University of Edinburgh.[19] Cullen not only meticulously saved and catalogued all the consultation requests he received from patients and doctors, but he also kept copies of all his responses to these letters. Initially Cullen's consultation notes were hand-copied by his secretary before being posted, but after 1781 Cullen had the luxury of using an early copy-machine designed by his friend, the inventor and engineer James Watt.[20]

To have both sides of a medicine-by-post correspondence is extremely rare, but to have such an extensive collection, as that of Cullen's letters, provides an almost unique opportunity to reconstruct the actual working dialogue between doctor and patient in a late-eighteenth-century practice. These letters offer, first of all, an invaluable record of the specific influence of Scottish Enlightenment medical philosophy on patient rhetoric within Scotland. However, because of the geographical and social diversity of Cullen's correspondents, these letters also represent broader trends in medicine-by-post outside the borders of Scotland and are not soley restricted to upper-class patients. Cullen's stature as a professor of medicine was unrivalled in the English speaking world, and his fame as a clinician – for example as an expert on environmental factors such as climate effects on health – brought him consultation letters from doctors and patients in Britain, the Continent, America, even Russia. In America one of his most admiring disciples was the famous Benjamin Rush of Philadelphia, a signatory of the Declaration of Independence. In addition to geographical diversity, Cullen's correspondence cuts across class. Both upper-class and various degrees of middle-class patients are represented here. Although Cullen was the physician to prominent Scottish Enlightenment figures and high-ranking Scottish families, a substantial portion of the letters he received were from midde-class citizens such as clergymen, soldiers, merchants, and also many women of middle-class background.[21] His consultation style is marked by a sympathetic ear and gracious response to all. Cullen's responses to women patients, regardless of class, were as serious, frank, and informative as those he wrote to his men patients. His tone remains consistently sympathetic and considerate, and only rarely can he be faulted for slipping into a patronising tone, and then usually when discussing a female patient with a spouse or physician, not in direct address to a women patient.

A word should be said about consultation-by-post protocol in regard to turnaround time from receiving a request to reply, and also in regard to customary fees. Cullen was assiduous in letter writing, putting aside time each morning for this purpose, and he responded expeditiously to all consultation requests, the usual turnaround time being within a day or two, and no more than a week.[22] Nonetheless, patients could become very restless awaiting a word from the doctor – perhaps in part an extension of the dramatic tone licensed by sensibility: 'I have waited with great impatience for some time past in hopes of hearing from you', writes Thomas Stapleton who hurries to explain that 'I have been exceedingly bad for these three weeks past, and still continue so.'[23] Another patient worried that 'Some time ago I wrote you mentioning so far as I could the Situation of my Complaints and inclosing [*sic*] a letter to you from Mr Lamont, both which I doubt has miscarried as neither have been favoured with an answer.'[24] This note followed the original inquiry by no more than seven days, though in that letter Mr Garthshore explained that 'I spit up an amazing Quantity of Slimy glutinous matter which makes Mr Lamont rather fond of vomiting which I think greatly increase the weakness of my Stomach.... I am convinced I write just now ignorantly but I know you will forgive as you will believe I am pretty anxious about my present situation.'[25]

Perhaps the concern occasioned by a less than an immediate reply from Dr Cullen is proof of the remarkable efficiency of his medicine-by-post practice. Patients accustomed to such service had reason to worry that the post might have 'miscarried'. Letters to Cullen from the Earl of Selkirk concerning his 9-year-old son, away at school, dramatically illustrates a distrust of the postal service at a time of parental angst. 'I am this far in my way to see my Son Daer who has had a Cold attended with feverishness hanging about him ever since about the middle of January', he writes to Dr Cullen in a note dated 10 April 1780 from Carlisle.[26] But within two days, the Earl feels compelled to send a second letter (this from Burrow Bridge) wondering whether it is the postal delivery or the doctor that has disappointed his expectation of a more immediate reply:[27]

Dear Sir,

I beg leave to give you the trouble of this from an anxiety lest a letter I wrote to you on Monday night at Carlisle should not go safe. It was not got to the Post Office till the man was on horseback, it was given to him with strict charge to put it in at Longtown, and to enforce his care, it was told him it was for a Physician, and concerning health. These fellows are sometimes forgetful of letters; and it is not impossible as the letter was thick, he might think there were some Scotch Notes in it, as it was about a consultation, in that case the letter would run some risk....

A dishonest postman might have found a guinea in the envelope, the usual fee for a consultation-by-post. However, in this case, the postman was honest and the fault, as a notation on the envelope informs us, was that the 10 April letter (postmarked Dumfries) was 'Missent to Kirkcubt' [Kirkcudbright]. By 17 April Cullen has advised: 'I think it will be proper to have him brought immediately to Hamstead, that is nearer Dr Fordyce. There is no advising with certainty upon such ailments but from the circumstances of the day.... Treatment must be expectant.'[28] This episode appears to have been resolved happily, but it makes clear that patients, or concerned family, might have good reason to become fretful if they had not heard back from the physician in what they considered a timely fashion.

Although the standard charge for consultation-by-post was a guinea, this was by no means fixed, and the fee also depended on patient's ability to pay.[29] One patient, Jane Webster, writes, 'I beg your acceptance of two guineas [for] your trouble which I have inclosed [*sic*] in this letter.'[30] Another patient comments in a letter to Dr Cullen that 'I am more ashamed to put you to the present trouble as you have generously given your advise without any fee or reward.'[31] Similarly, in a letter to a Mrs Likely Pitodry, who consulted him on behalf of a friend with a hearing problem, Cullen responded, 'You need not make apology for your fee for I am perfectly satisfied and without any further fee I shall willingly do you any service in my power.'[32] Cullen writes in another case, 'With respect to my fee... a draught upon him would imply my fixing my own fee which I never do, leaving it always to the circumstances and generosity of the patient.'[33]

Sensibility and customised cure

The dynamic association of sensibility with individualised doctor–patient communication, as seen in Scottish Enlightenment medicine, cannot be overemphasised. A blanket prescription, such as Cheyne had proposed for prevention and recuperation from the English malady – a national regimen of vegetable diet and exercise to fix the nerves – would not meet the expectations of the Scottish Enlightenment private patient who wanted exquisitely personalised medical attention to restore their sensibilities to their ideal, healthy state. In the matter of William Cullen's dietary advice to patients, for example, R. Passmore has observed that while there might be a 'sameness' in the recommendations, 'each letter is different and tailored to the circumstances of the patient.' Cullen, concludes Passmore, 'would have had little use for printed diet sheets.'[34]

The concept of sensibility introduced important changes in the doctor–patient relationship over the course of the eighteenth century. It had been apodictic among established doctors since the time of Galen that the physician must tailor his prescriptions and regimens according to the constitution of a given patient to effect cure. This tradition had remained vigorous into the first decades of the eighteenth century and was the cornerstone of the argument for established medicine over empiric and folk schools of medicine, in which the regimen was less customised to the individual patient. However, the development of iatromechanical medicine based on hydraulic physiology threatened the centrality of the patient's constitution in diagnosis and therapy. Treatment, in principle, could be determined mathematically. As we have seen in the medicine-by-post of the early-eighteenth century, the rhetoric of illness was largely influenced by the language of new science, and subjective patient experience contributed little on either side of medicine-by-post rhetoric. Nonetheless, professional survival in a medical commerce driven by patronage still required the physician to pretend to an exclusive knowledge of each patient's particular constitutional frailties. Patients seem to have been sufficiently flattered by such physician attention so as not to let their scepticism about inconsistencies in physician theory and practice interfere with daily medical care.[35] Still, the enthusiasm for iatromechanical medicine was doomed not only because its theoretical possibilities reached a dead-end but because a pure iatromechanical approach to disease ultimately failed to provide a rich doctor–patient discourse.[36]

By the close of the third decade of the eighteenth century, the neuroanatomical dissections of Thomas Willis and the theory of sensation expounded by Locke had reached the public consciousness and were producing a fresh medical vocabulary to replace iatromechanical ideas.[37] A rhetoric of nerves and sensations – what became the voice of sensibility – linked internal disorder to external causes, forcing a new doctor–patient rhetoric. Medicine-by-post under the influence of George Cheyne became, if not in and of itself cathartic, at least a type of prescription-by-example in which patients shared their experience of ill-health and its cure with a community of valetudinarians.[38] The doctor's role in Cheyne's successful model of practice, was to facilitate the interchange of patient narratives, which he complemented by his own professional authority. Paradoxically, at the very time that the medical case history was becoming more individualised through shared personal narratives, the perception of a pervasive national malaise – the English malady – allowed for therapeutic advice to be de-individualised. A national panacea of diet and exercise was applicable, with some modification, to any person susceptible to the ubiquitous symptoms of 'the spleen'. If such a turn in clinical practice was largely debunked by conservative physicians who hoped to preserve their private practices under the banner of Galenism, they found it exceedingly frustrating to defend against so popular a medical fad.[39] English patients had a long tradition of protecting their independence in the doctor–patient relationship, and George Cheyne's type of practice conformed nicely with popular inclinations to self-medication and home care.

For Scottish Enlightenment doctors to recover the professional authority implied in one-to-one medical consultation, it was necessary to restore the idea of the body needing interpretation, of medical diagnosis depending on semiotics.[40]

Sensibility – especially as elaborated upon with the idea of a 'sympathetic' collaboration of internal body organs which revealed the internal processes through pulse, movement, muscle tone, respirations, and so forth – required an interpreter rich in experience and himself of keen sensibility.[41] John Gregory said that 'sympathy produces an anxious attention to a thousand little circumstances that may tend to relieve the patient; an attention which money can never purchase: hence the inexpressible comfort of having a friend for a physician.'[42] It was sympathy which distinguished the 'gentleman physician' from the ordinary medical practitioner. Indeed, it was this very quality of sympathy in the physician character, of sensibility refined through education, that gave him the powers of fine observation and ability to interpret the semiotics of disease. It was, therefore, the amplification of the meaning of nervous sensibility by the principle of sympathy which firmly reasserted the necessity of a privileged therapeutic bond between patient and physician.

The rhetorical expression of sympathy, as described by Gregory, is exemplified in the consultation letters of William Cullen, extending to all ranks of society within his private practice. In communicating to a third party about a case of 'hypochondriasis' (so identified by Cullen in his index), he offers that 'I am heartily concerned to find Mr Ross's complaints have gained so much ground upon us and particul[y] to find that his own fears and apprehensions are so strong. They certain do him a harm and I am persuaded they are ill founded.'[43] Patients fully acknowledged and appreciated Dr Cullen's rhetorical niceties and the sense of genuine concern: 'I received your favour of the 2nd April', replied one grateful patient, 'which as every thing you ever said or wrote me did, gave me such satisfaction.'[44] This letter from Peterburg (a town two hundred miles outside Edinburgh) continues with the patient expressing concern that he may have offended Cullen's sensibilities by writing too frankly about a problem with venereal disease:

I am a little afraid tho from your not being quite so full and deccisive [*sic*] as I coud [*sic*] have wished, that in my last letters I have been rather impertinent and indiscreet – in troubling you with circumstances that may be deemed indelicate and invidious, and on the whole that you woud [*sic*] rather wish to discourage so indiscreet a correspondent while at such distance. Yet at the same time I cannot help thinking your humanity will forgive the man however you may blame his manner, when you consider the State I was in when I wrote both last times, so that any Patient in circumstances as I am to Dr Cullen must in any extremity look up to him with uncommon confidence, and write to him on his case more fully and with less reserve than to any other man on earth.

But I will not trouble you any farther with my conjectures – and impute the whole I would seem to complain of to my own peculiarities and the vast distance between us which makes correspondence on such cases very troublesome.

186

This is a truly revealing communication, in which we can see the patient's rhetorical effort to assume the role of the 'man of feeling' while requiring consultation on the 'indelicate' matter of venereal disease. The writer shapes his inquiry to the rhetorical framework of sensibility as he applies for help to a medical culture founded on the precepts of sympathy. He is appealing to Cullen's 'sympathy' to 'forgive the man however you blame his manner' because of 'the State I was in' as well as the 'vast distance' that necessitates written communication over a perhaps more informal face-to-face interchange.

In Enlightenment medicine-by-post, the emotional state is not uncommonly offered as excuse by the patient for some breach of epistolary etiquette – though such an excuse becomes, itself, formulaic within the context of the rhetoric of sensibility. In the case above, the patient was particularly anxious that he had been too bold in previous communications: 'Your returning half the fee I sent by Mr Spence is another incumbrance that makes me fearfull [*sic*] of my having been irksome to you.' But one does not doubt, in reading this letter, that Cullen is expected to reply in his usual sympathetic manner, and that the doctor–patient relationship is firmly based on a rhetorical protocol that guarantees such a response. Rhetoric becomes the substance of the therapeutic process, creating the environment in which healing can occur.

Sensibility and sympathy in medicine-by-post rhetoric in Enlightenment Scotland was, therefore, medical speculation turned to practical use in negotiating the diseases of patient and society, not simply a fashion for the physician to adopt in order to ingratiate himself with Enlightenment society. Similarly, an Edinburgh medical education differed importantly from the cerebral training of the 'gentleman physician' in the English universities in the way speculative medicine was combined with utilitarian purpose, even as concerned sensibility.

Medical education:
sensibility, speculative systems, and utility

On the surface, Cullen seemed to espouse a very different approach to medicine in the classroom than he did in everyday clinical practice – and therefore in his medicine-by-post. As a professor he was famous for advancing a systematic approach to medicine, and he developed a complete nosology on which he based his lectures and teaching method. On the other hand, in his private practice he allowed a more empiric approach, tailoring treatment to the individual.[45] I would argue, however, that it was the harmony of philosophical system and everyday practicality in Cullen that most embodied the ideal of the Scottish Enlightenment, and that this element he brought both to classroom, clinic, and private practice. If other professors at Edinburgh, such as James Gregory, questioned the validity of Cullen's particular systematic approach as an heuristic tool, the Edinburgh faculty were united in exemplifying the Scottish Enlightenment goal of joining philosophy to utility. The Edinburgh medical education was the reification of this ideal. Furthermore, it was this element in Scottish medical philosophy – coinciding with the socio–political agenda of 'improvement' – which in part, I believe, explains the eventual development of a more modest, less stylised, utilitarian medicine-by-post that made its appearance beside the more self-conscious, purposeful, dramatic rhetoric of this period.

The Edinburgh curriculum, unlike the curriculum of the English universities, provided a very organised and integrated exposure to the broad areas of clinical science. Lectures in anatomy and surgery, chemistry, and medical practice (all aspects of the diseased state and its cures) were the most popular. Additionally, lectures were offered in medical theory, the institutions of medicine (a compendium of subjects, the contents determined by the interests of the lecturer), materia medica (pharmacy), botany, midwifery (not required for graduation), and the clinical lectures at the Royal Infirmary of Edinburgh. Except for the infirmary lectures, which were presented twice a week at the patient bedside, all courses were offered five days a week so that students had the opportunity, if they desired, to attend the full spectrum of courses provided by the university. As Lisa Rosner informs us, 'this was the most extensive selection of medical lectures available at any university in Britain, a source of pride to the faculty and convenience to the students.'[46]

The bedside training at the Royal Infirmary, initiated by John Rutherford in 1748, was a unique offering of the Edinburgh curriculum as compared to the English schools. At least a third of the students came twice a week to hear a professor discuss a case currently on the wards. In addition, students could purchase tickets to 'walk the wards' at certain specified hours of the day. Dr James Gregory, the son of John Gregory and a colleague of William Cullen at the university, maintained that such regular scrutiny by students and fellow doctors at the Edinburgh Infirmary assured that the medical educators on the wards were always fully informed about the ward patients, up-to-date in medical knowledge, and scrupulous in regard to intellectual honesty.[47] Indeed, an Edinburgh medical training prepared its students to go out into the world and hang a shingle announcing competency in general medicine with far more legitimacy than graduates of the English universities, despite the continued snobbery of the Royal College of Physicians in London.[48]

By the second half of the century, when the English medical schools were on the decline, the Edinburgh medical school was considered one of the premier medical institutions in Europe.[49] The school was founded in 1726 and was one product of the national economic restructuring that followed the Act of Union with England in 1707. Edinburgh's prominent citizens understood the value of creating a medical institution that could compete with Leyden, thereby stemming the flow of its own students to the Continent as well as attracting English and foreign students to Scotland. The professors were appointed through the patronage of the Argylls and commanded great professional and social stature; they 'belonged to the most exclusive clubs' and 'were Whigs and moderates in religion'. The first professors had studied at Leyden under Boerhaave and based the early curriculum on that model.[50] However, as the school became established, its success became guaranteed by innovations such as courses being taught in English (rather than Latin) and the flexibility to attend only those lectures of interest to the student. Matriculation in a degree programme was not a requirement for attending courses. Medical education at Edinburgh was, therefore, eminently affordable since one paid only for the lecture one attended. The cost was three guineas per year for a course ticket, and the fact that professors' fees were a function of the number of student tickets sold served to encourage professors to make their courses as stimulating and practical as possible. Equally attractive was the fact that there were no religious restrictions here as there were at Oxford and Cambridge.

The philosophical approach to medicine promulgated by the medical school and its august professors was inseparable from the philosophical intentions of the Scottish Enlightenment as a whole but also should be seen as a continuum of seventeenth-century science and cultural movements. Much as Cheyne had incorporated, consolidated, and popularised the seventeenth-century mathematics of Newton, the anatomical dissections of Willis, and the epistemology of Locke (as I have shown in the previous chapter), so Scottish Enlightenment medical education complemented the optimism of Newtonian scientific method with a national vision matured out of the seeds of seventeenth-century Scottish antiquarians and natural philosophers. Roger Emerson has described these seventeenth-century intellectuals as the '*virtusosi*' who:

> [C]onceived of the economy of knowledge in 1700 in ways which led from natural histories of collections of carefully scrutinised facts to philosophical conclusions. Both Bacon and Newton had addressed the problem of how they could do so.... The systematic character of thought and the systematic teaching of philosophy in Scotland helped to make the moral sciences empirical studies.[51]

Seventeenth-century intellectuals were convinced that the application of Newtonian logic to all their endeavours would produce the fruits of knowledge about the true nature of human beings and society, to the end of discovering how best to use this knowledge to develop a culturally rich national identity. Emerson reminds us that 'the important Scottish moralists were to a man interested in, familiar with, trained to do or were pursuers of some science either professionally or by avocation.'[52] The inseparability of science and moral philosophy – and the desire to translate natural philosophy into practical benefit for mankind – is of the essence to Scottish medical philosophy during the Enlightenment.

One consequence, then, of the seventeenth-century legacy was a vision of institutionalising knowledge in the universities and through social commingling in clubs. A prominent figure among the *virtuosi*, Sir Robert Sibbald suggested as early as the 1680s that medical training should be incorporated into the university program; and this suggestion coincided with a larger vision to engender a more utilitarian and 'rigorous' approach to all areas of scientific and mathematical study.[53] Clubs were one form of institutionalising knowledge, and medicine had its own *virtuoso* club. Medicine, in the manner of so many other sciences, became the proper study of a gentleman. It was with such a point of view that many young men sought medical education at the University of Edinburgh once the medical school was inaugurated in the late 1720s.

In its first years, the Edinburgh medical school curriculum catered to the training of the 'gentleman physician'; it held medicine to be an 'art' founded on theoretical systems. However, once Scottish Enlightenment principles took hold, Edinburgh developed a curriculum that was much more a synthesis of the genteel and the practical in medical education. This innovative flexibility thrust the University into becoming the premier institution of medical education in the English-speaking world – and no one was more representative of this synthesis than William Cullen.[54]

The dramatic influence of individual educators in setting the path that medical education was to take in Scotland cannot be overstated. It was these doctors who put teeth into the ideal of combining theory with practice in medicine. For example, Alexander Monro *primus* and *secundus*, father and son, dominated anatomy at Edinburgh for most of the century. They brought surgery within the auspices of the university – unheard of in England – and combined medical lectures with surgical demonstration within the same course. Monro *primus*, a surgeon by training, taught iatromechanical principles yet was engaged equally in demonstrating, by dissection, the local spread of a pathological processes such as inflammation and malignancy. Furthermore, he made use of his anatomical discoveries to advise on the most appropriate surgical and medical treatments for various conditions. Monro *secundus* preferred the vitalistic account of physiology to the iatromechanical, but he extended his father's investigation of local pathological processes by elucidating the spread of disease along tissue planes. He also systematically applied autopsy findings to the physical exam in living patients, as in the case of differentiating hydrothorax from pericardial effusion by means of palpation of the heart, or by percussion of the abdomen in cases of ascites.[55] Monro's course was extremely well attended because he 'was not simply educating an elite group that once would have gone to Leiden', but was directing his lectures to a mix of 'apothecaries, dilettantes, surgeons, and others'. He 'was a physician who, in his surgical teaching, was using the most recent medical theory' and 'dealing sceptically with some of the most hallowed axioms of elite medical practice.'[56]

Although for some students the availability of teaching rounds in the Edinburgh Infirmary complemented the practical nature of the lectures in the school, it was primarily the lectures which provided the synthesis of theoretical and practical training that was so attractive to the student body.[57] Up to the mid-1760s, the university offered a diversity of courses, some pursuing the classical medical training of 'ornate and learned physicians' and other courses, in English, which emphasised practical matters of surgery and ontology.[58] But it was for professors such as William Cullen and John Gregory, beginning in the 1660s, to fully harmonise the theoretical with the practical within the body of their lectures. The spirit of 'improvement' inspired professors, such as Cullen, to use a systematic approach for pedagogic purposes while being 'prepared to organise their courses so that their practical applications were apparent.'[59] Christopher Clayson has remarked of Cullen that 'as professor of medicine it was his custom annually in the first lecture of the systematic course to describe the way in which "dogmatic" thought and practice must inevitably encompass the "empiric."'[60] Thomas Percival, who attended Edinburgh University, and was a member of the Medical Society in 1763, wrote in his *Medical Ethics* (1803) that '*Theoretical discussions* should be avoided in consultations, as occasioning perplexity and loss of time. For there may be much diversity of opinion, concerning speculative points, with perfect agreement in those modes of practice, which are founded not on hypothesis, but on experience and observation.'[61]

Cullen's fame was largely based on his ability to synthesise a system which 'presented a totally naturalistic account of health and disease based on the laws of the environment–organism relationship. For Cullen these laws were essentially those of sensibility and irritability.'[62] For example, Cullen associated hysteria mostly with warm climates and overheated rooms. The climate in Scotland was considered, therefore, especially beneficial for hysteric patients as compared to southern climes, including Scotland's immediate Southern neighbour: 'It is, I believe, common for a woman to threaten her husband with a fit in England, which I never knew or heard of here.'[63] The widespread acceptance of such teaching is evident in a letter to Dr Cullen from Dr Charles Blagden, who is seeking advice for a Mr Tillard, a patient with dyspepsia. Blagden writes that Mr Tillard 'brought it [his illness] on himself, as is commonly the case by Debauchery of every kind from his earliest youth, increased by the use of the strongest stimulants both in diet and medicine.' Still, the treatment Mr Blagden recommends, as the patient's primary cure, 'going into the Highlands of Scotland, to drink goat's whey, and be strenghthened by the invigorating air of that country.' He further adds, 'As he always shews great sensitivity to moisture, I apprehended that the most interior parts of the Highlands, at a distance from the Western coast, would suit him best....'[64] Blagden is certain that Cullen will approve of such advice. Indeed, these examples illustrate how Scottish Enlightenment medicine was able to offer a theory of environmentalism which gave direct scientific support to Scottish nationalism.

The Enlightenment concept of man as a reactive organism, who interacted intimately with his physical and social environment, created new career opportunities for the physician outside of traditional private practice; public service became respectable. Cullen, in his classroom, prepared students equally for a role in private practice or as the 'new social architects' who would concern themselves with the important Enlightenment projects of public and institutional health.[65]

At one extreme Cullen's lectures were part of a tradition that offered education to genteel physicians. At the other it provided a cultural and practical training for the new artisans of the medical world. Most students probably clustered around the middle of the spectrum, intent on becoming learned, but not elite practitioners, elegant but not afraid to use their hands. Cullen, it might be said, was the first mass medical educator in the vernacular.[66]

A model for the new type of physician was Sir John Pringle (1707–82), the Scottish physician who had worked with Cullen in improving the *Edinburgh Pharmacopoeia*. Pringle was highly esteemed for his work concerning military hygiene and was the author of *Observations on the Diseases of the Army* (1752) as well as articles on 'Gaol Fever'. Yet Pringle also carried on a prestigious private practice which included, among the patients, the fastidious James Boswell.[67]

Cullen, like Pringle, was a model of the Enlightenment physician who was able to combine an enormous private practice with a public medical role. In addition to his extensive teaching obligations, Cullen was an authority on various environmental issues, from farming practices (an extension of his work in chemistry) to institutional health. A letter from Dr Hutchinson of Dublin illustrates this aspect of Cullen's expertise:

You having so obligingly conducted me through the Edinburgh Infirmary in Octbr 1781, and answered so clearly a letter which I since troubld [*sic*] you with on the benefit of external Air to Hospitals, encourages me to apply to you again on that Subject viz to request you to inform me of whether it be custom in that Infirmary to allow Fires in all the Wards during *all* the Summer-Months? or if not – what are the Months during which they are disallowed? And if not allow'd in all the Wards in how many are they allow'd.

The Nurses, in some of the Hospitals which I sometimes inspect, plead the necessity... for keeping constant Fires in all the Wards – To me that method appears very precarious to health. The low price of Coals at Edinburgh doubtless induces you to allow fires there whenever you think it of the least use and not pernicious to health. If you favour me with an Answer on these points, Direct it to Sir Fras Hutchinson MP Dublin.[68]

Although the questions posed to Cullen by Hutchinson are of a utilitarian nature, the rhetorical tone of the letter is formal and courteous – indeed a prose that employs the vestiges of courtly prose, of obligation and favour. It signifies that the new role of the physician as public servant need not compromise respect for the profession; a qualified physician might serve equally the needs of elite society and the public at large without risk to his status as gentleman.

The expanding pool of students who could attend the Scottish university to study medicine, and the public and utilitarian contribution of the medical man, were both perfectly in keeping with the Scottish Enlightenment social ideology. However, such developments made it all the more necessary to safeguard the dignity and authority of the profession. The medical faculty made up of 'cultured' men, such as John Gregory and William Cullen, was diligent 'to impress on their students that medicine was a learned and genteel occupation.'[69] It was John Gregory, in his lectures on the *Duties and Qualifications of a Physician*, who emphatically stated: 'Perhaps no profession requires so comprehensive a mind as medicine.... [W]e have no established authority to which we can refer in doubtful cases. Every physician must rest on his own judgment, which appeals for its rectitude to nature and experience alone.'[70] The gentleman physician could be recognised by his reliance on sensibility to complement reason. It has been suggested by Laurence McCullough that Gregory was strongly influenced by David Hume's idea of 'sympathy', as when Gregory describes that 'sensibility of heart which makes us feel for the distresses of our fellow-creatures, and which of consequence incites us in the most powerful manner to relieve them.'[71] But Lisbeth Haakonssen has argued most convincingly Gregory could not have been influenced by Hume, and that his idea of sympathy was entirely in concert with the practical ethics and Common Sense moral philosophy of Francis Hutcheson, George Turnbull, and Thomas Reid, and which were already commonplace in Britain.[72]

It was moral character that identified the gentleman physician of the late-eighteenth century. The ideal physician, described by Gregory, 'possesses gentleness of manners, and a compassionate heart, and what Shakespeare so emphatically calls "the milk of human kindness"'. In addition to sympathy, that natural compassion for the patient, the doctor should display 'a species of good humour' that 'consists in a certain gentleness and flexibility, which makes him suffer with patience, and even apparent cheerfulness, the many contradictions and disappointments he is subjected to in his practice.' A physician, must 'support a proper dignity and authority with his patients', but if too rigid and absolute in his demands he will find the patient unwilling to cooperate, and 'a prudent physician should therefore prescribe such laws, as, though not the best, are yet the best that will be observed.'[73] This is a clear example of sensibility forming the basis for a utilitarian, effective, everyday medical practice.

The ideal Scottish Enlightenment doctor is a gentleman with medical and personal authority derived from education but also, more importantly, character. He is someone who shows sensitivity to both nature and experience; who has heart but also displays a manly, resilient spirit combined with a willingness to understand human limitations – both his own and the patient's – and to make practical compromise as is required of him for the good of his patient. It is important to Gregory that his audience of student doctors understand that 'men of the most compassionate tempers' are 'able to feel whatever is amiable in pity, without suffering it to enervate or unman them.' In fact, doctors who show true sympathy are those who have inured themselves to scenes of 'distress' and so gain 'a composure and firmness of mind so necessary in the practice of physick.'[74] Sensibility, thus ungendered – or at least reconfigured for masculine use – became a completely desirable trait that was in complete harmony with the Scottish Enlightenment social values outside the university walls.

Sensibility, sympathy and women Patients

Gregory was careful to distinguish, for his students, those attributes of sensibility which pertained specifically to the medical man: a manner and demeanour which conveyed great empathy and consideration for the patient without compromise to the important masculine qualities of self-discipline, reason, and moral authority. The correct display of sensibility in the Enlightenment male, and the particular adaptation of sensibility for the unusual demands made on the medical professional, was crucial in a culture in which sensibility had very definite associations with feminine character and physiology.[75] In the female body, for example, sensibility could manifest as hysteria and a paralysis in the ability to perform daily activities. A man who allowed the more feminine aspects of sensibility to overwhelm his constitution and character might also find himself disabled from attending to the responsibilities of work and family. Melancholia was a particularly serious consequence of unrestrained sensibility.[76]

Writers on the subject of Enlightenment sensibility, such as Jessie Ann Van Sant, John Mullan, and G.J. Barker-Benfield have been, therefore, very sensitive to its negative implications of sensibility. For Van Sant, the attributes of sensibility in women derive from a combination of metaphorical (literary and cultural) definition complemented by eighteenth-century nervous system physiology. Van Sant claims that the cultural ideal of the woman's body was one of 'immateriality', a being composed of such fine microscopic nerves and vascular structures as to be 'opposed to the material and sensual'.[77] Clarissa, towards the end of Richardson's novel, is the exemplum of this representation of the woman of sensibility, whose delicate physiology suffers the consequences of ravishment and who then, meticulously, casts off all the material and sensual aspects of life. The fact that Clarissa's physical decline occurs in parallel with an increasing remoteness from things material and sensual (literally, of the senses)[78] serves Richardson's spiritual–metaphorical purpose exactly as Van Sant describes. On the other hand, Barker-Benfield points out that what specifically upset Mary Wollstonecraft about the concept of sensibility as it applied to women was its very materialism, that 'when identified with "sensibility", women were reduced to an entirely physiological system', beings of 'refined' and 'delicate' reactivity deprived of intellect or soul.[79] Despite important differences, the common thread to both these views is the notion of women objectified through the physiology of sensibility.

A letter received by Dr Cullen from a distraught husband, concerning his 24-year-old wife, would seem, at first reading, to support the view of women patients as objectified through sensibility:

Dear Sir,

The long and kind letter you have favoured me with on the Subject of my niece gives me the boldness to write to you again on another case still more interesting to me, on which I stand much more in need of your advice. I mean that of my wife. For, you must know, that about two months ago, I married a lady with whom I had been in love since I was a child.... She is of sanguine temperament, but not plethoric, being rather pale, extremely fair and white. She is tall, well-made and now very lean, though when she was well, she had a great deal of *embonpoint*....[80] But 4 or 5 years ago, after much excess in Dancing, she became extremely weak.... After this she played a tragedy which moved her much, the consequence of which was the disease for which I consulted you, namely, fits of tension in the neck with great excitement of the imagination, followed by general relaxation and languor of both body and mind.... A little more than a year ago, she began to cough a little which she attributed either to cold or to singing... but two or three months after, having been exposed to some scenes exceedingly moving for her, from that moment she began to cough very much, she became lean and weak.... Her imagination is exceedingly susceptible of being much excited, and when in the course of conversation she has been much excited, she is worse not in the moment but some time after....[81]

Sympathy, in this case is a process of intense affect in a woman of delicate nerves, and the visible physiological effects produced describe a theatre of illness. The letter emphasises the theatricality of the medical scenario. The patient is pictured as a heroine of extreme susceptibility to imagination, of physical delicacy such that her constitution is weakened by scenes which move her, or even by the act of singing. Furthermore, the patient's 'imagination is exceedingly susceptible of being much excited' whether she is performer or audience. The patient–actress is one with the audience-culture in which she plays her role.

Yet there is a subtext in the letter which clearly aligns the male participants to the female patient through sensibility and sympathy. All three participants in the drama – patient, spouse, and physician – are attached to a larger world of polite society through the very rhetoric of sensibility, and the medical scene plays to a larger Enlightenment audience. As reflected in the opening words of the letter, sympathy is the glue which binds doctor, patient, and husband, through mutual regard for the civilised feminine qualities which have been appropriated to male sensibility. It is Cullen's 'kind letter' which emboldens the husband to write on a matter of intimate 'interest' to him. The husband narrator displays his credentials as a member of elite society through a language of feeling, describing his own vulnerability to the woman 'with whom I had been in love since I was a child', a language evocative of Lawrence Sterne but without the irony. Rather than the objectification of the woman patient, this letter suggests a continuum of sensibility, through sympathy, that joins the feminine to the masculine, and both to one society.

John Mullan has described sensibility as a double-edged sword, associated on the one hand with persons of refinement and taste, delicacy of feeling. passion, and (in males) high intellect – but these gifts were almost inevitably linked to a susceptibility to hypochondria, hysteria, and melancholia. Furthermore, there was a paradox that those traits so desirable in the social world, which signified a social being, were at the same time often a cause for withdrawal from society.[82] Barker-Benfield also has emphasised the dualism of sensibility, especially as it affected women. While the 'sensational psychology' of Locke implied that a woman's mind and character were the product of environment and cultural nurture (a 'tabula rasa'), not constrained by biology, the same nerve physiology was used to insist that 'women's nerves were normatively distinct from men's, normatively making them creatures of greater sensibility.'[83] This was associated with 'the aggrandisement of a certain kind of consciousness[,]... with the powers of intellect, imagination, the pursuit of pleasure, the exercise of moral superiority, and the wished-for resistance to men.' Yet these same gifts 'betokened physical and mental inferiority, sickness, and inevitable victimization.'[84]

But medicine-by-post of the Scottish Enlightenment suggests that late eighteenth-century patients and physicians regarded this duality as less problematic than mid-century patients who suffered the 'English malady' as a consequence of inappropriate diet and lack of exercise. In the late-eighteenth century, letters to Edinburgh doctors show that the physiology of sensibility is too intricately enmeshed in the idealised conduct of society to be considered undesirable. The medical consequences of extreme sensibility are not the 'fault' of over-indulgence and luxury causing diseased nerves (Cheyne's interpretation) but are 'the price to be paid for the refinements of civilization' and 'the result of fashion'.[85] Cullen's nosology classified diseases in terms of disordered sensation and movement (muscle and nerve conceived as a continuous unit), a disturbances of function rather than as a degeneration of nerves insulted by bad habits.

Within this more positive context, female sensibility was not so much 'the other' (non-male) sensibility, to-be-avoided, but a manifestation of sensibility that was part of a continuum of the visible spectrum of sensibility as it presented in both sexes within a civilised society. Male patients, as we will see in medicine-by-post letters later in this chapter, were quite as 'dramatic' in their rhetoric as female patients, but this was not a sign of being feminised or of inappropriate histrionics. The danger of indulging in the hypochondriacal state, especially for the male patient, was that it might eventuate in a state of melancholia and withdrawal from work and society. For the physician, however, there were aspects of 'female' sensibility that carried immediate risks to professional performance; it was a practical matter. For although sensibility was necessary to create a sympathetic bond with one's patient, the efficacy of the medical practitioner could be seriously impaired if he relinquished the 'masculine' control over feelings that might interfere with mental alertness and the ability to reassure the patient through quiet, 'masculine', authority.

The medicine-by-post letters of women patients in the latter part of the Enlightenment do much to dispel the idea that the women themselves felt particularly manacled by the rhetorical conventions of sensibility when it came to distinct physical problems that required medical attention. There appears to have been, for the eighteenth-century gentlewoman, a divide between the sensibility of the social world and that of her medical needs, a divide encouraged by the Enlightenment physician. Medicine-by-post may have provided a unique, liminal space in the world of the eighteenth-century woman, in which the rhetoric of sensibility served a special function: to encouraging doctor-patient communication through a rhetorical protocol of trust, in which actual physical symptoms could be described in detail without compromise to feminine character. This might be seen as the necessary counterpart of the role of the rhetoric of sensibility for the physician – providing a way to speak intimately without obfuscating gender roles necessary in society.

Medicine-by-post of the late-eighteenth century shows that woman patients could acknowledge a particular 'delicacy' of constitution without renouncing the physical reality of their bodies. The many letters to Dr William Cullen from woman patients do not evidence a need for rhetoric that plays to a stereotypical ideal of the female body; rather, women patients express medical concerns within the confines of the rhetoric of sensibility in a language remarkably pragmatic. Furthermore, the voice of medical self-observation by these women asserts the presence of an intellect that resists objectification, either as a body devoid of feeling – as in the new science rhetoric – or as a welter of fine feelings and nervous disorders devoid of body.[86]

The character of medicine-by-post written by a woman patient is well illustrated in the 'Case of Mrs Major Ross'. We have preserved, in the Cullen archives, both a letter from the patient and his response to her.[87] In this interchange, a letter from Mrs Ross – apparently written to her own doctor with the understanding that Cullen would be consulted – describes flagrant gastrointestinal symptoms that are driving her to near distraction. She attributes these symptoms to a constitutionally 'weak stomach'. I have provided a long abstract of this letter below to show how successfully the patient is able to represent herself as having a very material body – no coyness here in the description of some very unattractive symptoms – while enclosing her medical narrative within the frame of sensibility and having a 'delicate constitution'. The letter also confirms that sensibility was not regarded, by doctor or the patient, as a form of moral failing or the consequence of a fault in character:

All my complaints seems to proceed from a very weak Stomach, as I have every possible Stomach complaint. Sometimes I have a weighty and gnawing pain at the pit of my stomach and immense quantities of Wind Comes off it. The physicians who attend me say that I sometimes pass Bilious stuff but that I am not sensible of – what I feel most is that every thing that I eat (and my diet is as plain as possible) turns sour[.] I feel constantly as if I have Vinegar in my mouth. I have almost every day bad gripes and purging, the latter comes particularly at a certain time and carries off that affair. When I have not the purging I am costive.... [F]rom my stomach growing so much weaker every now and then I have a Bowl complaint [*sic*] most so violently as the one you attended me in long ago and it comes either by the purging being checked or by lasting too long and then I pass like the mucus of my bowls and an inflammation is threatened. I trust when my stomach is strengthened the Bowl complaints will be less frequent as they put me into agonies that I cannot express, but in the meantime I should like to know how to treat them when I am violently seized. Sometimes they give opiates – sometimes physic to carry away the sharp humour that occasions them[.] I trust that Dr Cullen will think of something to remove this Stomach Complaint that has been so long rooted. To get rid if it I would follow any course of medicines and adhere to any Regimen. And you can tell him I have a great deal of Resolution and perseverance. Be so good as to mention to him that I used to be subject to St. Anthonies [*sic*] Fire, and that any thing healing used to bring it on....

Mrs Ross is able to embellish on the frailties of her physical body through a subjective language which at once pleads the urgency of her situation while refusing to deny strength of character. She attributes all her problem to a 'a very weak stomach', and is put 'into agonies that I cannot express'. Yet she is sure to provide great clinical detail in her letter and insists on her 'Resolution and perseverance', rejecting any notion of a particularly female helplessness.

An increasingly prominent feature of late-eighteenth-century medicine-by-post patient rhetoric, evidenced in the above letter, is drama and a boldness of expression that, I would argue, is a consequence of the more firm acceptance, in both social and medical circles, of sensibility as a positive attribute. Sensibility provides less a conventional rhetorical style for patient letters than a rhetorical matrix for individual expression. Patient hypersensibility is taken for granted – by both male and female patients alike – and what the medicine-by-post correspondent wants to convey most to the doctor in respect to subjective feeling, is the absolute distress of their condition and the urgency of obtaining relief. Without leaving the framework of sensibility, medicine-by-post experiments, in this period, with language that more directly states the case of the patient as individual.

Dr Cullen's answer to Mrs Ross validates her feelings and her mode of writing about her illness. The physician's rhetorical stance is sympathy combined with practicality and respect for the patient's intelligence. He fully acknowledges Mrs Ross's interpretation of her symptoms and addresses them in detail. In particular, Cullen is able to remark on the matter of constitutional weaknesses without suggestion of fault in the patient's character or habits:

> I have considered the case of this Lady with all the attention that the particular regard I have for her no other can possibly engage.
>
> I am of the Lady's own opinion that her ailments consist especially in a weakness of her stomach but I am sorry to add that this weakness in some measure runs through the whole of her constitution, and I mention this to insinuate that the mending a constitution requires time and pains. I hope however that Mrs Ross may soon be considered mended, and the first step must be to avoid those things that may hurt it, and I am strongly persuaded that both drinking Bath waters and bathing in them have been hurtful and if continued might be pernicious to her... [Yet] I don't think the great City of London to be very proper for valetudinous persons....

In his seven-page consultation note, Cullen does not require that Mrs Ross leaves Bath, but he advises, 'Besides the cold baths I would prescribe a medicine for strengthening her stomach and the whole of her constitution. Thus I have prescribed [?] powder... which is here enclosed. Of this Electuary she is to take the bigness of a hazlenut twice a day....' He encourages Mrs Ross to drink 'a few glasses of Lime water' daily but to avoid several types of food and drink including malt liquor. The rhetorical tone of the consultation is entirely different from Cheyne's, who would have exhorted Mrs Ross to undertake a prodigious change in habits and supported such advice through the example of other valetudinarians whose health was restored by adhering to Cheyne's abstemious regimens. For late Enlightenment physicians, however, sensibility was to be preserved, and the corrective to disorders associated with it was quantitative rather than qualitative.

Cullen's manner of writing to women patients, or about them, concerning nervous disorders emphasises the physiological over the psychological. Responding to Mayor Hamilton at Murdeston about his wife's 'nervous stupor', Cullen remarks:

I am very sorry to find my agreeable acquaintance Miss Hamilton complaining. It is not exactly the same complaint I was formerly advised about; but it is upon the same foundation of weak nerves, and is only in another shape a nervous complaint. I hope it shall have no consequence farther than the present uneasiness, and even that I hope we shall discuss very soon.

Upon perceiving the first approach of any stupor let her take a tea- spoonful of the cephalic drops in a little water; and if that does not prevent the fit in a quarter of an hour she may take another dose and at a like interval of a third. The same course is to be taken if a fit comes without warning....

Cullen says that 'it is extremely difficult to restore such a constitution as Mrs Hamiltons's', but he hopes to strengthen her partly through treatment with 'some bark in powder' he has provided. He then adds:

There is commonly a costiveness attending all nervous complaints, and it very much encreases [*sic*] them. If there is any thing of that kind in this case it must be obviated by an Anderson's pill, Sacred Tincture, or Elixir or other such medicines that possibly Miss Hamilton may have been in use of.[88]

When Cullen urges behavioural changes (an infrequent recommendation), they are far more likely to be recommended to one of his male patients, especially those with hypochondriacal symptoms than to one of his women patients. Similarly, when women patients record the fact of a 'weak constitution' in their letters, they tend not to dwell upon this subject but on the particular symptoms for which they are seeking consultation.

A series of letters to and from a Mrs Frances Fontescue illustrate the manner in which the language of physical symptoms trumps the rhetoric of sensibility. If women patients do not extricate themselves from the particular bonds and associations of sensibility assigned to their sex, it is also evident that they are not gagged by the conventions of sensibility to such a degree that the utilitarian reasons for seeking medical consultation become obscured by propriety and the need for delicacy:

Sir,

I have received your prescriptions[89] and I have apply'd the healing Syrup which proves beneficial to the Tongue and throat, and has dispersed the Humour to the inside of my jaws and lips where I can bear it much better; The whole of my Complaints exists in these parts at least principally, My Nerves were always weak particularly my Hands; My appetite is good, and I sleep tollerably [*sic*] well. My Chief Diet has been Milk, Hartshorn jellys and Calves feet Veal and Mutton Broths; I drink Asses Milk Morning and

Evening, for three Months, My Physician Ordered me Cows Milk, I am Now drinking Lime Water and Milk but have not yet found any benefitt [*sic*]. I have taken great quantities of Medicine but to No good purpose Nor can any of the faculty yet Employ'd Certify the Complaint more than by guess. I shou'd be glad to be inform'd if I may Eat white Meats or Broths. Milk agrees with me very well. I have drank No Wine or anything strong these twelve months. I had a pea[90] arise in my thigh but it never discharged and causing me great pain I had it taken out. My leg is not quite well But the discharge from it is but very small. I have a particular tingling in the Tips of my fingers. Insted [*sic*] of the glisters recommended by you I have Hitherto made use of Castor Oile [*sic*] and Syrrup [*sic*] of Roses[91] which have found to answer the purpose. Wou'd you Sir recommend Exercise as my Hopes of relief are dependant [*sic*] on you Sir. I hope you will Excuse my taking up so much of your time in the stating of my Case.[92]

It is evident that Mrs Fontescue is in no way deferential towards the physicians who have treated her in the past; one detects a note of sarcasm when she writes, 'Nor can any of the faculty yet Employ'd Certify the Complaint more than by guess.' Her own physician, William Thompson, and others have offered 'great quantities of Medicines but to No good purpose.' In a letter from her own physician to Cullen, we discover that Mrs Fontescue has not asked Thompson to serve as intermediary with the famed Edinburgh consultant but has decided she is quite capable of providing Cullen herself with all the clinical information he needs. Thompson is clearly a bit put out when requested, close to a month after Mrs Fontescue's January letter, to offer his own account of her case:

Sir,

I am sorry I was not acquainted with my patient and friend Mrs Fontescue's intention to consult you about the state of her health, otherwise I would gladly have done myself the honour of writing to you, and giving you the best accot I could of the present, and also some former complaints which she has been liable to....[93]

In the meantime, Dr Cullen responded to Mrs Fontescue's note within ten days of her own. The opening paragraph contains admonishments to persist in diet and to have patience in expecting cure that recalls the consultation letters of George Cheyne. However, there is a certain evident restraint in Cullen's rhetorical manner (without loss of authority) which differs from the rigorous (if respectful and deferent) rhetoric of Cheyne:

Confirmed in my former opinion I must persist in the advice

– A general fault of the blood to be cured by Diet can only be cured in great
length of time – I must therefore desire you not to despair of your milk Diet
and I should not yet for some time have you take even of the lightest animal
foods – I would even have you sparing of broths – When the Season advances
a little and becomes much milder than at present[,] daily exercise in a
Carriage or on horseback may be of great Service to you –

Keeping the Belly reg^r most necessary and as long as the Stomach bears it,
none more proper than Castor Oil.

No Internal meds can be of use – and if you digest milk tolerably, I would
not even add the Lime Water to it. – I am glad to find that the Syrup I
advised has relieved your tongue and throat and I hope it will relieve your
Cheeks and lips also, but you should sometimes intermit the use of it and
only take to it again when your mouth happens to become worse[.]

I still think you might have benefit from an Issue and still would have you
try it in another place, as on the inside of the leg a little below, the knee; but
if it is disposed to inflame and give little matter, it must be let alone – [94]

Consistent with the tone of his lectures, Cullen qualifies his advice, and
he urges but does not insist on the patient's compliance: riding 'may' help,
or 'I think you might benefit from an Issue'. There are no warnings about
dire consequences in failing to follow through on regimen: 'I should not yet
for some time have you take', or 'I would even have you sparing of
broths.' He 'persists in the advice' but does not insist. The rhetorical tone is
in keeping with the patient's letter – acknowledging 'a general fault of the
blood' but staying with practical regimens and paying heed to the patient's
own observations on her response to treatments already tried.

Therapy is negotiated not to achieve authority within the doctor–patient
relationship (as with Cheyne), but because it is intrinsic to the relationship.
Miss Fraser of Inverlochy consults Cullen on a matter categorised by Cullen
as 'Fever and Flux.' In the previous month, she had written to Cullen
regarding pain in her left breast, and now writes in follow-up:

The pain in My Breast, tho it has been for the last four weeks More
unenterupted [*sic*] yet has been less Violent and rather Constant Uneasiness
across the Breast and high up – the Shooting pain through to the Shoulder
has been Gone for four weeks.

A looseness has mostly been a Complaint all this autumn and winter – and
more particularly Violent from the Middle of last month till a week ago –
and Indeed it has reduced the both, in Strength and Flesh[.] A very uneasy

Sensation has come on – both in the Night and afternoons of late... a palpitation of the heart which Prevents Sleep – [95]

The letter continues with a discussion of diet and drink, that 'malt liquor shall be given up'. Although she has tried to exercise by horseback riding, in the six days prior to this letter she has been 'unable to leave my room', and suffers from 'looseness' which is a 'Weakening Enervating Complaint'. The letter concludes with comments on her tolerance for medication: 'A Blister has always been a most severe and painfull aplication [*sic*] to me – and for the time, it is unhealed up Intirely deprives me of Sleep – However if this desired shall be obeyed.' Cullen's consultation voice is authoritative only in the command of medical knowledge; when he prescribes for Miss Fraser, Cullen uses his authority for reassurance and not for dominance. He is both charming and sympathetic, attentive to the patient's customary pleasures when recommending sacrifice of some favourite beverage:

I now understand better the State of Miss Frasers bowels and perceive that the tendency to looseness is still to be apprehended and gaurded [*sic*] against....

No malt Liquor not even Porter. She has given me a reason why she should abstain from Wine – and if she needs any Cordial it should be Spirits and Water.

I am sorry to take away tea which she seems attached to, but I still think it very improper – I would allow a little very weak and especially if she will take a little Cinnamon infused in it – I cannot advise Chocolate but Cocoa is very proper and safe....

I am glad her breast is easier; but if any pain should return the Blister must not be dispensed with – [96]

Cullen is politely apologetic, without any hint of either intimidation or deference – 'sorry to take away tea which she seems attached to' he writes, though the letter is clearly to a third party, most likely another physician, and not requiring any pretence for the sake of the patient. The rhetoric successfully merges genuine feeling with professional authority and practicality.

Cullen's consultation letters are marked by a respect for the patient's own experience. Cullen's letters contrast to Cheyne's in approach to patients. Cheyne's letters, especially to women patients, characteristically evidence frustration or an obsequious deference to patients who insist on their own ways – as when the Countess of Huntingdon impulsively changes her diet. Cullen, however, philosophically believes in the need to tailor medical treatment based on empirical observations of the patient. If Cheyne's correspondence reveals a necessary give-and-take in the doctor–patient tug of war for power, a game played to maintain clients, Cullen's medicine-by-post, in contrast, reveals a process of co-operation between elite expert and patient. Importantly, failure of medical treatment results in a doctor–patient conversation and not in the assumption of moral weakness and failure on the part of the patient.

Cullen is not alone among his contemporary Edinburgh medical colleagues in showing regard for the patient's narrative and medical judgment. Richard Lainberg from Newcastle-upon-Tyne refers two women patients to Cullen with a letter remarking: 'As the ladies who deliver this will be much better able personally to relate the particular Symptoms of their disorders from the commencement, than any Narrative I could possibly give, would do – I therefore refer that matter entirely to themselves.' Lainberg then confines himself primarily to advising Cullen on the treatments he has tried, thus far, to treat a bladder problem in one lady, and abdominal symptoms and 'Pleurisies' in the other. [97] Another doctor, William Ingham from Newcastle, wishes consultation on a Miss Mary Clutterbuck, and comments:

> Sir
>
> For an account of Miss Mary Clutterbuck's Case prior to 4 [*sic*] and 6th of February last I must refer you to herself as I never visited her till then, when I found her strongly affected with Hysteria; she cough'd incessantly and gave signs of great oppression and Uneasiness in her Chest – Her friend who had been accustom'd to see her in these convulsive Paroxysms inform'd me that upon these Occasions a great Variety of antispasmodic Medicines had been us'd but nothing ever reliev'd except copious Bleedings.... [98]

It is noteworthy that Dr Ingham expects that the 'account' of symptoms from Miss Clutterbuck will be reliable and meaningful even though she is 'strongly affected with hysteria' at the time. The patient's state of mind is not considered unreliable in view of her gender or her condition of hysteria. It is clear that the 'hysteria' consists of predominantly physical symptoms though the origins of these symptoms are left to Dr Cullen's judgment. It is also significant that Dr Ingham makes use of Miss Clutterbuck's female acquaintance to complement the patient's own narrative. The female patient is given voice and there is no evidence of a male voice, even professional, superimposed on the patient's own, nor is there any tone of condescension.

Cullen's consultation note to Dr Ingham shows serious concern for the patient and genuine interest in her condition. Revealing here is Dr Cullen's desire to reduce the quantity of bleedings received by the patient and his scepticism about the usefulness of antispasmodics. In private practice, Cullen was careful not to overtreat – he distrusted the safety and efficacy of polypharmacy – and very attentive to individual patient needs. And in regard to venesection, Guenter Risse has observed from the consultation letters that Cullen 'was conservative about bleeding, only occasionally recommending the withdrawal of four to six ounces, perhaps to be repeated in one or two days.'[99] All these elements are apparent in his somewhat pessimistic note to Ingam regarding Miss Clutterbuck:

> Her complaints have been long obstinate; and they may still prove tedious not without much danger.
>
> They seem entirely spasmodic; but connected with, if not dependent upon a turgescence of blood rendering them violent and dangerous. The last circumstance has directed her temporary relief but has not I believe contributed to cure. I mean the large and frequent blood lettings. They have been unavoidable but will increase the anasarca and probably render it fatal. Every time blood is let, diminish the quantity taken and thus by degrees, get quit of the necessity of bleeding so largely. I would rather allow a fit to continue, than persist in such profusion of blood –
>
> I have little confidence in Antispasmodics....[100]

Cullen was convinced that bleedings contributed to a 'plethoric state', but he also seems to have judged that even the 'delicate wealthy patients' could re-establish their losses by an adequate diet, which was readily available to them.

By contrast, over half of the fever patients under Cullen's care at the Royal Infirmary underwent a standard vigorous venesection – two to three times the amount of blood removed as compared to the those in his private practice – although their ability to replenish losses by diet was usually compromised by their socio–economic state. Risse has concluded that Cullen must have determined that the 'robust' labourer, or soldier, or lower-class woman, had a hardier (less delicate) constitution than patients from the upper ranks of society and therefore was able to withstand more aggressive, by-the-book, therapy than the upper-class patient. Furthermore, aggressive treatment was encouraged by the desire to move patients in and out of the Infirmary expeditiously to preserve its efficacy as a teaching service.

The example of Cullen's different approach to venesection in his private practice and infirmary patients is symptomatic of a broader attitude of physicians with regard to private-practice patients and patients on the teaching wards. Risse observes that the individual needs of patient–patrons, and their constitutional condition, took precedence in Cullen's therapeutic decisions over the nature of a particular disease entity; therapy was gentler and more adjusted to individual patients. However, the purpose of the teaching ward was to serve didactic purposes, and focus on the disease entity itself took precedence over the individual patient in the clinic. This attitude was encouraged by the 'need for accountability in a charitable and public institution such as the Edinburgh Infirmary' where 'diagnostic labels were always required on admission or at discharge.'[101]

While Risse's distinctions of private and Infirmary practice in the case of Dr Cullen (and these seem to hold true generally) should not come as a surprise, it must also be pointed out that the types of illness seen among the poor differed greatly from those of the upper-class patients in a medicine-by-post practice. For example, fevers would be far more common than hypochondriacal disorders, and the treatment of fevers called for more aggressive measures. Although Risse suggests that 'precise diagnostic labels' were uncommon in private practice communications – so as not to offend the patient and to remain tuned to matters of individual constitution – Cullen, in fact, meticulously classified his private-practice cases within the folios of his consultation letters. Medicine-by-post cases are regularly identified at the head of the (copied) letters, and in indexes, with such designations as 'dyspepsia', 'hypochondriasis', 'dropsy', 'nervous stupour', or with more specific diagnoses such as 'stricture of the gullet', 'debility from abortion', or 'syphilis'. Risse's useful observations therefore might be extended to suggest that Cullen, while remaining equally attentive to medical diagnostic categories in both private and Infirmary patients, was particularly sensitive to the demands of rhetorical style in his private letters to his upper class patients.

While an important element of that rhetorical style was discretion, discretion was not, for practical reasons, an excuse for subterfuge. One letter, in which Cullen advises on a case of venereal disease affecting a wife, strongly supports the idea that Cullen appreciated rhetorical niceties while eschewing any form of medical dishonesty in the name of sensibility. Cullen is scrupulous in maintaining discretion – not naming the patient anywhere in his notebook or on the copied letter as he does in more usual cases (including cases of venereal disease), but the heading 'syphilis' is distinctly penned across the top of the letter in the folio. The letter makes it clear that the concern here is not for the husband's interests but for the welfare and dignity of the patient herself:[102]

> Having now all the circumstances of the case very fully before me I can be
> more explicit in my opinion and advice. I wished to have got clear of any
> Suspicion of Venereal Infection but am Sorry I cannot nor can I say that it is
> yet entirely washed out. However disagreeable this opinion may be to the

patient it is not so bad as amusing a person with false security and allowing a pernicious mischief to remain in the body.... I am persuaded that it is necessary to throw in a little more mercury.... I would advise the bigness of a small bean of the ointment formerly employed to be anointed on the thigh at bedtime.... [A] close watch must be kept over the month and as soon as any Copper taste or other unusual nauseous taste is observed or the least taint on the breath is perceived the ointment must be intermitted for several nights and only returned to as these Symptoms wear off. This is not only necessary to prevent any discovery of bystanders, but is also prudent with respect to cold as it is never safe to push the Mercury far without close confinement....

I perceive how desirable it is to manage this matter without confinement and I think it may but I would however advise that in cases of wet and colder weather the Air is avoided as much as possible and especially when the Mercury has come the length of producing sweats or of threatening the mouth.... I must conclude with observing these are many circumstances in this affair that touch me with much concern and if I can on any occasion or with regard to the smallest doubt or difficulty be of further Service I shall from my heart give the best advice I can.

Perhaps no other letter in the extensive collection of Cullen's correspondence so completely exemplifies how physician sensibility – being in 'sympathy' with the patient – is put in the service of the female patient, enabling the physician to respect her 'feelings' both in the literal sense of her physical symptoms produced by disease and unpleasant medicines, and the emotional feelings produced in reaction to an embarrassing illness.

Susan Staves has shown, in an unpublished paper, that there were many instances in the eighteenth century in which a wife infected with venereal disease through the illicit activities of her husband was kept in the dark about her condition. A medical man might take it upon himself to disguise the actual condition of the wife, or else there was a complicit agreement between husband and doctor to not reveal the true diagnosis to the spouse. Such subterfuge was occasionally necessary to convince an anxious husband to bring his wife to the doctor for necessary treatment. She would be told that she had some minor gynaecological infection, such as *fluror albus* ('the whites', a kind of vaginitis). Alternatively, to assuage the husband's guilty conscience, a spouse might be reassured by the doctor that she had been cured entirely of venereal infection when this was not the case – a sanguine attitude on the part of eighteenth-century physicians which Staves has labelled 'therapeutic optimism.'[103] It served both the medical man's reputation and husband's embarrassment to believe in mercurial cures. But clearly this was not Cullen's manner. He was not indifferent to the inconveniences of therapy, or the social implications of public discovery of venereal disease, and he would in no way compromise his integrity, or that of the patient, by deluding her 'with false security'. Cullen insisted on joining extreme sensibility with absolute therapeutic honesty.

Other letters to and from women patients are entirely consistent in the elements exemplified in the above examples: the acceptance of 'weak constitution' but not at the cost of the material body. Nor does the reactive sensible female body signify the absence of an intelligence that deserves regard. But whereas the letters here contain an intrinsic drama in the rhetoric because of the undercurrent of sensibility, one can detect that letters from some women patients in the 1780s begin to show a diminishment in the drama of sensibility as practical considerations, still individualised, take precedence in doctor–patient letters. It is noteworthy that it is the letters from women patients where one first detects the effective shedding of sensibility in favour or a more direct discourse focused on the physical and the practical needs of the patient. It is also noteworthy that it is in the letters from male patients where one sees the most dramatic expression of the rhetoric of sensibility – especially in cases of hypochondria.

Hypochondria: solitude, the passions, and staying in touch with the social world

Cheyne worried that many of his patients, especially women, suffered from want of healthy distractions. Indeed, for Cheyne it was the exclusion of women from the business of the marketplace – their restricted role as consumers of luxury items – that he felt promoted a tendency to 'Hysterick Disease.'[104] Similarly, the self-imposed retreat of the scholar and the poet was an invitation to hypochondriacal symptoms, but only in so much as isolation encouraged unrelieved mental exertions. Participation in the social world was not mandatory for cure of the English malady; solitary diversions would suffice, such as exercise, entertaining, or tasteful reading.[105] It is also true that one way to signal recovery from the English malady was to 'go public' with an epistolary personal case history, a narrative letter that served as example to others and as recommendation of Cheyne's regimen. However to announce one's recovery to the 'public' is not the same as needing society for cure. Cheyne explained that his indulgence in the 'Egotism' of detailing his own case history was the need for 'Vindication' of his regimen and to refute the 'sneers' and scepticism by the 'Truth'. He also believed that others who had symptoms with 'some Resemblance to mine' could benefit.[106] Cheyne actively encouraged and orchestrated the public recommendation of his regimen through letters, but he did not subscribe to the idea of epistolary catharsis as cure of the English malady, or advise, the need to resume public life and society to achieve cure. In fact, just the reverse, as it was his own extreme effort to conform to the London social scene to which Cheyne ascribed the ruin of his health.[107]

For Scottish Enlightenment doctors, however, patients were not cured till they showed signs of re-entering and being in harmony with their society – in a true state of sympathy, within and without. The intimate, and paradoxical, relationship of private illness to public life is well-illustrated by hypochondriasis, a condition which particularly in its more extreme form of melancholia was characterised by the patient's withdrawal from society into a world of private physical and mental distress. Hypochondriasis was attributed to physical causes brought on largely by participation in the material pleasures or intellectual over-stimulation available and encouraged within a highly sophisticated and prospering society. But although the symptoms – primarily those of low spirits, anxiety, and gastrointestinal distress – were considered the consequence of an overwhelming of the senses by external stimulation, a critical step towards cure was one's return to society and distraction from morbid self-absorption.

Cullen, in a letter dated 5 November, 1789, writes to James Sandilands, seventh Lord Torpichen, to warn him that his brother Alexander may be succumbing to a 'love of Solitude', the major impediment to the cure of hypochondriasis. However, he adds that if this tendency be overcome, the prognosis is excellent:

> I have again and again considered Mr Sandiland's complaint, and a hundred such have occurred to me before. They are very distressing but no ways dangerous. They are commonly obstinate and tedious, arising from the symptoms which stand in the way of the very measures which should be attempted for their relief. Such is especially the love of Solitude which indulged, festers and aggravates every uneasiness attending the disease. When this love of Solitude, and aversion to company can be got the better of, I hold that the disease may be readily cured. Although the disease appears especially in the state of the mind, I am certain that it is founded on the state of the body, and that the state of the mind is as involuntary as the figure of a man's face....

What ails the mind in such a condition was not the fault of character or psychology but physical disturbance. Still, medicinal cures promise only transient relief, and 'I am persuaded', writes Cullen, that the patient's condition 'depends upon a general languor in the motions of his Nervous System.' Therefore, he continues:

> his remedy must depend upon measures which may excite, and for some length of time, steadily support the activity of his System, and the only

means that I know, or have ever found effectual for this purpose, is constant and habitual exercise, which may be carried on without fatigue, and with as much as possible interruption of thought, or train of thinking.[108]

A land journey is recommended, but only on condition that it provides physical exercise, 'in the open air and on horseback'; travel 'must not be conducted in an indolent way, and therefore not in a Carriage.' The patient should seek new scenery for greatest stimulation, but he must also be 'warmly cloathed and guard well against all causes of cold.'

Cullen urges that Mr Sandibanks be 'constant and steady in the pursuit of his Journey, and that he will avoid no circumstances that can render it as amusing as possible.' But it is in a follow-up letter to Lord Torpichen, five days later, in which Cullen adds his most important prescription: 'What I think would be of most benefit to Mr Sandilands is his admitting of a companion who might obviate his irresolution and constantly solicit his exertions.' It is the society of others which can set the hypochondriac patient to rights again, even though it was the accoutrements of society-at-large that may have precipitated illness and even defined it as a fashionable condition.

While Continental authors of this period, like Tissot, worried increasingly about the dark underside of sensibility – the spiral of symptoms into deep melancholia, Scottish physicians for the most part took a more sanguine view of disorders arising from sensibility. Without ignoring the perils of such disorders, they were optimistic about the prognosis for their patients to be restored to health and society.[109] For example, there is good reason to suppose that Cullen had reason to prescribe to Adam Smith, in 1760, for symptoms of hypochondriasis associated with overexertion from work on the *Theory of Moral Sentiments.* Cullen's prescription was rigorous, 'to ride at least five hundred miles' over a period of months if he was to 'survive' the upcoming winter.[110] Like Cheyne, Cullen believed in the value of diverting the mind from self-absorption and melancholy through physical exercise. However, Cullen did not on principle discourage 'occupations of business suitable to a person's circumstances and situation in life, if neither attended with emotion, anxiety nor fatigue.'[111] More practical and realistic than Cheyne, Cullen was also very sensitive to the limitations imposed by social position and finance on the abilities of patients to follow through with prescribed regimens intended to effect the external influences of the non-natural on their systems. Smith had the privilege of making some alterations in his life and wrote to Cullen that he intended to resume work at the Custom house 'for the sake of relaxation and a much easier business.'[112] While Cullen's advice to Smith reveals a continuity in eighteenth-century medical thought about the treatment of hypochondriasis, his philosophical attitude about the condition, and Smith's view, suggests a more ready acceptance of hypochondriasis as the consequence of exceeding the limits of one's natural role in life more than a fault in judgment – a slippage rather than a gross disregard of healthy habits. Nonetheless, David Hume disregarded 'any Excuse' from his friend Smith about poor health as long as Smith gave excuses which smacked of 'Subterfuges invented by Indolence and Love of Solitude.'[113] Persons of sensibility must guard against being overwhelmed by the passions.

However, within the vitalistic framework, even 'the passions' shed much of their negative connotations as relating to sensibility. The passions became respectable in terms of representing natural reactions that served to protect the body – part of a Providential design to protect the organism from environmental dangers, as long as those passions are not carried to extreme. This favourable view of the passions is illustrated by Geoffrey Sill in 'Neurology and the Novel: Alexander Monro *primus* and *secundus*, *Robinson Crusoe*, and the Problem of Sensibility'.[114] 'For the vitalist', such as Monro *secundus*, Sills explains, 'the nerves are seen to regulate the body through the passions, which may cause the organism to respond in some way other than mechanically to a stimulus.'[115] In this view, sensibility is given a moral character through medical physiology. In Defoe's work, Crusoe responds to passions that ultimately rescue his physical being from disaster, and in retrospect sees these spontaneous reactions as the gift of Providence intending to save him. In the novel of sensibility, it was this underlying concept of physiology, the trust of one's reaction to things, which gave characters the 'capacity to make moral distinctions through feeling rather than reason.'[116] Of course, it is always a given that excess of passion, capitulation to pure passion without judgment, can mislead one into dangerous situations and disorders of body and mind.

The absolute belief in the inseparability of mind and body in illness was being challenged by the end of the eighteenth century by new theories of mental illness which postulated conditions of mental derangement occurring independently from the influence of the body.[117] Nonetheless, as Cullen's letter to Lord Torpichen indicates, the concept of mind–body interaction remained very strong. The patient, Alexander Sandilands, respects Cullen's authority and accepts his prescription to travel, yet a letter to Cullen from Newcastle-upon-Tyne is not encouraging and the patient questions Cullen if the mind should not be credited with a greater role in his condition:

> I cannot say that the Journey hitherto has produced any happy effects; on the Contrary my appetite is not nearly so good as before I set out, and my nights so restless that I am obliged every night to get up and pass hours in a Chair in the dark, and am almost distracted with an inexpressible flutter of spirits....

I am persuaded that these uneasinesses, are... arising not so much from bodily infirmity as perturbations of mind produced by indulging certain extravagant but very harassing thoughts.[118]

While the patient here challenges his physician's emphasis of the body over the mind, at least in his own case, he nevertheless discovers no more reason to fault himself, accepting Cullen's sentiment that 'the state of the mind is as involuntary as the figure of a man's face.'

James Gregory (1753–1821) was a younger colleague of Cullen at the University of Edinburgh (and 43 years his junior). His response to Lord Meadowbrook about a cousin suffering from melancholia is much more grim in its prognosis than Cullen's, largely because the mind by this time (1812) is seen to endure pathology separate from the body. Mere physical exertion cannot suffice for cure:[119]

My Dear Lord

I am very sorry to say that after carefully perusing the inclosed [*sic*] Documents, I think just unfavourably as you do of your unfortunate Cousin's Situation.... Supposing it certain that [he] had unequivocally the *Diabaetes*, it must be equally certain that he has got perfect and obstinate hypochondriasis, approaching very near, if not absolutely amounting to partial Insanity, or what we, in our Slang, call Melancholia. It is infinity to one that such inveterate Hypochondriasis, or Melancholia, never will be cured; and abundantly probable, that sooner or later, it will become general and furious Insanity....

I see no reason to expect any good to him either from a long Sea Voyage or from bringing him to Europe[.] Caelum non Animum mutant qui trans mare currunt.[120]

Gregory's letter shows that psychological disorders were now regarded as a pathological state separate from the body, but blame is not attached to the condition of melancholia. The pathology only invokes pathos. Gregory's letter also exemplifies the mutual respect that educated gentlemen in Enlightenment Scotland paid to each other. Here, the physician takes time to elucidate his thinking for his friend and to educate the non-physical in the nature of melancholia and its rhetoric. The theoretical is combined with the practical, and education with sympathy.

Sensibility, confidentiality, and a new medical ethics

If to be cured was to return to 'public' life, illness itself was becoming more private for the upper- and middle class in the second half of the century. The public expression of private illness, while still present, was overshadowed now by a distinctly public sphere of voluntary hospitals and interest in urban and military health. Private patients needed to be differentiated from patients who required public charity and who were, literally, 'on view' to both a medical and non-medical audience. The wards of hospitals were opened up to students of medicine and surgery, while private citizens continued to find amusement in the well-established pastime of sightseeing tours of Bethlem and other mental asylums.[121] If the culture of sympathy demanded that doctors at least should recognise that institutional patients had feelings, there was still an obvious differentiation made between the 'private' and the 'public' patient in respect to the right of confidentiality.

The new medical ethics as codified by John Gregory and Thomas Percival were a mix of the pragmatism and 'gentlemanly' sensibility.[122] Gregory taught his students that the physician's ability to observe patient confidentiality was an essential sign of a physician's good character by evidencing genuine sympathy for the patient:

A physician, by the nature of his profession, has many opportunities of knowing the private characters and concerns of the families in which he is employed.... [H]e is often admitted to the confidence of those, who perhaps think they owe their life to his care. He sees people in the most disadvantageous circumstances, very different from those in which the world views them.... Hence, it appears how much the characters of individuals, and the credit of families, may sometimes depend on the discretion, secrecy, and honour of a physician. Secrecy is particularly requisite where women are concerned. Independent of the peculiar tenderness with which a woman's character should be treated, there are certain circumstances of health, which, though in no respect connected with her reputation, every woman, from the natural delicacy of her sex, is anxious to conceal; and, in some cases, the concealment may be of consequence to her health, her interest, and to her happiness.[123]

A more private doctor–patient epistolary communication was required in the context of an entirely new, modern, medical ethic which was supplanting the code of 'honour' with professional standards based on 'gentlemanly sensibility – perhaps ultimately revealing the desire to be more gentlemanly than those to the manner born.'[124]

The instantiation of the new medical ethic was the hospital, in which the individual autonomy of the physician had to be integrated into the 'collective autonomy attendant upon collaborative self-regulation.'[125] Thomas Percival's *Medical Ethics* was conceived, in great part, to fill the need for a collective professional ethic within the institutional setting.[126] As Lisbeth Haakonsssen explains, 'Percival's own medical ethics reflects the revolution in medicine brought about by the advent of the voluntary, or charity hospital, and, likewise, the dilemmas which arose from the conflict between the demands of a nascent experimental medicine and the physician's duty of benevolence.'[127]

Percival, in Manchester, translated Gregory's rules of discretion for private patients into pragmatic application on the hospital ward where poorer patients, with diseases once treated at home, were now moved into the public space of the infirmary. Percival insisted that 'the familiar and confidential intercourse, to which the faculty are admitted in these professional visits, should be used with discretion, and with the most scrupulous regard to fidelity and honour.'[128] Percival allowed that in this institutional setting, in which medical students were instructed and medical decisions often made by consultation, patient privacy must be compromised from time to time. The limits of 'discretion' were dictated by the circumstance in which confidential information was intended to be 'used' for didactic purposes as well as to justify the existence of the institution to its supporters.[129] However, Percival clearly intends that:

> In the large wards of an Infirmary the patients should be interrogated concerning their complaints in a *tone* of *voice* which cannot be *overheard*.
>
> Secrecy, also, when required by peculiar circumstances, should be strictly observed. And females should always be treated with the most scrupulous *delicacy*. To neglect or to sport with their feelings is cruelty; and every wound thus inflicted tends to produce a callousness of mind, a contempt of decorum, and an insensibility to modesty and virtue. Let these considerations be forcibly and repeatedly urged on the hospital pupils.[130]

While the rhetoric conveys a paternalistic attitude towards the ward patient (and women patients in particular) Percival's instructions must be understood within the context of Enlightenment sensibility as an earnest, liberal, endeavour to suspend social class and gender as obstructions to the doctor–patient relationship within the hospital walls. As Robert Baker observes, 'Percival's urging of *condescension* and *tenderness* emerge as radically egalitarian attempts to secure for the sick poor the same sort of psychological relationship that Gregory had urged as morally requisite for sick private patients.'[131] That Percival was compelled to make a case for the confidentiality of the patient in the hospital is evidence that Enlightenment physicians normally distinguished between the confidentiality owed their own private-practice clients and that accorded to the hospital patient. Those patients who could afford to pay the one or two guinea fee to consult a physician by post in the latter years of the Enlightenment would have expected that confidentiality which had now become basic to the medical ethics of the doctor–patient relationship.

Cullen's great discretion concerning the lady patient who suffers from venereal disease demonstrates delicacy of feeling and respect for privacy. He advises against the slightest excess in mercury treatment in order 'to prevent any discovery of bystanders', but he also protects the patient's confidentiality by removing her name from the letter in his folio of patient letters. We can see that sensibility, with its rhetoric of sympathy, is not only about feeling for the patient but also has become a foundation for modern medical ethical theory. Medicine-by-post letters document the new medical ethic philosophy in practice, within the intimacy of the private doctor-patient relationship. It is not surprising that Enlightenment medical ethics, so dependent on the rhetoric of sensibility, should display itself so prominently in the written word of patient and doctor – in the absence of bodies which, by signifying other aspects of societal behaviour and manners, complicate meaning that is so clear on the page.

Sensibility as drama – rhetorical hyperbole in medicine-by-post

It would be incorrect to assume, however, that a growing presumption of confidentiality in medicine-by-post interrupted the need for dramatic self-expression. Illness was more performative than ever. While the doctor was now beginning to recognise clear obligations to patient confidentiality as part of a developing modern medical ethic, the patient, equally, had increased license to express his or her feelings within the doctor–patient relationship. As Matthew Bramble writes to Dr Lewis in *The Expedition of Humphry Clinker*:

> If I did not know that the exercise of your profession has habituated you to hearing of complaints, I should make a conscience of troubling you with my correspondence... Yet I cannot help thinking, I have some right to discharge the overflowings of my spleen upon you, whose province it is to remove those disorders that occasioned it[.][132]

But while patients may have started to expect confidentiality on the part of their doctor, they retained the right to share their health problems with acquaintances. When Frances Burney wrote to her sister about her mastectomy, she assumed the letter would be passed on to various acquaintances even though she would have preferred to limit the news of her surgery.[133] Privacy and confidentiality were not the same in matters of health. Confidentiality was the discretion expected of one's physician, but privacy about health matters was an option for the patient and not in any way a societal expectation.

Sensibility, divorced from its negative connotations, was a useful flag for patients to wave before their physician during times of illness in order to demand special attention – as in the case of the fictional Matthew Bramble. This was not the dramatic narrative of remorse for the consequences of high living (à la Cheyne) but a theatrical, dramatic rhetoric that signalled a clinical condition of constitutional dismay specific to patients of exquisite sensibility. It was a rhetoric that was in and of itself intrinsic to the constellation of symptoms – not only descriptive but evidence of a disordered body.

As such, sensibility was accompanied by distinct forms of rhetorical gesturing. Letters to doctors became marked by extreme personal drama – several ratchets in intensity above even that of the confessional tone exhibited by Cheyne and his clientele – and by a pervasive irritability and crankiness; all in a very self-conscious rhetorical style. Mr James Dallas of Edinburgh complains to Cullen that 'the Irritability or Irascibility attacked me [and] caused me to curse swear blaspheme and toss all the papers in [*sic*] the Floor which was followed by a dejection of two hours.... [W]hen in Bed Tears are my relief.' He concludes, 'It is the irascible Temper... my great Curse and that only exists when the Nerves are weak. I am as with Vapour: weak as any delicate female.'[134]

In fiction, this kind of rhetorical drama by patients is exemplified in the letters of Matthew Bramble to Dr Lewis in Smollett's *The Expedition of Humphry Clinker*. Bramble is the quintessential irritable and demanding patient. His letters correspond in tone and, in some instances, duplicate almost word-for-word actual medicine-by-post of the period, including Smollett's letters to his own doctors.[135] For example, the following communication written to Dr Cullen by Mr Charles Wedderburn might almost come from the quill of Matthew Bramble on one of his excursions to an English spa:

> It took us ten days to reach this place having our own chaise and horses, during that time the weather was hot, and I had a good deal of pain travelling but at night it was so violent I cou'd obtain no rest without 30 drops of laudanum – on arrival at Buxton I attended scrupulously to the directions you was pleased to give me as to Bathing and drinking the Waters... ; the effects of it at the beginning were violent and disagreable [*sic*] – the weather was most unfavourable... [and] there is no fit place under cover here to walk.... Another Effect the Waters and Bath have produced, was sickishness and reaching [retching] to vomit one morning and after that I had some bilious hot stools, that almost excoriate the parts.[136]

217

Compare this letter to Matthew Bramble's account to Dr Lewis of his arrival at Harrigate spa:

Dear Doctor,

Considering the tax we pay for turnpikes, the roads of this country constitute a most intolerable grievance.... I have suffered more jolting and swinging than ever I felt in the whole course of my life, although the carriage is very remarkably commodious and well hung, and the postillions very careful in driving....

As for the water, which is said to have effected so many surprising cures, I have drunk it once, and the first draught has cured me of all desire to repeat the medicine. – Some people say it smells of rotten eggs, and others compare it to the scourings of a foul gun.... As for the smell, if I may be allowed to judge from my own organs, it is exactly that of bilge-water; and the saline taste of it seems to declare that it is nothing else than salt water putrefied in the bowels of the earth.... My stomach could hardly retain what it received. – The only effects it produced were sickness, griping, and insurmountable disgust. – I can hardly mention it without puking.[137]

Charles Wedderburn and Matthew Bramble are constitutional and rhetorical twins. They are scrupulous reporters on their own conditions and tireless commentators on the environment as it tests their every fibre. These sufferers are marked by cranky dispositions and delicate stomachs, and by an entrenched scepticism amid their pleas for medical salvation. In modern medical parlance such rhetoric would identify the 'help-rejecting' patient, the perpetual sufferer who clings to his or her discomfort for secondary gains – most significantly, because the patient's identity, and voice, has become one with the pain he or she endures.

Carol Houlihan Flynn, in *Running Out of Matter*, has said of Smollett that, in his own case of consumption and disgruntled experiences with Continental physicians, he 'provokes the hardships that reward his notorious resistance to accommodation.' It is apparent that 'his sentiments can, indeed must hurt to be felt, and provoke in the process a motion that depends upon irritability.'[138] His sense of vigour depends upon the discomfort which excites irascibility and proves his sensibility. To his physician, Dr John Moore, Smollett reports:

I have not lately lost any Ground; but on the contrary, have gained some flesh since coming to Bath.... I do not, however, flatter myself that I shall continue to mend, for I have always found myself better for about a month after any change of air, then I relapse into my former state of Invalidity. My Disorder is no other than weak Lungs and a Constitution prone to Catarrhs,

with an extraordinary irritability of the nervous System.... My greatest
Misfortune is my being so extremely susceptible of cold that I can hardly stir
abroad without Danger. The acrimony of my Juices is owing to the Scurvy
which has produced a very ugly Eruption on my right hand. Nothing agrees
with me so well as hard Exercise, which, however, the Indolence of my
Disposition continually counteracts. If I was a Galley slave and kept at hard
Labour for two or three years, I believe I should recover my Health intirely.[139]

To be cured would be to extinguish the life of sensibility. And the
rhetoric of Smollett's letters, like Matthew Bramble's, is infused with drama
fuelled by the energy of discomfiture and the resignation to an eternally
valetudinarian state. To his other doctor friend, the famous William Hunter
(who had been apprenticed to Cullen in Glasgow), Smollett writes:

> I trouble you with this Intimation as in Duty bound that you may know I
> am still crawling on the face of the Earth, and that I am even in a Condition
> to crawl on all fours as the use of my right hand is in some measure restored.

> [...] I was verily persuaded that the cursed ulcer on my Forearm was become
> cancerous, and that the sore was a Judgement of God upon me for the
> ridiculous use I had made of that wretched member in writing such a Heap
> of absurdities in the Course of my Authorial Probation.... Meanwhile, I can
> sit without agony and sleep without opiate.... I am almost stupified with ill
> Health, Loss of memory, Confinement and solitude, and I believe in my
> Conscience the Circulation would have stopped of itself if it was not every
> now and then stimulated by the Stings of my Grub street Friends, who attack
> me in the public Papers.[140]

The Scottish Enlightenment physician, faced with such a challenging
patient, was prepared to respond in a rhetoric characterised by
understanding, reassurance, and personal consideration. The antithesis of
this ideal of the doctor is represented by Tobias Smollett, in the *Travels
Through France and Italy* in the person of the arrogant Dr Fizes, 'the
Boerhaave of Montpellier' of whom Smollett complained to William
Hunter: 'I found he had a set of Phrases and Prescriptions which he applied
to all Cases indiscriminately.'[141] Dr Fizes is foreign and 'other', but mostly he
is the epitome of the smug, affected, classically-trained doctor whom
Smollett derides in England as well as France (as in *The Adventures of
Ferdinand Count Fathom*) – the stereotypical physician of satire.[142]

Cullen's epistolary bedside manner, like that of Smollett's ideal physician,
exemplifies calm authority touched by modesty, a voice of compassion
joined to the extreme reassurance that authority can supply. A response to a
letter from Thomas Stapleton, of Carlton, is typical of Cullen's tone in

answering a patient who has written to him with great intensity of feeling and strong opinions about his own condition. The opening lines of this note should be familiar as they served earlier in this chapter to illustrate how the anxious patient expected a prompt reply to a request for consultation. The rhetoric that follows the letter's opening lines begs us to reconsider those lines not just as a salvo of impatience in awaiting Cullen's response, but as part of a histrionic whole:

> Dear Sir-
>
> I have waited with great Impatience for some time past in hopes of hearing from you. I have been exceedingly bad for these three weeks past, and still continue so; my greatest pain seems to me, to be about the entrance of the stomach and causes a Prodigious quantity of wind; I am in constant pain.... I am very clear the whole proceeds from some obstruction at the Entrance of the Stomach, but let it proceed from what it will, it gives me great pain, and makes me very miserable; I would suffer over again with pleasure all the usual complaints that attend mankind as the small pox just to be quit of my present uneasiness, which is, and has been for some time past my daily companion and what is worse, I almost dispair of ever being better, unless removed by you. I go to town on the 13th where it will give me great pleasure and satisfaction to hear from you, and have your opinion....[143]

While Stapleton acknowledges Cullen's authority – Dr Cullen is, perhaps, the only physician who can relieve his distress – at the same time, Stapleton expresses his own quite definite opinion of his medical disorder without the least hesitation or apology. Cullen's letter of 30 December – identified at the top as a case of 'dyspepsia' – shows remarkable restraint and respect for both the patient's fears and opinions:[144]

> Sir,
>
> It is possible there may be a fixed ailment tumour or constriction about one or other orifices of the Stomach and if there is I shall not be able to do you much service but such an ailment is a meer possibility and I see no reason for supposing it. On the other hand there are many strong reasons for supposing that your pains are owing to the recurrence of Spasms which very often can be prevented and cured and tho you have suffered long and severely I hope you need not yet dispair of a remedy.
>
> Whether these Spasms depend upon the weakness of the Stomach alone or the weakness of this, is owing to a gouty disposition which does not take its proper course, I shall not determine, but own that I am much inclined to the last Supposition. It is not however necessary to determine, because, upon

either supposition my advice, will be the same and it is to restore and support the tone of the stomach, and thereby both to prevent the recurrence of Spasm and to dispose the gout as well as we can to take its proper course.

For these purposes I trust to a Single Medicine which has indeed in some measure been employed in your case already, but it neither has been in the form I think best, nor in the quantity in many cases I have found found [*sic*] necessary to render it successfull [*sic*].

There follows extensive directions and a recipe. However, as indicated in this letter, Cullen was very much a proponent of using one medication at a time and was instructing his students against the all-too-common use of polypharmacy.[145] It is worth noting that Cullen takes time to instruct his patient also – explaining his diagnostic and therapeutic rationale in Enlightenment fashion, and using such exposed reasoning to inspire confidence in a cure. Yet the rhetoric of 'sympathy' is not lost and, in fact, sets the spirit of the entire communication: 'and tho you have suffered long and severely I hope you need not yet dispair of a remedy', writes Cullen most prominently at the start of his letter.

Dramatic declarations of suffering, as an epistolary device to show sensibility, frequently crossed Cullen's desk. The symptoms of these patients were usually those of benign peptic disorders, or more specifically what a twentieth-century doctor would ascribe to acid reflux or a spastic bowel. The Reverend Elliot is near blasphemy when he pleads with Cullen:

I have had such a disagreeable acidity, pain, and burning heat upon my Stomach so as to render every thing in this world and even life itself insupportable.... To conclude, if you can do nothing for me; I must soon go hence or drag out a miserable existence for a few weeks; I wou^d gladly have waited on you, but cannot bear the horse under me, it raises such a burning in my stomach and I am immediately seized with a nausea and sickness in a Chaise.[146]

The dramatic stakes are yet higher in this plea from Mr Cowmeadow, 'Lecturer of her Late Royal Highness, Princess Amelia, at Berlin':

Sir, I suffer since 19 years the greatest torture a poor mortal is able of suffering, and you Sir are now the only hope I have left.... I have Consulted some of the first physicians in Europe, but in vain, they all agree it is an hypocondriacal [*sic*] sickness attended with... irritability of the nerves. I have continual rumbling of wind in my stomach, and belching upwards which lasts for hours together, my head is then giddy, my pulse low, and intermitting and the greatest Dejection of spirits and every thing I see around me seems to be gloomy, and void.... I beg of you to be so kind to send me your advice as soon as possible, for I would give worlds if I had them to get rid of this many headed hydra.[147]

Sensibility, here, gives licence to uninhibited rhetorical expression – to extreme exclamations of personal torment that almost pass into the absurd. Cowmeadow is not, after all, succumbing to consumption; he is describing a rather typical case of dyspepsia, common to eighteenth-century patients.[148] If this letter were penned by Sterne's Yorick (in *A Sentimental Journey*), one would assume the irony, but the language would be perfectly in keeping with Yorick's hyperbole. Such language, however, is written in earnest, as in the following letter:

> Enclosed you have my melancholy Case described by Dr Douglas in Kelso, melancholy Case it undoubtably is so that Dr Cullen would pity me to the utmost was he witness to half the Agony I just now endure. I have been troublesome to you on some former occasions but absolute Necessity forces me to apply to you again hoping for your compassionate Advice.[149]

For the most part, Cullen only rarely questions such extremities of patient self-expression, though in the case of Mr Cowmeadow, Cullen expresses some surprise that so many consultants have failed to be of service.[150]

However, even Dr Cullen must occasionally set limits on such extreme patient rhetoric and self-indulgence. In the case of Mr Wedderburn – the medicine-by-post twin of Matthew Bramble – who so fully detailed the inconveniences of travel and the trials of the Buxton baths, Cullen does not encourage the patient's inclination to self-medication with laudanum, an opium derivative. 'At night', writes Wedderburn, I should get no rest without 30 or 40 drops of Laudanum':

> I had left it off on my beginning the Bath here – but Captain Scott, telling me you had not found fault with it in his case, I presumed you wou'd think it at least not very detrimental in mine.... Wherein I have deviated from your good advice given in so very gracious a manner as bespoke much humanity and anxiety for my recovery, I hope you will be pleas'd to pardon me as invalids are eager to try every thing for relief.[151]

One side effect of sensibility that greatly troubled eighteenth-century physicians was the obvious increase in self-medication with pain-killing drugs and patients justifying this habit on the basis of a delicate constitution. It was a growing trend among fashionable society that was vigorously criticised by late eighteenth-century medical writers such as Thomas Beddoes and Thomas Trotter.[152] Cullen shared this concern and responds to Wedderburn:

Your Evening doses of Laudanum I should not have advised, but the...

pain would have probably made me indulge you in them, but if you can either get rest and ease without them I would wish them to be moderated and if possible avoided altogether, but must leave this to your own discretion. I dont expect you will quit of them while you remain at Buxton, but when you again get into a course of travelling I hope you may. Your case and that of Capt. Scott are very different.[153]

Cullen's response demonstrates his ability to be critical of a patient's behaviour without departing from the rhetorical niceties of sensibility. He gently but definitely admonishes the patient for his all-too-free use of the laudanum without being unduly authoritative or in any way insensitive to the patient's distress.

Rarely, Cullen does show a degree of impatience in his replies to certain correspondents, as when Dr Armitstead consults Dr Cullen from Lancaster regarding his own case, questioning the benefits of treatment advised by the famous John Hunter, (brother of William Hunter):

Dear Sir

As I now have a full Trial of the warm Sea bathing, and as the situation of this place begins to be exceedingly unpleasant, I thought it proper to give you an account of the operation and effects of Mr J. Hunters remedy. When I first came here I found my self exceedingly weak. It was with the greatest difficulty and resolution, I was able to be got into the Tub. The first bath I had heated to betwixt 80 and 90, and the feelings I experienced while in it were such, as I really can not describe. There seemed to be an unacountable affectn of the whole of the Thoracic Viscera, particularly of the Lungs. [T]he circulation is hurrd on in a most rapid manner, and I had a taste arose from the Lungs while in the Bath which I never before experienced. I regulate the heat and the time to my own feelings and I generally come out stronger than when I went in...[154]

The letter, which proceeds for yet another two pages, includes endless queries, and concludes by asking Dr Cullen if he thinks it would be useful 'to try an Artificial Sea Bath at Harrogate [*sic*].' Cullen's response is polite but official:

You give me more questions than I can easily answer, and such a complicated history of particulars that I cannot consider and judge of with any clearness, and the only proper advice for your future conduct should be from Mr John Hunter the Author of your late conduct. It is he only that can give you a proper opinion with regard to your Harrowgate scheme.[155]

One suspects that Cullen is less bothered by the tone of Dr Armitstead's inquiry than by the fact that Dr Armitstead is second guessing such an established physician as John Hunter. It also seems that Cullen is annoyed by the unnecessary complexity and imprecision in Armitstead's inquiry.

On the few occasions that I have discovered Cullen to be less than perfectly kind in his letters it has been mainly when he was chastising other physicians for not being more attentive to professional etiquette. A striking example of this is Cullen's response to a note from Dr James Wood, who had requested consultation on a Mrs Mercer:[156]

> Dear James
>
> I have yours concerning Mrs Mercer a case attended with more difficulties than I can easily solve. I am not satisfied with any opinion you have given concerning the seat of the disease, nor can I venture to ascertain it. I am rather surprised that you have not told me whether the original tumour be increased, or to what size since the Month of April, nor do you tell me what has happened with respect to the original symptoms of Evening fever and some sweat breaking out. You perhaps have not mentioned the circumstances because they had no influence upon your own judgement, but you should have allowed me to have mine also, and indeed you have given me no [?] what is likely to be the event, or the more or less sudden event of this disease, which, however, I think is of some consequence....
>
> I don't like for several reasons your opinion that you are to receive no benefit from Consultation. It may be well founded, but it is not civil to say so to a physician whom you consult.

Dr Wood is clearly stung by Cullen's reprimand, and he replies most apologetically:[157]

> Dear Sir,
>
> I received your letter this morning respecting Mrs Mercer, and I must begin my answer by assuring you that I meant nothing uncivil to you by any expression in my letter. The personal obligations which I owe you, and the high opinion which I entertain of your abilities, would prevent me from being guilty of such rudeness.

But such interchanges are highly exceptional in the large collection of Cullen's correspondence. For the most part, Cullen took as a matter of course in his everyday medicine-by-post the extreme rhetorical hyperbole of the upper-class Enlightenment patient.

A more modest rhetoric

In the final decades of the eighteenth-century a remarkably modest rhetoric that eschews drama, and which concentrates on the substantive issues of illness, makes its appearance side-by-side with the more dramatic rhetoric of medicine-by-post. This alternative rhetorical voice was genuinely individual because it was not restricted by either the formal rhetorical demands of new science – as in medicine-by-post of the first decades of the century – or the hyperbole of sensibility. It is a more flexible and independent mode of expression that reflects the great variation of the writers who now participate in medicine-by-post. It is as if the personal expression of illness has assumed a comfortable rhetoric that is a balance between, or an amalgam of, the extremes of new science objectivity and the hyperbole of sensibility.

In the Cullen collection of letters, this kind of patient rhetoric becomes more evident towards the close of the century, though the roots of this it may be found in the letters from women patients discussed earlier in this chapter – women patients who had a particular need to circumvent the mould of sensibility to obtain the practical benefits of medical consultation. Nonetheless, those letters still betray the conventions of sensibility even as the writers tried to overcome the limitations imposed by the rhetoric. In the medicine-by-post that appears in the 1780s, however, the language is clearly less governed by style and much more directed by immediate medical need. But this in no way implies a return to the impersonal, objective, language of new science. Indeed, personal narrative and individual voice flourish in patient letters to doctors of this period.

It would require a separate study to locate the origins of the more individualised, 'liberated' patient rhetoric of the last decades of the Enlightenment, but I would like to propose a few possibilities. First, as has been emphasised, Scottish Enlightenment philosophy and its medical counterpart emphasised the practical application of knowledge, and it is not unlikely that the relative importance of the letter to accomplish its medical purpose may have superseded stylistic considerations that had prescribed the nature of patient correspondence during the earlier decades of medical sensibility. The increasingly dramatic and emotive rhetoric of sensibility in the second half of the century allowed for a more direct statement of patient need, a rhetoric more readily adapted by a larger and more varied patient population. Freed from the limitations of proving sensibility through rhetoric, a larger proportion of the middle class took advantage of medicine-by-post consultation without embarrassment because of their limited education or social position. Such middle-class patients may have been less self-conscious about those stylistic considerations which dictated to the pens of fashionable upper-class patients.

Significantly, if William Cullen may be taken as representative of the ideal of the late eighteenth-century Enlightenment doctor, such efforts to expand the rhetorical possibilities of medicine-by-post were in no way discouraged by the medical establishment. Cullen's responses to inquiries written by patients with evidently more limited writing skills are as sensitive and attentive as his responses to the effulgent rhetoric of sensibility of his upper class clientele. Medicine-by-post, in fact, might be said to document one aspect of the democratisation of private practice at the close of the Enlightenment. This conjecture is supported by what we know about Thomas Percival's efforts to democratise medicine within the hospital in the first years of the 1800s. More significantly, my speculations about the changes in medicine-by-post rhetoric are supported by the patient letters of the period.

The alternative medicine-by-post rhetoric of which I am speaking took the form and tone of the familiar letter. The doctor, once given due respect, is addressed almost as friend. However, while this 'familiar' consultation letter was not limited to social equals, neither did it signal social presumption arising from a feeling of patient entitlement. Just the reverse. The modest rhetoric of these letters seems to have arisen out of a confidence that doctors of the late-eighteenth century had become better listeners, attuned to patient need without high drama or affectation. Many of the letters of this category in Cullen's practice were written by women. Their letters easily combine clinical detail with expression of personal need, as in this letter from Jane Webster:

> Sir, from your generall Character in this Country, and the oppinion I entertain of you I am very disirous of having your sentiments on my own Case. I shall be as particular as I can but if I am no sufficiently so you will impute it to my want of experience in these matters.
>
> I am about 44 years of age with dark hair, a darkish Complexion and a warm temper, of the middle size as to height or rather less than that, but of a very Corpulent habit.... I now walk generaly 4 miles before breakfast, and 2 or 3 in an evening, and I have moderated my Diet.... The question I wish you to determine upon is whether or no you would advise me to continue the plan I am upon.... [I] beg the favour of as speedy an answer to my querys as is consistent with your other engagements.[158]

Cullen writes back that 'corpulence certainly disposes to violent diseases. You should persist in your present measures till you make your body still lighter by two stone or more. For in a woman of middle size, anything above 12 stone is too much.' He provides a detailed regimen including advice all-too-familiar to twentieth-century patients, to exercise and to 'Cheat appetite by bulk of light things especially vegetable.'[159] The interchange is one of extreme directness on the part of both patient and physician, and there is never a question that Dr Cullen has been careful in 'listening' to the patient.

While Jane Webster was able to offer Dr Cullen two guineas for his services, patients of less financial ability consulted him just as freely. Such letters are filled with misspellings, grammatical solecisms, and colloquialisms, identifying the writer as untaught in the niceties of polite English prose. Such is the case in this letter from Mrs Likely Pitodry, who writes to Dr Cullen from Aberdeen on behalf of a friend.[160]

> Sir – as the young Lady who called at your House in Edenburgh with a weakening in her hearing said you was pleas'd to desire her to writ(e) you how the Medicine succeeded – as a friend of hers I avail myself of your goodness and take the Liberty to writ(e) you[.] she got the Medicine from your Apothecary as you desired it was Carefully droped in to her Ears at Night for ten or twelf days but as she felt no advantage from it I thought it better to give it over.... [S]he said you was very good and told her particularly how to apply the Medicine.... [A] few lines from you when perfectly convenient I would esteem as a particular favour.[161]

Cullen's reply, though in genteel prose, shows not hint of condescension:

> Madam: [re] Miss – I remember very well the young Lady who applied to me some months ago for a cure of deafness, and I will with the utmost willingness give her every relief in my power.... On the other page of this sheet that it may be easily cut off and sent to the Apothecary I have given a prescription of a medicine which I hope shall be more powerful than the former.... After a trial of two weeks I beg to hear from you again....[162]

In a subsequent note, Cullen reassures Mrs Pitodry: 'You need not make no apology for your fee for I am perfectly satisfied[,] and without any further fee I shall willingly do you any service in my power.'[163] Dr Cullen was ever the gentleman-physician.

This new patient voice does not supplant the rhetoric of sensibility but co-exists with it, much as patients today employ many different voices to solicit medical attention. Yet Cullen does seem to be responding, in Jane Webster and Mrs Pitodry, to a new patient voice for which his recommendations to Riddoch and Erskine would not be appropriate. Within the body of Cullen's consultation letters, I am suggesting, is evidence of a new rhetoric in medicine-by-post that points to a redefinition of doctor–patient relationship, its being freed of eighteenth-century conventions and fashion, though born of it – not the product of scientific advance, but of eighteenth-century speculative medicine and Enlightenment philosophy.

Notes

1. J. Boswell, *Boswell's Life of Johnson*, 6 vols., G.B. Hill (ed.), (New York: Bigelow, Brown & Co., 1921), iv: 304

2. Robert Whytt, professor of medicine at Edinburgh from 1747, was extremely influential in his theories of nervous system function. He rejected iatromechanism but he also rejected Haller's distinction between nerve sensibility and muscle irritability – the idea that muscle might contract with stimulation independent of the nervous system through an intrinsic reactive property that Haller called the *vis insita*. Whytt posited a 'sentient principle' that directed all responses in a purposeful way, and since it was a 'feeling agent', it was considered as residing in the nervous system. Most of the actions of the sentient principle were unconscious, though some, as the need to urinate, were conscious. Whytt's theories established the concept of an integrated system of body function.

   Cullen thought Whytt's 'sentient principle' too abstract and instead postulated a similarly co-ordinated and purposeful nervous system, but based on 'an excited state of an aethereal fluid in the nervous system'. For Cullen there was a hierarchy of body function, in which sense came before will, brain, nerve, and finally muscle. Sense enjoyed this important place because, as Cullen explained, one's will does not come into play unless stimulated to do so – for example, 'Unless I see you before me... I will not open my mouth to speak.' It is sensory stimulation that keeps the body awake. See W.F. Bynum, 'Cullen and the Nervous System', in A. Doig *et al.* (eds), *William Cullen and the Eighteenth Century Medical World*, (Edinburgh: Edinburgh University Press, 1993),157. Also, in same volume, see R.E. Kendell, 'William Cullen's Synopsis Nosologiae Methodicae', 216–33.

3. See J. Mullan, *Sentiment and Sociability: The Language of Feeling in the Eighteenth Century* (Oxford: Clarendon Press, 1988), 229; and regarding earlier eighteenth-century, less cohesive, models of the 'body unified in its sensitivities', see 228–32.

4. See A.J. Van Sant, *Eighteenth-Century Sensibility and the Novel: The Senses in Social Context* (New York: Cambridge University Press, 1993), in particular Chapter 5, 'The Centrality of Touch', 83–97. Van Sant describes how a tradition of visible pathos (sight as source of pathos) was conflated with eighteenth-century nerve physiology to create a new dimension of psychological 'feeling' which was internalised: 'Sensibility... translates all sensory experience into a form of touch.' A particular visual image becomes less crucial in and of itself than the 'internal vibrations it activates' (96).

5. M. McKeon, 'Historicizing Patriarchy: The Emergence of Gender Difference

in England, 1660–1760', *Eighteenth-Century Studies*, 28, (1995), 314.

6. C. Lawrence, 'The Nervous System and Society in the Scottish Enlightenment', in B. Barnes and S. Shapin (eds), *Natural Order: Historical Studies of Scientific Culture* (Beverly Hills: Sage Publications, 1979), 27.

7. *Ibid.*, 20. After the Union with England (1707), there was a national economic and cultural vacuum which alarmed the Scottish elite and inspired them to a goal of national 'improvement'. Lawrence divides the Enlightenment project into three periods, 1707 to 1720s as a time of 'economic depression and social fragmentation'; 1720 to 1750, the revival of prosperity and cultural activity marked by the change from a commercial to an agricultural economy by the ruling oligarchy, with tight controls on land and labour; 1750 to 1780, a flourishing society in the hands of gentry and intellectuals who were mostly Whig, pro-English, and followers of a moderate Presbyterian church. The House of Argyll became the dominant ruling clan and its patronage determined professorships at the University of Edinburgh and its medical school. The socio–economic changes occurring in lowland Scotland had their 'counterpart in the programme of cultural improvement that burgeoned among the intellectuals of the capital.... One important facet of this improving ideology was the cultivation of manners and polite literature', and 'refinement, delicacy, and moderation were the key synonyms for culture by mid-century.' A fruitful symbiotic relationship existed between the landed gentry and Edinburgh intellectuals, the latter becoming 'the articulators of a specifically *Scottish* cultural identity.' In this context, highland society was regarded as backward and savage in comparison to the 'civilized values' of the lowlanders.

8. *Ibid.*, 34–5. For an explanation of the French medical theory of vitalism and individual glandular responsiveness to environmental stimulation, see A.C. Vila, *Enlightenment and Pathology: Sensibility in the Literature and Medicine of Eighteenth-Century France* (London: The Johns Hopkins University Press, 1998), 66–73.

9. Mullan, *op. cit.* (note 3), 237.

10. G.J. Barker-Benfield, *The Culture of Sensibility: Sex and Society in Eighteenth-Century Britain.* (Chicago: University of Chicago Press, 1992), 15.

11. Van Sant says that 'the problem of defining sensibility arises in part from the ease with which writers' of all genres, including medical texts, 'modulated between physiological systems and between literal and metaphorical terms'; Van Sant, *op. cit.* (note 4), 11. Cullen believed strongly that the empirical lessons of bedside observation, only became understood, useful, and applied, if the observer approached the patient with some 'system' in mind – a system which could be tempered by the empirical experience. In this, Cullen was clearly adopting the philosophy of his friend, David Hume. While some of Cullen's students and colleagues (among them James Gregory and Sir John

Pringle) questioned the usefulness and desirability of Cullen's elaborate nosology, the medical rhetoric of the period seems to have regularly blended the speculative with the practical, as Cullen did, but with less deliberateness and self-awareness than Cullen. See M. Barfoot, 'Philosophy and Method in Cullen's Medical Teaching', in Doig *et al.*, *op. cit.* (note 2), 110–33 and, especially, 122–24. In the same volume, see C. Clayson, 'Cullen in Eighteenth Century Medicine', 92; Clayson explains how Cullen described how 'dogmatic' thought and practice must inevitably encompass the 'empiric'. A specific example of Cullen's teaching philosophy is illustrated in his early chemistry courses in which he joined theories of chemistry to practical use in agriculture, for which see, J.R.R. Christie, 'William Cullen and the Practice of Chemistry', also in Doig *et al.*, *op. cit.* (note 2), 98–109.

12. There were, of course, alternative medical options available to the patient from 'irregular' ('unorthodox' or 'fringe') medical healers, including vernacular cures, homeopathic preparations, and charlatan recipes. However, among the 'regular' physicians, those who had at least a smattering of medical education (or experience in a surgical apprenticeship), and who followed prevailing medical practice, treatment remained centred on bleeding and the standard vomits, cathartics, diuretics, and febrifuge preparations. See W.F. Bynum and R. Porter, *Medical Fringe and Medical Orthodoxy 1750-1850* (New Hampshire: Croom Helm, 1987).

13. I am using 'national' in the sense of a people united by blood and customs; politically, Scotland no longer had its own Parliament after the Act of Union with England in 1707.

14. James Gregory (1753–1821) was professor of the theory of medicine and successor to the senior chair held by Cullen; he was the son of Cullen's colleague, John Gregory (1724–73), who authored the *Lectures on the Duties and Qualifications of a Physician* (1770). James had a very successful private practice and some of his medicine-by-post correspondence is included in this chapter.

15. C. Lawrence, 'Ornate Physicians and Learned Artisans: Edinburgh Medical Men, 1726–1776', in W.F. Bynum and R. Porter (eds), *William Hunter and the Eighteenth-Century Medical World* (New York: Cambridge University Press, 1985), 175. In America, many of the founding members of the College of Physicians of Philadelphia had been students of Cullen in Edinburgh. J.M. O'Donnell claims that the influence of Cullen on such doctors as Benjamin Rush was not a particular system of teaching as much as 'the imaginative cultivation of the art of teaching' itself, with his emphasis on the clinical experience as the final and most important determinant of diagnosis and therapeutic decision regardless of any didactic system. See O'Donnell, 'Cullen's Influence on American Medicine', in Doig *et al.*, *op. cit.* (note 2), 243.

16. Both Cullen and Smith supported Hume's bid for the chair of moral philosophy, although he was ultimately refused the position on the grounds of his religious scepticism.

17. Clayson, *op. cit.* (note 11), 89. The biographical material in this section is large drawn from his chapter in Doig *et al., op. cit.* (note 2), 87–97.

18. The collection of Cullen's correspondence at the Royal College of Physicians of Edinburgh is divided into 'Letters to Cullen', stored loose in 17 boxes, and the Consultation Letters [CL] which are bound in 21 volumes by year(s). 'Letters to Cullen' will be designated in subsequent footnotes by sender, date, postmark, box number (in Roman numerals), and letter number. Cullen's 'Consultation Letters' are cited as CL, and are sorted into volumes by date, so that citations refer to the date of letters and the letter number (often corresponding to page number) in the volume of consultation letters inclusive of those dates. All of Cullen's letters are from Edinburgh. I am especially indebted to the Burroughs Wellcome Fund for sponsoring my research of the letters of William Cullen at the Royal College of Physicians in Edinburgh, and to Iain Milne, Librarian of the RCPE, for his more than generous assistance in this project.

19. Risse's original study of this collection of consultation letters was '"Doctor William Cullen, Physician, Edinburgh": A Consultation Practice in the Eighteenth Century', *Bulletin of History of Medicine,* 48 (1974), 338–51. More recently, in a most instructive essay, Risse has compared Cullen's private practice methods (as evidenced in medicine-by-post) to Cullen's medical management of the hospital patients seen on the wards of the Royal Infirmary of Edinburgh (the source material for the latter are 183 case histories preserved in four student notebooks); see Risse, 'Cullen as Clinician: Organisation and Strategies of an Eighteenth Century Medical Practice', in *W.C and ECMW, op. cit.* (note 2),133–51.

20. Watt's copy-machine involved pressing a thin, blank, moistened paper over the original letter which was written with a special ink developed by Watt; the ink was absorbed from the original document onto the moistened paper and produced a mirror image which was read through the thin copy paper. See Doig *et al., op. cit.* (note 2), *op. cit.* (note 2), 69 (fig. 53).

21. Poorer patients would not have the education to participate in a medicine-by-post correspondence. Cullen saw such patients through the Royal Infirmary in his role as teacher. Risse has noted that in the case of private patients, Cullen focused on the patient rather than the disease and took a more holistic approach. Although he was 'the foremost medical nosologist of his time', he 'frequently eschewed precise diagnostic labels' in his private practice. Therapy was tailored to the patient's constitutional make-up, and severe therapies, such as blood-letting, were kept to a minimum. The Infirmary patients, on the other hand, were regularly tagged with diagnostic

labels and treated more uniformly and aggressively than the private patients. 'Hence, in this institutional setting', concludes Risse, 'the patient was less important than the disease.' Part of the explanation for this difference in approach, however, may lie in the fact that a register of specific disease types admitted to the Infirmary was obligatory for bureaucratic as well as didactic reasons; also, the patients admitted to the Infirmary were largely suffering from acute (often infectious) disease rather than chronic conditions. See G. Risse, 'Cullen as Clinician', *op cit.* (note 19),145–6.

22. *Ibid.*, 135–6.
23. Thomas Stapleton to William Cullen, 6 December 1774, Carlton; Box I, 202. Garthsore has been advised by Mr Lamont to take Elixir of Vitriol but has deferred until he hears from Cullen as he considers this to be a 'Dangerous medicine'. Mr Lamont's note to Cullen, dated 28 October 1774, is confined to clinical symptoms and treatments, though Lamont hazards a diagnosis of 'worms'.
24. James Garthshore to Dr Cullen, 4 November 1774, Alderston; Box I, 191.
25. James Garthshore to Dr Cullen, 28 October 1774, Alderston; Box I, 184.
26. Hamilton Douglas, Fourth Earl of Selkirk, to William Cullen, 10 April, 1780, Carlisle; Box VII: 44.
27. Selkirk to Cullen, 12 April 1774, Burrow Bridge; Box VII, 47.
28. Cullen to Selkirk, 17 April 1774, Edinburgh; CL, XI: 4–5.
29. Risse, *op. cit.* (note 19), 136.
30. Jane Webster to Dr Cullen, 11 September 1780; Box VII, 126.
31. Jo. Rogers to Dr Cullen, 28 March 1774, Kelso; Box I, 155.
32. Cullen to Mrs Pitodry, May 1789; CL, 152. In a letter to Mr Cowmeadow, Lecturer of her Late Royal Highness Princess of Amelia at Berlin, dated 16 September 1789, Cullen writes: 'With respect to my fee... a Draught upon him would imply my fixing my own fee which I never do, leaving it to the circumstances and generosity of the patient'; CL, 304–5.
33. Dr Cullen re: Mr Cowmeadow, 16 September 1789; CL, 304–5. Compare to Thomas Percival's recommendations in his *Medical Ethics,* in which he advises a two guinea fee for the initial consultation-by-post, but also recommends that subsequent correspondence 'may justly be regarded in the light of ordinary attendance, and may be compensated, as such, according to the circumstances of the case, or of the patient' (43).
34. R. Passmore, 'Cullen and Dietetics', in Doig *et al., op. cit.* (note 2), 169–70.
35. Patient scepticism was voiced quite amply in the form of a prodigious number of satirical representations on the profession on stage, cartoons, and painting, as well as in everyday conversation and private letters; see Chapter 1.
36. See B. Mandeville, *A Treatise of the Hypochondriack and Hysteric Diseases* (London, 1730), reproduction of 2nd edition (New York: George Olms

Verlag, 1981). In the 'Preface', Mandeville mentions that the reader may wonder why the author should write a dialogue in which 'two Persons should discourse for half an Hour about a Science, which they both profess not to understand, as the Doctor and his Patient do about Mathematics' (xxi). Within those pages, Mandeville demonstrates, as the chapter headings preview for the reader, 'Why Mathematicks can be no Help in the Cure of Diseases' and that 'A Scheme to bring purging and emetick Medicines to mathematical Certainty' will always be 'fruitless'.

37. See G.S. Rousseau, 'Nerves, Spirits, and Fibres: Towards Defining the Origins of Sensibility', *The Blue Guitar*, 2 (December, 1976): 125–53. Rousseau emphasises that it takes several decades before a revolution in thought (in Kuhnian terms) becomes a generally accepted paradigm incorporated into a culture. Hence, the work of Locke and Willis would not be expected to have had more widespread influence in medicine until the early decades of the eighteenth century. See Chapter 3 on Dr George Cheyne for details on the influence of Willis and Locke.

38. As noted in the previous chapter, Cheyne's readiness to share his personal narrative of illness was in large part the source of his popular success and his claim to authority on treatment of the English malady. James Boswell, inspired no doubt by Cheyne's example, was able to use personal case history to give authority to his opinions and advice in his *London Magazine* column, 'The Hypochondriak' (1777 to 1783).

39. For example, recall the anecdote about the prestigious Dr Richard Meade (in the previous chapter), his upset with the church minister who insisted on following Cheyne's diet despite Meade's advice to the contrary.

40. See J.F. Burnum, 'Medical Diagnosis Through Semiotics: Giving Meaning to the Sign', *Annals of Internal Medicine*, 119, 9 (1 November 1993), 939–43; see also K.M. Hunter, *Doctor's Stories: The Narrative Structure of Medical Knowledge* (New Jersey: Princeton University Press, 1991).

41. See Vila, *op. cit.* (note 8), ch. 2, 'Sensibility and the Philosophical Medicine of the 1750s–1770s', 43–79. Vila describes French philosophical medicine as a 'sort of literature', dominated by the theme of sensibility and the method of semiotics:

> How does it [philosophical medicine] operate, if not via an elaborate series of discursive tableaux of sensibility in action? ... [We] have seen how such tableaux could be deployed to cover every aspect of medical theory and practice: the construction of the body as a reactive animal economy, the coding of signs for deciphering that body, the organization of medical facts into a reasoning body of knowledge, and finally, the depiction of the inspired medical observer engaged in diagnosis.... [T]he moment of medical diagnosis

hinges upon a dramatic, dynamic body-to-body engagement between two personas who represent opposite ends of the sensibility spectrum. One person is the patient, whose sensibility is pathologically disturbed; the other is the heroic médicin philosophe, whose sensibility is both exquisitely developed and exquisitely mastered. Out of the intercommunicative interplay between those two diametrically opposed types of sensibility is born a medico–philosophical fact, which captures sensibility and puts it into words. (63–4)

42. J. Gregory, *Lectures on the Duties and Qualifications of a Physician* (London, 1772), 19.
43. Cullen to uncertain recipient, re: Andrew Ross, Esq., 26 December 1774; CL: Vol. II, 151–3.
44. Unidentified correspondent to Cullen, 14 August 1774, Peterburg; Box I, 169.
45. Cullen treated Infirmary patients more in accordance with the dogmatic ideas of the classroom. His purpose in the infirmary setting, as Risse points out, was didactic, with emphasis on disease over patient. In private practice, however, Cullen focused more on the individual than the disease. Nevertheless, in the case of ward patients, Cullen taught the importance allowing bedside lessons to alter dogmatic principles. See Risse, 'Cullen as Clinician', *op. cit.* (note 19), for the difference in Cullen's approach to private and infirmary patients; also see Clayson, *op. cit.* (note 11).
46. L. Rosner, *Medical Education in the Age of Improvement: Edinburgh Students and Apprentices 1760–1826* (Edinburgh: Edinburgh University Press, 1991); R. Porter, *The Greatest Benefit to Mankind* (New York: W.W. Norton, 1997), 47; also Lawrence, 'Ornate physicians', *op. cit.* (note 15), 153–75.
47. G.B. Risse, *Hospital Life in Enlightenment Scotland: Care and Teaching at the Royal Infirmary of Edinburgh* (New York: Cambridge University Press, 1986), 251 and 268–9.
48. Porter, *op. cit.* (note 46), 290–1.
49. In England, a student seeking an education in the practical aspects of medicine had to turn to offerings outside the universities, to private anatomical lectures (such as those of William Hunter) or bedside experience within hospitals that now welcomed students to 'walk the wards.'
50. Lawrence, *op. cit.* (note 6), 23–4. On the politics and patronage of Edinburgh appointments, see R.L. Emerson, 'Medical men, politicians and the medical schools', in Doig *et al.*, *op. cit.* (note 2), 186–215. Also, on the role of the Scottish *virtuosi* in forming the core of Scottish Enlightenment thought by introducing seventeenth-century natural philosophy and Continental philosophy to Scotland – elements which became

institutionalised in the Scottish universities of the eighteenth century – see R.L. Emerson, 'Science and the Origins and Concerns of the Scottish Enlightenment', in *British Journal for the History of Science*, xxvi (1988), 333–66.

51. Emerson, *Science, ibid.*, 348.

52. *Ibid.*, 350–1.

53. *Ibid.*, 353.

54. Lawrence, *op. cit.* (note 15), 153–76.

55. The spread of breast cancer was of particular interest to Monro *secundus*.

56. Lawrence, *op. cit.* (note 15), 167.

57. The clinic had few teaching beds and the rounds were always overcrowded to the point that students complained of not being able to hear the professors on rounds. For practical experience many students preferred London where there were private schools of anatomy. But London had no equivalent to Edinburgh with regard to the variety and organisation of lectures in medicine and the particular combination of theoretical and practical contents of the lectures.

58. The ontological (Platonic, rationalist) model of disease considers each disease as a discrete entity with its own natural history which exists in its own right, irrespective of its actual clinical presentation in an individual patient. It is a model of disease that invites nosology along the line of botanical classification. It stands in contrast to the 'physiologic' (Hippocratic/Galenic/empirical) model of disease which focuses on the temporal disease process within the patient. In the 'physiologic' classification of disease, the patient history is the basis for categorisation, creating a virtually endless list of disease based on each individual response and making it hard to draw the line even between normal and abnormal states. See O. Temkin, 'The Scientific Approach to Disease: Specific Entity and Individual Sickness', in A.C. Crombie (ed.), *Scientific Change: Historical Studies in the Intellectual, Social and Technical Conditions for Scientific Discovery and Technical Invention, from Antiquity to the Present* (New York: Basic Books., 1963), 629–58.

59. Lawrence, *op. cit.* (note 15), 174.

60. Clayson, *op. cit.* (note 11), 91. Michael Barfoot describes more precisely the manner in which Cullen was a sceptical dogmatist when it came to medical practice – a blend of dogmatist and empiricist, though more of the former. He believed, along with Hume, Smith, and Hutton, that the mind could never be entirely free of 'system', and that 'true facts were not to be acquired independently of analogical reasoning but by means of it.' However, Cullen was equally prepared to have his theory modified by bedside experience. Hence, there was a 'dialectical relationship between theory and fact in general found throughout his writing'; M. Barfoot, 'Philosophy and

Method', in Doig *et al., op. cit.* (note 2), 122.

61. T. Percival, *Medical Ethics, or a Code of Institutes and Precepts Adapted to the Professional Conduct of Physicians and Surgeons* (Manchester, 1803), 36.

62. Laurence, *op. cit.* (note 15), 171.

63. Cullen's conception of the effects of environment are discussed in detail by Bynum, *op. cit.* (note 2), 156. The quotation from Cullen, found in Bynum's chapter, is from J. Thompson (ed.), *The Works of William Cullen*, 2 vols. (Edinburgh: William Blackwood and Sons, 1827), 2: 505–6.

64. Mr C. Blagden to William Cullen, 29 July 1774, Gray's Inn; Box I, 164.

65. Lawrence, *op. cit.* (note 15), 171. For a more comprehensive description of Cullen's nosology and system of teaching, see M. Barfoot, 'Philosophy and Method in Cullen's Medical Teaching', in Doig *et al., op. cit.* (note 2), 110–32; also, in the same volume, W.F. Bynum, 'Cullen and the Nervous System', 152–62, and R.E. Kendall, 'The Synopsis Nosologiae Methodicae', 216–33. More on Cullen and his specific view of the nervous system discussed below.

66. Lawrence, *op. cit.* (note 15), 173.

67. Boswell sought Pringle's advice in 1769 during a recurrence of gonorrhoea. See journal entry dated 2 September 1769, in J. Boswell, *In Search of a Wife: 1766–1769*, F. Brady and F.A. Pottle (eds), (New York: McGraw-Hill, 1956), 269–70, an entry by Boswell dated 2 September 1769.

68. Francis Hutchinson to Dr Cullen, 19 June 1789, Dublin; Box XVI, 95.

69. Lawrence, *op. cit.* (note 15), 170.

70. Gregory, *op. cit.* (note 42), 13–14.

71. *Ibid.*, 19. For a detailed discussion of the derivation of Gregory's concept of sympathy from Hume, see L.B. McCullough, 'John Gregory's Medical Ethics and Humean Sympathy', in R. Baker, D. Porter, and R. Porter (eds), *The Codification of Medical Morality: Historical and Philosophical Studies of the Formalization of Western Medical Morality in the Eighteenth and Nineteenth Centuries* (2 volumes): *Volume 1, Medical Ethics and Etiquette in the Eighteenth Century* (Boston: Kluwer Academic Publishers, 1993), 145–60.

72. L. Haakonssen, *Medicine and Morals in the Enlightenment: John Gregory, Thomas Percival, and Benjamin Rush* (Amsterdam: Rodopi, 1997), 11–2 and 70–4.

73. Gregory, *op. cit.* (note 42), 19–23, *passim*.

74. *Ibid.*, 20.

75. See Barker-Benfield, *op. cit.* (note 10), ch. 3, 'The Question of Effeminacy', esp. 132–41.

76. Mullan, *op. cit.* (note 3), 216–28.

77. Van Sant, *op. cit.* (note 4),106–7.

78. See discussion of Samuel Richardson's novel *Clarissa* in Chapter 1, in particular her final moments and the diminution and loss of her senses.

79. Barker-Benfield, *op. cit.* (note 10), 1–2.
80. Embonpoint: corpulence; stoutness; fine condition
81. [?] November, 1774, Geneva; Box I:186 (partial letter, unable to make out signature).
82. Mullan, *op. cit.* (note 3), 201–40.
83. Barker–Benfield, *op. cit.* (note 10), 27.
84. *Ibid.*, 35–6.
85. Bynum, *op. cit.* (note 2),155.
86. I did not make a count of the number of letters penned by women patients in the 17 boxes of 'Letters to Cullen', but letters from women patients are abundant and, I would estimate, make up near a fifth of the letters seeking Cullen's medical advice. A significant number of letters received by Cullen were, not surprisingly, from male physicians requesting consultation for their female patients, and it is worth noting that such consultation request on behalf of women patients convey the patient's needs in a clinically objective but also personally interested manner, with extremely rare suggestions of paternalism or a demeaning of the patient's concerns because of gender. See examples in text.
87. So headed in the folio where Cullen preserved consultation letters; see note 20 below for details on the collection and interpretation of citations from the collection.
88. Cullen 'To Mayor Hamilton at Murdeston', 31 October 1770; CL, II: 6–8
89. This prescription is dated 13 December 1779; CL, X: 132. This 'prescription' is mostly of interest in that is appears hastily penned – the handwriting is much less neat than most of the copies which were written by a secretary, words are run together and lines crossed out. It is likely this was Cullen's own hasty scrawl, and it is signed 'W.C.'. The note seems less a prescription than a brief note on the case for future reference:

> An erysipelatous affection of perhaps the whole but especially the upper parts of the alim:canal. Internal medicines can do little and I must especially to a Diet [*sic*]. I am not informed of any thing of this kind; but [?] for it has been already wout [without] effect, I would advise a diet consisting entirely of milk and vegetables....

> Obviate costiveness by glysters. Applications to the mouth may perhaps give some relief but the choice of the best I must leave to former trials.

> Formerly upon slight information I ordered a Rx for this which I have often found useful but as there is no mention made of it ['I must beg to be tried; and with caution' is crossed out] I fear it has

not been transmitted. When it is let it be used with due caution. W.C.

90. Pea-size lump.
91. Probably syrup of rosehip. However, a 'conserve of roses' was a jelly made out of *Rosa Damascena* mixed with vitriol and sugar, and this was used as a mucolytic gargle but also as an analgesic which had a mild laxative effect. See J.W. Estes, *Dictionary of Protopharmacology: Therapeutic Practices, 1700–1850* (Canton, MA: Science History Publications, 1990), 167.
92. Mrs Frances Fontescue to Dr Cullen, 12 January 1780, Cook Hill; Box VII, 6.
93. William Thompson (physician) to Dr Cullen, 17 February 1780; Box VII, 28.
94. Cullen to Mrs Frances Fontescue, 22 January 1780; CL, X: 147. An 'issue' is an artificial ulcer, eg. created by incision, to allow drainage of pus.
95. The first letter from Miss E. Fraser to Cullen is from [?] November 1780; Box VII: 135. In that she describes an 'uneasy pain in the left side Shrieking [*sic*] through from the left breast to the shoulder.' This subsequent letter to Cullen is dated 5 December 1780; Box VIII: No.167.
96. Letter headed 'For Miss Fraser of Inverllochy', 11 December 1780; CL, XXI: 117.
97. Richard Lainberg to William Cullen, 19 January 1780, Newcastle-upon-Tyne; Box VII: 11.
98. Mr William Ingham to William Cullen, 20 August 1780, Newcastle; Box VII: 110.
99. Risse, 'Cullen as Clinician', *op. cit.* (note 19), 146.
100. Cullen to William Ingham, 26 August 1780; CL, XI: 59–60. In Cullen's nosology, which he used for didactic purposes in the classroom, 'spasm' is differentiated according to whether it affects animal function (the voluntary muscles as in epilepsy), the vital organs (causing, for example, palpitations of the heart or asthma), or the natural muscular organs (uterine, gastrointestinal) resulting in colic or hysterical symptoms. Cullen's nosology, difficult to grasp today, classified disease on the basis of disorders of sensation and motion; muscles and nerves were seen by him as a continuum and this view lent itself to this unusual nosology. For example, dyspepsia was included among 'neuroses' because it involved dysfunctional movement of the stomach. For more on this, see Bynum, *op. cit.* (note 2), 152-162. 'Anasarca' is defined in Johnson's *Dictionary* as 'A sort of dropsy of the whole body.'
101. Risse, 'Cullen as Clinician', *op. cit.* (note 19), 141.
102. Cullen to [?], probably to physician, 4 June 1768; CL, I:14–15.

103. S. Staves, 'Married Life, Venereal Disease, and Therapeutic Optimism' (unpublished).

104. Mullan, *op. cit.* (note 3), 220.

105. See Chapter 3, especially in reference to Cheyne's advice to Richardson on exercise and his urging to make up a list of books fit for 'Pamela's Library.'

106. G. Cheyne, 'The Author's Case', in *The English Malady* (1733), R. Porter (ed.), (New York: Routledge, 1991), 362; see also Porter's 'Introduction' to same, xxxix–xl.

107. See Chapter 3.

108. 5 November, 1789; CL: XXI, 335–7.

109. Regarding Tissot, see Vila, *op. cit.* (note 8), 94–107. That sensibility was a double-edged sword – at once the driving force of a more perfect civilisation but, simultaneously, the Achilles heel of a society – was a subject of concern and lively debate both in Britain and on the Continent. But in Scotland during the final decades of the eighteenth century, the philosophical attitude towards sensibility, as I am hoping to show here, was perhaps more consistently positive than it would be anywhere else during the Enlightenment.

110. M. Barfoot, 'Dr William Cullen and Mr Adam Smith: A Case of Hypochondriasis?', in *Proceedings of the Royal College of Edinburgh*, 21 (1991), 208. The quotation is taken from a letter of Adam Smith to Lord Shelburne written in 1760.

111. *Ibid.*, 211. Quotation is from Cullen's *First Lines of the Practice of Physic*, 4th edition, 4 volumes (Edinburgh: Elliott & Cadell, 1784), Vol. 3, 268.

112. *Ibid.*, 211. The letter from Adam Smith to William Cullen, quoted in Barfoot, is dated September 1774 and is found in *The Correspondence of Adam Smith*, E.C. Mossner and I.S. Ross (eds), (Oxford: Clarendon, 1987), letter no. 143.

113. *Ibid.*, 210; quoting from letter from Hume to Smith, letter no. 129.

114. G. Sill, 'Neurology and the Novel: Alexander Monro *primus* and *secundus*, *Robinson Crusoe*, and the Problem of Sensibility', in *Literature and Medicine*, 16, (1997), 250–65.

115. *Ibid.*, 261. Monro's 'living principle', as described by Sill, 'stops short of animism, in which the organism is governed by an in-dwelling spirit, but it goes beyond mechanism, in which the body operates in response to external objects or secretions from the brain.'

116. *Ibid.*, 251.

117. See R. Porter, 'Barely Touching: A Social Perspective on Mind and Body', in G.S. Rousseau (ed.), *The Languages of Psyche: Mind and Body in Enlightenment Thought* (Clark Library Lectures 1985–1986), (Berkeley: University of California Press, 1990), 45–80.

118. 23 November 1789, Newcastle-upon-Tyne; Box XVII: 32.

119. Porter, *op. cit.* (note 117), 71 ff.

120. 'Wednesday Night April 1812, St. Andrew's Square', to Allan Maconochie, Lord Meadowbrook (1714–1816); University of Edinburgh Library manuscripts, microfilm m. 1070–34. Underlined words are, in fact, underlined in the letter, not in italics. The Latin quotation is from Horace, and translates, 'Those who cross the sea may change the sky [or scene] but not the soul [or spirit].'

121. Porter, *op. cit.* (note 46), 287–99. See the always interesting speculations of Michel Foucault, 'The Politics of Health in the Eighteenth Century', in P. Rabinow (ed.) *The Foucault Reader* (New York: Pantheon Books, 1984), 273–89. On the particulars of the charity hospital, see M.E. Fissell, *Patients, Power, and the Poor in Eighteenth-Century Bristol* (New York: Cambridge University Press, 1991). On public 'sightseeing' of asylums, see R. Porter, *Mind-Forg'd Manacles: A History of Madness in England from the Restoration to the Regency* (New York: Penguin Books, 1987).

122. M.E. Fissell, 'Innocent and Honorable Bribes: Medical Manners in Eighteenth-Century Britain', in *Codification, op. cit.* (note 71), 19–45.

123. Gregory, *op. cit.* (note 42), 26.

124. R. Baker, 'Introduction' to *Codification, op. cit.* (note 71), 7.

125. *Ibid.*, 9.

126. See R. Baker, 'Deciphering Percival's Code', in *Codification, op. cit.* (note 71), 179–211.

127. Haakonssen, *op. cit.* (note 72), 32.

128. Percival, *op. cit.* (note 61), 30.

129. The charity hospital, and like institutions, were designed to treat particular types of conditions that affected the lower classes of society, and which often carried moral implications embarrassing to the greater public – unwed mothers, venereal disease, lunacy. The state also had an interest in maintaining a healthy labour force and sound military, and the clinics and infirmaries therefore served political and economic interests as well as being the incubators of new medical knowledge. An absolute prohibition on using confidential information from patients within such settings would have confounded their purpose and discouraged financial support by private citizens and the government. What happened within the walls of the new medical institutions was of great interest to private citizens and the public at large. Patients needed to be 'recommended' for care, but doctors also were expected to justify admissions based on the likelihood of benefit (cure) and the value of a particular patient for didactic purposes. See Risse, *op. cit.* (note 47).

130. Percival, *op. cit.* (note 61), 11.

131. Baker, *op. cit.* (note 126), 195.

132. T. Smollett, *The Expedition of Humphry Clinker*, T.R. Preston and O.M. Brack, Jr. (eds), (Athens: The University of Georgia Press, 1990), 34.

133. See Chapter 5 of this book, which discusses Burney's letter in detail.

134. 12 January 1789, Edinburgh; Box XVI: 6.

135. Tobias Smollett (1721–71) was born in Dumbarton, Scotland. He attended Glasgow University and became surgical apprentice to the very reputable William Stirling and John Gordon. After going to London but failing in aspirations to produce his play, *The Regicide*, he joined the British navy in 1740 as surgeon's mate on a man-of-war. After extreme disillusionment with naval service, Smollett returned to London in 1744 to establish a private surgical practice in Downing Street. However, his medical practice was thwarted by being a Scotsman in London, and like other Scottish physicians (who had not attended the English universities), he was unable to attain professional recognition – an arrogance of British medicine that Smollett represented with biting satire in his novels such as *The Adventures of Ferdinand Count Fathom* (see chapter 1, above). Smollett purchased his MD degree (a common practice) for £28 Scots in 1750 so he could officially call himself Dr Smollett. However, despite this and moving his medical practice to new locations in London, his practice never flourished. When his writing career took off after *The Adventures of Roderick Random*, Smollett spent proportionately much less time in medicine, though medicine played a great role in his novels. His health was complicated by an asthmatic condition and, later, tuberculosis. He therefore had much opportunity to experience suffering as a patient and be under the care of a number of, to him, most incompetent physicians with inflated egos whom he portrayed in *Travels Through France and Italy* (1766), a memoir in epistolary form (see Chapter 1) and personal letters, as illustrated here.

136. Box XVI: 109, 7 July 1789, Buxton.

137. Smollett, *op. cit.* (note 132), 158–9.

138. C.H. Flynn, 'Running Out of Matter', in *Languages of Psyche, op. cit.* (note 117), 179.

139. Tobias Smollett to 'Mr Moore, Surgeon in Glasgow North Britain', 13 November 1765, Bath; from *The Letters of Tobias Smollett*, L.M. Knapp (ed.), (Oxford: Clarendon Press, 1970), Letter 97, 125–7.

140. Smollett to Dr William Hunter, 24 February 1767, Bath; *ibid.*, 132–3.

141. Smollett to Hunter, 6 February 1764, Nice; *Ibid.*, 120–3.

142. See Chapter 1 for further details regarding Smollet, *The Adventures of Ferdinand Count Fathom.*

143. Thomas Stapleton to William Cullen, 6 [8?] December 1774, Carlton; Box I, No. 202.

144. Cullen to Stapleton, 30 December 1774; CL: vol II, 148–50.

145. See C. Clayson, *op. cit.* (note 11), 95. Clayson writes that 'Cullen's general

approach to medicine fits well with his benevolent personality. The burden
of his consultation letters indicates that balance and moderation in all
human activities were essential. Moderate meals secure health and promote
long life. In therapy he favoured only one drug at a time.'

146. Reverend Elliott to Dr Cullen, 14 August 1789, Towberry near Bambro; Box
    XVl, No. 135.

147. Cowmeadow to Dr Cullen, 1 September 1789, Berlin; Box XVI, No. 140.

148. In modern medical parlance, Cowmeadow suffers from reflux esophagitis
    (severe heartburn) and a spastic colon.

149. Jo. Rogers [*sic*] to Dr Cullen, 28 March 1774, Kelso; Box I, No. 155.

150. Cullen to Mr Cowmeadow, 16 September 1789; CL: 304–5. This letter is
    very faded and difficult to read, but one can make out the sense of the letter.

151. Charles Wedderburn to Dr Cullen, 7 July 1789, Buxton; Box XVI, No. 109.

152. See R. Porter, 'Consumption: Disease of the Consumer Society,' in J. Brewer
    and R. Porter, *Consumption and the World of Goods* (New York: Routledge,
    1993), 58–81.

153. Cullen to Charles Wedderburn, 14 July 1789; CL: 240–1.

154. Dr Armitstead to Dr Cullen, 6 September 1789, Lancaster; Box XVII: No.
    6. John Hunter was of equal fame as a medical man as his brother, William
    Hunter, was in surgery.

155. Cullen to Dr Armitstead at Lancaster, 16 September 1789; CL: No. 309.

156. Cullen to James Wood, 28 July 1789; CL: 254–5.

157. Dr Wood to Dr Cullen, 29 July 1789, Perth; Box XVI, No. 122

158. Jane Webster to Dr Cullen, 11 September 1780, York; Box VII:126.

159. Cullen to Jane Webster, 16 September 1780; CL, vol XI: p. 69

160. For the distinctions between eighteenth-century common and polite
    (courtly) prose, see C. McIntosh, *Common and Courtly Language: The
    Stylistics of Social Class in 18th-Century English Literature* (Philadelphia:
    University of Pennsylvania, 1986). This is discussed more fully in Chapter 3
    in regard to correspondence of Dr George Cheyne.

161. Mrs Pitodry to Dr Cullen, 24 February 1789, Aberdeen; Box XVI: 21

162. Cullen to Mrs Pitodry, 6 March1789; CL, Vol. 21: 99–100, .

163. Cullen to Mrs Pitodry, [?] May l789; CL, Vol. 21: 152

5

Literary Applications
of Medicine-by-Post

I believe I do amiss in writing so much, and taking too much upon me:
but an active mind, though clouded by bodily illness, cannot be idle.
Now I resume my trembling pen.

> Miss Clarissa Harlowe to Miss Howe
> Samuel Richardson, Clarissa [1]

The changing rhetoric of medicine-by-post over the course of the eighteenth century signified a shift in how patients and their doctors viewed the experience of illness. New rhetorical forms epitomised and reinforced evolving doctor conduct and simultaneously defined the reciprocal moral obligations of the patient in the therapeutic process. Enlightenment medical speculation combined with societal self-image and contemporary philosophical ideology produced a common language used with equal facility by the medical man and his clients. The public was well-educated on the notions of sensational physiology through the popularisation of Newton's *Opticks* and Locke's *Essay Concerning Human Understanding*, and they were regularly exposed to the rhetoric of medical theory through popular magazines. It is not surprising that literate members of British society – those who would engage in correspondence with their doctors – would negotiate medical experience using the fashions of contemporary medical rhetoric. It follows that this same borrowing would be mirrored in the novel and other literary genres.[2] Aileen Douglass observes, in her study of Tobias Smollett's representation of the sick and traumatised body, that 'medical and fictional writing shared, to at least some extent, the same audience.'[3]

Although I have joined the development of specific medicine-by-post rhetorical styles to particular decades, fashions overlapped during watershed periods. For example, the novelists Samuel Richardson (1689–1761) and Henry Fielding (1707–54) were contemporaries who differed radically in their representations of illness and their adoption of medical rhetorical conventions. While Richardson embraced the rhetoric of medical sensibility modelled in the writings of George Cheyne, Fielding's novels remained firmly entrenched in the rhetoric of iatromechanical persuasion.

243

Richardson's last novel, *The History of Sir Charles Grandison* (1754) was completed the same year in which Fielding composed his final work, *The Journal of a Voyage to Lisbon*; but while Richardson remained devoted to Cheyne's medico-spiritual philosophy and language, Fielding regarded the Bath physician as a figure of ridicule, especially in the matter of his rhetorical idiosyncrasies. In a *Champion* article of 17 May 1740 (No. 80), Fielding imagines Colley Cibber, the English Poet Laureate, put on trial for his abuse of the English tongue, but a 'critic' testifies that Cibber's faults must be judged favourably compared to the famous Dr Cheyne:

> the English language has had more violence done it by a very great and eminent physician, who is MD CR EdS and FRS, than by the prisoner at the bar, for though the prisoner certainly left several sore places in it, yet the condition he left it, it might be understood, and sometimes expressed itself with vigour; but the MD &c. hath so mangled and mauled it, that when I came to examine the body, as it lay in sheets in the bookseller's shop, I found it an expiring heavy lump, without the least appearance of sense.[4]

Fielding was eager to distinguish himself from his literary rival, Richardson, in every respect – moral, philosophical, social, and rhetorical. Although Fielding was as eclectic in his sources of medical advice as any other eighteenth-century patient, he dismissed the 'nervous sensibility' of Cheyne and Richardson as foolish, even in his one sentimental novel, *Amelia* (1751).[5]

In *The Journal of a Voyage to Lisbon*, Fielding clearly shows his adherence to the principles and rhetoric of iatromechanical medicine. The author dispassionately describes his own bloated and dissipated body. The intention of his detailed report is not to elicit sympathy at the end of life but to represent, graphically, the ongoing physical decline of his body with the same objectivity that he describes his own past accomplishments as a magistrate: 'I relate facts plainly and simply as they are, and let the world draw from them what conclusions they please.'[6] While Fielding encourages the reader to see the author's wasting as a metaphor for societal ills, the account remains grounded in the reality of medical detail, in shifting fluids and wasting limbs: 'I saw the dropsy gaining rather than losing ground; the distance growing shorter between the tappings.'[7] Even his jaundiced eyes do not colour experience but are a physical fact like any other: 'I was now, in the opinion of all men, dying of a complication of disorders' he writes, but assures the reader that this journal is not to be compromised by sentimentality.[8]

Fielding describes his illness variously as a 'gout', 'dropsy', and 'jaundice'; in modern pathological terminology, his condition is clearly a cirrhosis of the liver complicated by ascites, the accumulation of a massive amount of fluid in the abdomen. His doctors resort both to instrumentation (the trochar) to remove fluid directly and to various nostrums, including the Duke of Portland's medicine, Ward's pills, and even (with the author's expressed scepticism) Bishop Berkeley's tar-water. In addition to the ship's surgeon, Fielding consults his own favourite surgeon, John Ranby (Principal Sergeant-Surgeon to the King), and asks advice of the popular 'irregular' physician Joshua Ward, some unnamed 'Physical friends', and the 'very eminent' William Hunter.[9] Despite this very eclectic array of medical opinion, the author's own medical descriptions remain firmly rooted in new science rhetoric with its aura of clinical detachment.

We recognise that these final months must have been a most miserable time for Fielding, yet we are never invited to read spiritual meaning into illness or to overreact to Fielding account: 'By Dr Joshua Ward's advice I was tapped, and fourteen quarts of water drawn from my belly. The sudden relaxation which this caused, added to my enervate, emaciated habit of body, so weakened me, that within two days I was thought to be falling into the agonies of death.' But recovery follows and 'I began slowly, as it were, to draw my feet out of the grave; till in two month's time I had again acquired some little degree of strength; but was again full of water.'[10] Tom Keymer has pointed out, most cogently, that Fielding, the author–patient, 'turns a cool scrutiny on the repulsiveness of this decay' of his body, that he 'measures his periodic draining of excess fluid' with a 'statistical rigour chillingly reminiscent of the bills of mortality used by Defoe to punctuate and calibrate his reports' in *Journal of the Plague Year*.[11] In a remarkable passage, in which Fielding relates his dreadful state as he is hoisted up the ship's side with a makeshift winch, his clinical objectivity would dissolve quickly into pathos if it were not for the author's insistence on a 'cool scrutiny' reinforced by tongue-in-cheek humour:

> I presented a spectacle of the highest horror. The total loss of limbs was apparent to all who saw me, and my face contained marks of a most diseased state, if not of death itself. Indeed, so ghastly was my countenance, that timorous women with child had abstained from my house, for fear of the ill consequences of looking at me.[12]

Fielding takes the same rhetorical tone that we saw in the medicine-by-post letters of Shallett Turner to James Jurin concerning Shallett's consumptive symptoms – as if the patient were the physician standing at his own bedside: 'I think my illness grows upon me, and I observe my self to waste and fall away in flesh very much.'[13] Keymer has observed rightly that, 'It is as though the act of writing, of subjecting pain to the control of a measured language, enables Fielding to confront his predicament with a directness impossible in daily life.'[14] .

In *Tom Jones,* illness and injuries, and even death, serve only as brief interruptions in the progress of the plot, defining character only in that truly good people – those without hypocrisy – make little fuss about such things. When Captain Blifil fails to return home for dinner one evening – the reader knows he has succumbed to a sudden apoplexy contemplating the fortune that would befall him on the death of his brother-in-law, Mr Allworthy – Mrs Blifil flies into a histrionic display of anxiety while her brother only grows more subdued with concern. A Lady companion advises Mrs Blifil that 'her Brother's Example ought to teach her Patience, who, though indeed he could not be supposed as much concerned as herself, yet was doubtless very uneasy, though his Resignation to the Divine Will and restrained his grief within due Bounds.' Mrs Blifil responds: 'Mention not my Brother... I alone am the Object of your Pity.'[15] When Tom breaks his arm rescuing Sophia from a riding accident, he reassures her: 'If I have broken my Arm, I consider it as a Trifle, in Comparison of what I feared on your Account' (200). Sophia herself is only aggravated by the Surgeon attending her after this mishap who multiplies reassurances about his skill in bleeding patients until '*Sophia* declared she was not under the least Apprehension', adding 'if you open an Artery, I promise you I'll forgive you' (203). Later in the novel, Tom disregards, for many pages, what is clearly a severe head injury after Ensign Adderly has hurled a bottle at our hero in a dispute on Sophia's moral virtue.

When Mr Allworthy comes down with a cold and fever, we are told that 'This he had, however, neglected, as was usual with him to do all Manner of Disorders which did not confine him to his Bed, or prevent his several Faculties from performing their ordinary Functions' (240). In this case, however, Allworthy is forced to his bed and to call for the doctor, and the narrator reminds us that, 'surely the Gentlemen of the Æsculapian Art are in the Right in advising, that the Moment the Disease is entered at one Door, the Physician should be introduced at the other' (240). The doctor warns the patient that he is 'in very imminent Danger' (241) – a habit of professional pessimism, the narrator advises, which is shared by the physician and the 'wise General' who know it is best to overestimate the foe so that 'by these Means the greater Glory redounds to them if thy gain the Victory, and the less Disgrace if by any unlucky Accident they should happen to be conquered' (249). Allworthy, however, thoroughly at peace with himself, and untroubled by the prospect of mortality, 'received this Information with utmost Calmness and Unconcern' (241). He attends to the practical matters of saying farewell to his family members and clarifying the intentions in his will. Allworthy's calm resignation presages the mood of *The Journal of a*

Voyage to Lisbon and Fielding's own stoical acceptance of his failing body. Illness in *Tom Jones* then, as in the case of the beloved Allworthy, is only a mechanical failing of the body that underscores what we already know about the virtues or vices of a character. Hypocrisy is confirmed, simplicity and honesty appreciated. In contrast to the fulsome attentions of the surgeon bleeding Sophia, Fielding praises the authentic medical knowledge and humanitarian qualities of his friend, the surgeon John Ranby, who is 'the first Character in his Profession,... [a] very generous, good-natured Man, and ready to do any service to his Fellow-Creatures' (468).

In Fielding's only sentimental novel, *Amelia* (1751), Fielding also represents the best in the medical profession in the character of the doctor who attends the heroine who has fainted upon learning that Booth intends to repair to his regiment in Gibraltar:

> Of all Mankind the Doctor is the best of Comforters. As his excessive Good-nature makes him take vast Delight in the Office; so his great Penetration into the human Mind, joined to his great Experience, renders him the most Proficient in it; and he so well knows when to sooth, when to reason, and when to ridicule, that he never applies any of those Arts improperly... and which requires very great Judgment and Dexterity to avoid.[16]

Although stricken by the grave news of Booth's departure, Amelia's physical disturbance is transient and made light of by the excellent doctor who 'principally applied himself to ridiculing the Dangers of the Siege, in which he succeeded so well, that he sometimes forced a Smile even into the Face of *Amelia*.' The heroine is allowed only a very brief hysterical fit and quickly pulls herself together. Meanwhile, the men in this story – despite the serious tone of the novel as compared to Fielding's other works – dismiss their various physical wounds with much the same indifference of the protagonists of sound character in *Tom Jones*, who make light of physical hurts and accept even severe illness with a benign resignation.[17]

In the fiction of Fielding and Defoe, infirmity and physical trauma mostly serve to illuminate basic character traits, and in their non-fiction works, illness becomes a metaphor for the character of a society. But in Samuel Richardson's novels, illness is inextricably entwined with character development, a test of character more than a revelation. It therefore serves Richardson's novelistic intention that bodily hardship should become more metaphorical than physical and an ultimate challenge to personal morality and individual strength of character. Van Sant suggests that Richardson borrowed from the experimental models of medicine in which truth about the nervous system is discovered through painful stimuli: there is a 'revelation of the heart through entrapment and trial' in *Clarissa*.[18]

Ultimately, Clarissa's terminal illness is an escape from that very physical world in which she has been put to such a cruel test; illness is transformed by the language of sensibility, in which a shock to the nerves is sufficient to explain the slow and progressive release of life from the heroine's body. Clarissa is increasingly defined by the departure of physical sensation and desire. For Clarissa there is no pleasure in food, a subject of great importance to Fielding in *Tom Jones* and in *The Journal of a Voyage to Lisbon*. Instead, for Clarissa, eating is translated into an act of obligation to others. Mr Goddard, the apothecary advises:

> The lady... will do very well if she will resolve upon it herself. Indeed you will, madam. The doctor is entirely of this opinion; and has ordered nothing for you but weak jellies, and innocent cordials, lest you should starve yourself. And, let me tell you, madam, that so much watching, so little nourishment, and so much grief as you seem to indulge, is enough to impair the most vigorous health, and to wear out the strongest constitution.

> What, sir, said she, can I do? I have no appetite. Nothing you call nourishing will stay on my stomach. I do what I can: and have such kind directors in Dr H. and you, that I should be inexcusable if I did not.[19]

The food offered to Clarissa itself becomes metaphorical for her condition, 'Weak jellies and innocent cordials' with hardly any substance or body. Yet, as discussed in Chapter 1 of this book, Clarissa is determined to meet her moral obligation to doctor, friend, and even her cruel family, by being a compliant patient. It is, also, a religious obligation that Clarissa feels she must not intentionally precipitate her own demise. As in the medical writings and medicine-by-post of George Cheyne, diet becomes a moral obligation for the well-being of physical body but goes hand-in-hand with the spiritual fortitude necessary to endure physical trials in the patient of sensibility.

Clarissa is keenly aware of the mind–body connection of her illness. She writes to Mrs Norton that her current state should not be attributed to 'gloominess or melancholy' even though 'it was *brought on* by disappointment (the world showing me early, even at my first *rushing* into it, its true and ugly face).' Furthermore:

> I have as humane a physician (whose fees are his least regard) and as worthy an apothecary, as ever a patient was visited by. My nurse is diligent, obliging, silent, and sober. So I am not unhappy *without* : and *within* – I hope, my dear Mrs Norton, that I shall be every day more and more happy *within.*[20]

Richardson, through Clarissa, instructs the reader that a person of delicate nerves is subject to real illness through the shocks of experience – physical and mental – but that the soul can rise above bodily cares. That same complex relationship of mind and body which pervades the writing of Cheyne is ubiquitous in Richardson's novels.

A dualism of mind and body asserts itself in states of morbidity, and as the epigraph to this chapter indicates, the mind resists idleness just because the body is debilitated. At the same time, body and soul must each be attended to in illness; neither can be neglected without impunity.

There is a temptation, however, when considering Richardson's representation of illness, to minimise the physical. Richardson provides us with a gruesome account of the 'dreadful agonies' suffered by the soulless Belton on his deathbed. He is 'never free of these horrible pains in my stomach and head.' Belton suffers from 'convulsions, terrible convulsions! for an hour past. Oh Lord! Lovelace, death is a shocking thing! By my faith it is!' writes Belford, and at the final moments:

> He is now at his last gasp – rattles in his throat: has a new convulsion every minute almost. What horror is he in! His eyes look like breath-stained glass! They roll ghastly no more; are quite set: his face distorted and drawn out by his sinking jaws and erected eyebrows, with his lengthened furrowed forehead.... [21]

Belton, in contrast to Clarissa, rages against the medical profession which can provide him no relief. His pain is unremitting and disfigures his body because the needs of the soul have not been consulted and nurtured; he is distressingly unprepared for either infirmity or his own mortality because he has been a 'free-liver', a term used by both Richardson and Cheyne.[22] Belford turns Belton's final illness into an allegory much approved by the attending physician:

> [T]hat the 'seeds of death are sown in us when we begin life,' and if the flower of life is not to be choked prematurely by the 'rampant weeds' that persist in our bodies, we must know our own constitutions and 'root out by temperance, the weeds which the soil is most apt to produce; or at least keep them down as they rise: and not, when the flower or plant is withered at the root, and the weed in full vigour, expect that medical art will restore the one or destroy the other.'[23]

This is certainly a page from Cheyne.

Clarissa's illness is not without physical symptoms, and these are also detailed by Belford. But Clarissa's moral spirit, and her ready acceptance of the limits of the physical body, compensate for bodily discomfort and increasing frailty. In her last days there is no disfigurement but only a supple beauty associated with serenity, even though it is made clear that Clarissa must endure much in the way of physical hardship:

> I am thinking... what a gradual and happy death God almighty (blessed be his Name!) affords me! Who would have thought... I should be so long a dying! – But see how little by little it has come to this. I was first taken off from the power of *walking*: then I took a *coach* – a coach grew too violent an exercise: then I took a *chair* – The prison was a large DEATH-STRIDE upon me – I should have *suffered longer else!* Next, I was unable to go to church ; and a *less* room will soon hold me [her coffin] – My *eyes* begin to fail me, so that at times I cannot see to read distinctly; and now I can hardly *write* or hold a pen – Next, I presume, I shall know nobody, nor be able to thank any of you.... And thus by little and little, in such a gradual sensible death as I am blessed with, God dies away in us, as I may say, all human satisfactions, in order to subdue his poor creatures to Himself.[24]

The measured downward spiral in physical self-sufficiency culminates in the inability to write; as death nears, Clarissa says that, 'my fingers' ends seem numbed – have no feeling! ... 'Tis time to send the letter to my good Mrs Norton,' a letter she has intended to be forwarded at her imminent demise.[25] Clarissa, then, remains a woman fully conscious of her physical body even as she is about to depart that body. It is fitting in a medicine of 'nervous sensibility' that the last sensations to be relinquished in this 'gradual sensible death' are purely of the nervous system – the feeling in her fingers and the ability to recognise those about her. In the death scene tableaux, Clarissa says that 'My sight fails me! – Your voices only...'. Finally there is only the touching of hands of those in the room, till at last she is 'holding up her almost lifeless hands for the last time,' calls the name of Jesus, and expires. Touch is the critical sense of the eighteenth century, and it is with touch and the loss of touch that Clarissa leaves the physical world.[26] Richardson's novel is, finally, a supreme example of the use of the melding of actual medical convention with literary convention.

In *Clarissa,* it is only in death that the heroine is able to reclaim her rightful place back within the society that has rejected and abandoned her in life. Richardson's other major heroine, Pamela, from his earlier novel *Pamela, or Virtue Rewarded* (1940), also seeks a secure place in society, but in a class above her own station. Like Clarissa, Pamela suffers intolerable abuse at the hands of a rake who assumes his behaviour is condoned, ignored or even admired by the society he moves in. While an episode of illness is not crucial to Pamela's narrative, yet it clearly serves to accentuate her ongoing moral conflict in her trials with Mr B. Frustrated in her attempt to escape the grounds, injured and in despair, Pamela even contemplates suicide by throwing herself into a stream. She considers that '*these bruises* and *maims*' may exculpate the sin in God's eyes, so that 'spotless and unguilty' she would surrender her life. But she turns from this extreme action and limps over to a wood-house where she is found and returned to the house, and where she 'fainted away, with dejection, pain, and fatigue' and becomes 'very feverish, and aguishly inclined'. The importance of this illness is that, though brief, it serves to punctuate Pamela's moral crisis; it marks the start of a new moral maturity that finally earns her a place in upper-class society by demonstrated virtue of character: without suicide she will prove that she 'is no hypocrite, nor deceiver; but really... the innocent creature she pretended to be!'[27]

Despite important differences, in both *Pamela* and *Clarissa* illness constitutes a private space that speaks back to contemporary society in the form of a moral exemplum. Although Richardson's main interest lies with the moral and spiritual fortitude of his protagonists, it is misguided societal values that create the severe trials experienced by both heroines. In this respect, illness in the novel of sensibility is no longer, as in Fielding or Defoe, primarily a 'public' mode of social comment (serious or satirical), but rather illness has become – to invert Fielding's claim for *Joseph Andrews* – more a measure of the individual than the species.[28]

The late eighteenth-century novel, like the medicine of the period, is a reinvented amalgam of the public and the private space. Personal illness and societal health are intertwined more tightly than at any other time in the century, such that illness no longer stands outside the mainstream – as a crisis, a metaphor, or a moral trial – but it stands adjacent to the everyday activity. One consequence is that in the works of Burney, Smollett, and other late Enlightenment novelists, a cure is signalled most surely by the return of the patient, in some fashion, to their society, a condition not at all relevant in the works of Defoe, Fielding, or Richardson. In some cases, as in Burney's *Cecilia*, societal health is simultaneously restored with that of the patient.

In *Cecilia, or Memoirs of an Heiress* (1782) Burney details three episodes in which main characters fall ill and require the services of the 'worthy' and humane' Dr Lyster. In all three cases a physical illness is precipitated by a combination of psychological and social upset, confirming a continued belief in the intimate connection of mind and body as well as the individual and society. In each episode there is dramatic perturbation on the part of concerned family, friends, and lovers, and the physician must use his skills to tend to their emotional and social needs as much as to the physical and social status of the patient. Throughout, the doctor remains a voice of reason and practical advice amidst the hysteria of those close to the patient. Illness in this novel takes on a social significance that is probably more important than the personal physical suffering of the patient.

In the first event, Delville catches a cold after escorting Cecilia back to the Delville mansion through a fierce summer storm during which he stands between her and the full force of the hailstones. As they make their way to the house, Delville expresses his passion for Cecilia, but she is only confused and upset by his alternately tender and aloof attitude towards her, so she determines to find her own way back to the Delville mansion alone. Cecilia and Lady Honoraria, who also had been exposed to the foul weather, are inconvenienced by minor colds, but over the next days 'the health of Delville seemed to suffer with his mind, and though he refused to acknowledge he was ill, it was evident to everybody that he was far from well.'[29] Subsequently, Delville 'acknowledged in answer to his mother's earnest enquiries that he had a cold and head-ache: and had he, at the same time, acknowledged a pleurisy and fever, the alarm instantly spread in the family could not have been greater.' The exaggerated response of the protective parents is noted by Cecilia: 'she believed his illness and his uneasiness were the same,... while the terrors of Mr and Mrs Delville seemed so greatly beyond the occasion that her own were rather lessened than encreased [*sic*] by them' (482). Enter Dr Lyster who immediately establishes himself as a gentleman-physician of great tact, good humour, and much heart. While Delville tries to dismiss his illness as trivial, insisting he is well enough to play the role of physician himself if only he had the training, Dr Lyster answers, 'What with such a hand as this?... come, come, you must not teach me my own profession. When I attend a patient, I come to tell how he is myself, not to be told' (483). When, in great agitation, Delville's mother cries, 'He is, then ill!... oh Mortimer, why have you thus deceived us!' and her husband is about to send for more consultants, Dr Lyster's responds unperturbed, 'What now?... must a man be dying if he is not in perfect health? we want nobody else; I hope I can prescribe for a cold without demanding a consultation?' He insists, 'let us all sit down, and behave like Christians: I never talk of my art before company. 'Tis hard you won't let me be a gentleman at large for two minutes' (483).

Dr Lyster assumes his place not only in society, but, as it turns out, in the family's deepest emotional concerns. He is next called when Mrs Delville has suffered an apoplexy when her son refuses to give up Cecilia – 'Grief and horror next to frenzy at a disappointment unexpected ... striking her hand upon her forehead, cried "My brain is on fire!" and rushed out of the room.' She is found 'extended upon the floor, her face; hands and neck all covered with blood!' (680). Dr Lyster reassures Cecilia that Mrs Delville will recover and then reveals (after some distracting humour) that he knew 'from the moment I attended Mr Mortimer in his illness at Delville-Castle... that the seat of his disorder was his mind' – that passion for Cecilia which the doctor now discourages because of the extreme anguish such a match would cause

252

Deville's parents.[30] Yet it is also Dr Lyster who, while attending Cecilia through her madness, fever, and near death at the close of the novel – a time of emotional frenzy for Delville and other of Cecilia's friends – is the main force in reconciling father and son and arranging for a happy conclusion. Burney has seen fit for Dr Lyster – the healer of social as well as physical disorder – to announce the moral of the story: that 'The whole of this unfortunate business... has been the result of PRIDE and PREJUDICE' (930). Throughout the extremes of emotional response to events and to illness, Dr Lyster retains a sympathetic heart and a rational head, a kind authority, and a sense of the larger social scene. He is the ideal of the Enlightenment physician at the close of the century, and in manner and tone that greatly resembles Dr William Cullen as reflected in his consultation letters (see Chapter 4).

The drama that attends illness in *Cecilia* perfectly reflects the intense expression of sensibility that flourished in the second half of the eighteenth century, while in Delville senior we can see elements of that irritability, even irascibility, so characteristic in the novels of Tobias Smollett. Not only is Delville quick on the servant bell to call in other consultants for his son, but he himself is suffering 'a severe fit of the gout', and Dr Lyster tells Cecilia, 'I found him in an agitation of spirits that made me apprehend it would be thrown into his stomach' (690). But it is characteristic of Dr Lyster that he should be as sympathetic and attentive to Mr Delville's histrionics as to the needs of his other patients; he is prepared for the full range of human response to illness, including the commotion it causes among family and friends. Importantly, like the novelist, he is skilled at recognising how social disturbance participates in causing physical distress.

While the character of Yorick in Lawrence Sterne's *The Journal to Eliza* (1767) parodies the extremes of the 'man of sensibility', Yorick articulates many sentiments familiar to the reader who follows the rocky recuperation of the cranky Matthew Bramble in Tobias Smollett's, *The Expedition of Humphry Clinker*. When Yorick is told by his doctors that he suffers from lues, his indignation about the 'imputation' of venereal disease recalls a similar vigorous posturing in the case of author Smollett, himself a patient, exclaiming against the diagnosis of tuberculosis by the 'insolent' Dr Fizes.[31]

In *The Journal to Eliza*, Yorick reports with great consternation:

> The Injury I did myself upon catching cold upon Jame's pouder, fell, you
> must know, upon the worst part it could, – the most painful, and most
> dangerous of any of the human Body – It was on this Crisis, I call'd in an
> able Surgeon and with him an able physician (both my friends) to inspect my
> disaster – 'tis a venerial Case, cried my two Scientifick friends. – 'tis
> impossible. at least to be that, replied I – for I have had no commerce

whatever with the Sex – not even my wife, added I, these 15 years – You are *****, however my good friend said the Surgeon, or there is no such Case in the world – what the Devil! said I without knowing a Woman – we will not reason about it, said the Physician, but you must undergo a course of Mercury, – I'll lose my life first, said I, – and trust to Nature, to Time – or at the worst – to Death, – so I put an end with some Indignation to the Conference; and determined to bear all the torments I underwent, and ten times more rather than, submit to be treated as a *Sinner*, in a point where I had acted like a *Saint.* Now as the father of mischief would have it, who has no pleasure like that of dishonouring the righteous – it so fell out, That from The moment I dismiss'd my Doctors – my pains began to rage with a violence not to be express'd, or supported. [E]very hour became more intolerable – I was got to bed – cried out and raved the whole night – and was got up near dead, That my friends insisted upon sending again for my Physician and Surgeon – [32]

Yorick is not mollified by the information that the infection may have 'laid dormant 20 Years' in the blood. The doctors, in frustration, forego debate with the patient, 'wherein I was so delicate' (142). But within a few days, Yorick confesses, 'I fear I have relapsed', and 'I'm still to be treated as if I was a Sinner – and in truth have some appearances so strongly implying it.' But if he had any real doubts, of course he would immediately visit Montpellier, 'where maladies of this sort are better treated and all taints more radically driven out of the Blood.' Yorick concludes that he will go to Montpellier in any case if symptoms persist, 'for the bettering my Constitution by a better Climate,' adding dramatically that 'I write this as I lie upon my back – in which posture I must continue, I fear some days – If I am able – will take up my pen again before night' (149). In the style of late-eighteenth-century medical rhetoric in medicine-by-post letters, Yorick is not only insistently dramatic but has read up enough to know the best places and climates to seek for cure.

Yorick's offence at the presumptive diagnosis of syphilis by his doctors also recalls Matthew Bramble's outrage with 'the famous Dr L___n, who is come to ply at the Well for patients.' In Smollett's epistolary novel, Jery Melford muses on the character of his uncle: 'I think his peevishness arises partly from bodily pain, and partly from a natural excess of mental sensibility; for, I suppose, the mind as well as the body, is in some cases endued with a morbid excess of sensation.'[33] Jery describes in some detail his uncle's discomfiture at receiving the unsolicited consultation from Dr L___n. Bramble is singled out at the baths and diagnosed with a 'dropsical habit' which is likely to proceed to an 'confirmed *ascites*' ; furthermore, ventures the mountebank physician, Bramble may well be exhibiting a case of oedema, gout, or even *lues venera*. For the latter Dr L__n offers his own fail-proof pills. With the same vehemence as Yorick reacted to his doctors, Bramble writes to Dr Lewis that Dr L__n is obviously a charlatan, yet Bramble compulsively returns to the episode in the baths, wanting reassurance from his own doctor that all is well – perhaps, as we discover later, because he is now worried about the consequences of his years of free-living (20 April, Hot Well; 24–6). Bramble, however, remains true-to-character: 'It makes me sick to hear people talk of the fine air upon Clifton-Downs: how can the air be either agreeable or salutary, where the dæmon of vapours descends in perpetual drizzle?' (17 April, Clifton; 13). Despite the great differences in their personalities, it seems that in matters of health and illness the fictional characters Bramble and Yorick share a most similar dramatic rhetoric, one in keeping with actual medicine-by-post letters of the period as seen in many of the more dramatic letters from patients to Dr William Cullen (see Chapter 4).

Smollett and Sterne, as late-eighteenth-century authors, share with Fanny Burney the view of illness as inseparable from the social environment. However, both Sterne and Smollett are more attuned to the effects of physical environment than Burney, and both are distinctly wary of becoming overly incorporated into society at the loss of one's own individuality, even eccentricity. As Aileen Douglass explains in *Uneasy Sensations: Smollett and the Body*, Smollett's novels are primarily interested in the necessary conflict between the individual body and the societal body. Smollett is uncompromising in reminding his readers of the physical reality of the body – so regularly and violently abused in his novels; and to this inescapable fact of physicality Smollett opposes the artificial, abstract notions of the body that societal institutions try to impose on the individual. In his novels, the body is relentlessly subject to its environment: to climate, to economic conditions, to culture, and to both large- and small-scale social interactions. In the *Travels through France and Italy*, the author simultaneously asserts the universality of physical experience in peoples of different countries while detailing how specific cultures temper physical being in unique ways. In *The Expedition of Humphry Clinker*, Matthew Bramble regularly alludes to the direct relationship of his immediate social environment to the state of his health; a medical downturn may be precipitated by proximity to a noxious public who populates a particular spa town during the 'season', or else by the vexations caused by his immediate family, and especially by the intrigues of the females in his entourage.[34] In all this, Smollett's view of illness remains entirely consistent with Scottish Enlightenment medicine with its intense interest in environment and society as integral and inseparable from matters of individual physiology and health, so well illustrated in the medical lectures of William Cullen to his medical students in Edinburgh.

Although Smollett would not enjoy comparison to Sterne, and while Sterne would abhor any suggestion of similarity with Tobias Smollett – whom he satirised as the impossibly splenetic and 'jaundiced' Smelfungus of *A Sentimental Journey* – these authors clearly share medical ideas about the manifestations of sensibility and the relationship of health to environmental and social circumstance. Yorick's physical body in *A Sentimental Journey* is, like Bramble's in Smollett's novel, a most sensitive barometer of his environment; for both characters, illness is an assertion of their uniqueness at the same time that they define themselves through membership within society. Illness is therefore a form of social commentary for both Sterne and Smollett that differs noticeably from the circumscribed upset to daily routine (even if in a major way) that we read about in Defoe or Fielding, or the isolated test of character as it is for Richardson, in whose novels societal ills are merely the backdrop to personal experience. Even Richardson's famous friend, Dr Cheyne, while diagnosing an 'English Malady', accepts as matter-of-fact the environmental state of affairs created by national wealth and diet and directs his medical advice to the individual rather than to the society at large. For Richardson and Cheyne, sensibility and illness remains largely a private affair while for the late-eighteenth-century writer – as for Sterne, Smollett, and Burney, each in their own way – private illness and personal sensibility must regularly reckon with the larger environment.

I began this chapter with Fielding's personal testimony of illness, *The Journal of a Voyage to Lisbon*, and I would like to conclude with another personal testament, Frances Burney's account, written to her sister, Esther, of her mastectomy which took place 30 September 1811. The significance of Burney's extended letter – 'this miserable account, which I began 3 Months ago, at least'[35] – is that it contains all those elements characteristic of medicine-by-post in the last decades of the eighteenth century: the idea of illness as narrative drama, as something to be shared; the rhetoric of sensibility combined with a firm sense of utility and practicality; the frank language (by a woman) about the experience of her body; and the awareness of illness as integral not only to one's immediate family and friends but reflecting the qualities of the larger society in which one lives.

A postscript to the initial pages of Burney's letter, posted to Esther before the remainder of the letter was completed, is revealing. She writes, 'I have promised my dearest Esther a Volume – & here it is: I am at this moment quite Well.... Read, therefore, this Narrative at your leisure, & without emotion – for all has ended happily. I will send the rest by the very first opportunity....' (615). Burney regards the 'miserable account' of her illness as a 'narrative' to be read as such. Despite her claim that 'I fear this is all written – confusedly' (614), the letter to Esther is crafted as finely as any novel; it is an account that is intended to have enormous emotional effect on its readers. Indeed, Burney is well aware that her 'narrative' is not for her sister's eyes alone, but will be passed on to other acquaintances: 'you will lend it also to my tender & most beloved Mrs Angerstein,... I leave all others, & all else, to your own decision' (615). Burney's combines excruciating objective clinical detail with her own emotional terror as the subject of the surgery to create one of the most startling and dramatic accounts of surgery ever rendered to paper:

> Yet – when the dreadful steel was plunged into the breast – cutting through veins – arteries – flesh – nerves – I needed no injunctions not to restrain my cries. I began a scream that lasted unintermittingly during the whole time of the incision – & I almost marvel that it rings not in my Ears still! so excruciating was the agony. When the wound was made, & the instrument was withdrawn, the pain seemed undiminished, for the air that suddenly rushed into those delicate parts felt like a mass of minute but sharp & forked poniards, that were tearing the edges of the wound – but when I felt the instrument – describing a curve – cutting against the grain, if I may say, while flesh resisted in a manner so forcible as to oppose & tire the hand of the operator, who was forced to change from the right to the left – then, indeed, I thought I must have expired. (612)

The all-too-vivid description of the mastectomy captures the exquisite pain experienced by the patient with an effect that discredits any suggestion of 'confusion' on the part of the writer. The effect is calculated. Furthermore, the shock of the surgery is augmented by the deliberately paced medical history of the events in the months, days, and hours preceding the operation. The reader is put through intolerable suspense – reliving with Burney the agony of multiple consultations as the doctors determine whether or not to operate, and then keep their patient in the dark as to the actual hour of the mastectomy in order to spare her, so they believe, the anticipation! Burney is both detached observer and heroine of her narrative, a mind at once detached from the body but imprisoned within it.

The continued public nature of illness is not only demonstrated by Burney's instructions to her sister to share her letter with others, but also in the opening section of the letter in which Burney says that she realises that any idea of keeping this matter private is impossible. However, this fact does not negate Burney's original desire to have her illness remain a private matter – restricted, at most, to a very few of her dearest acquaintances. She had hoped to protect her aging parents from the shock of the news, and therefore had remained quiet till now, but she wonders 'how can I hope they will escape hearing what has reached Seville to the South, and Constantinople to the East?' Burney realises that her secret is surely not safe when 'I heard that

M. d Boinville had written it to his Wife' (598). She uses the fact of public knowledge about her case as a reason to set the record straight, from her own hand – much as Cheyne argued that it was better that he should give the public an accurate account of the medical history of some of his private patients and, of course, their cure through his hands, before some unauthorised pirate printer did so. It is also clear from the start of Burney's narrative that numerous friends have been invited by M. Arblay to advise her on seeking medical attention for the breast lump which Burney has denied as a serious problem. Close women friends, we discover, have offered their services throughout the patient's ordeal and have supported her emotionally, but also practically – bringing dressings for after surgery, or helping Burney to attend to family business. It is, therefore, only the physician who is required to maintain absolute confidentiality within the new medical ethic, and this is because of the special regard he must show for the patient's feelings, not because private illness has gone underground as a social topic.

The language of Burney's narrative combines rigorous objectivity with high emotion and also makes unabashed use of the rhetoric of sensibility. The latter is especially well conveyed by Burney's description of the surgeon, M. Larrey, who performs the role of the physician of sensibility in his every word and gesture. M. Larrey is introduced as:

> [O]ne of the worthiest, most disinterested, & singularly excellent of men, endowed with real genius in his profession, though with an ignorance of the World & its usages that indices a *naiveté* that leads those who do not see him thoroughly to think him not alone simple, but weak. They are mistaken; but his attention & thoughts having exclusively turned one way, he is hardly awake any other (601).

When combined consultation confirms Burney's worst fear, surgery, 'the good Dr Larrey, who, during his long attendance had conceived for me the warmest friendship, had now tears in his Eyes; from my dread he had expected resistance.' He proposes recalling the famous accoucheur M. Dubois, for yet another opinion, even though M. Larrey, 'this modest man,' Burney explains, is himself the 'premier chirugien de la Garde Imperiale, & had been lately created a Baron for his eminent services!' (603).

Modesty and friendship is accompanied with the utmost sensibility. The surgeon 'hid himself nearly behind my sofa' as the verdict for surgery is conclusive (604). Burney learns sometime after the surgery from M. Larrey that he was advised by M. Dubois that the cancer was probably too advanced for surgery to be beneficial, and that 'M. Larrey was so deeply affected by this sentence, that... he regretted to his Soul ever having known me, & was upon the point of demanding a commission to the furthest end of France in order to force me into other hands' (607). But ultimately, M. Larrey sends a letter to his patient to expect surgery and that she should 'rely as much upon his sensibility & his prudence, as upon his dexterity & his experience' (608). Near the end of the twenty minute ordeal, Burney, whose vision has been blocked by a veil draped over her head, makes out the voice of 'Mr Larry... in a tone nearly tragic, desire every one present to pronounce if anything more remained to be done;... & again began the scraping!' It is '*very* principally meant for Dr Larry,' for his benefit and relief, that Burney exerts herself at the end of the operation to say, 'Ah Messieurs! que je vous plains!' [Ah, Messieurs! How I pity you!] (612–13).

Sensibility is not limited to M. Larrey, but pervades the scene, as in the fragile emotions of Burney's husband, M. Arblay, whom the patient protects from the horrors of the surgery in every way possible. Even the severe accoucheur, M. Dubois, while demanding that faithful servants leave the room where he prepares the patient for surgery, is forced to drop his authoritarian aspect entirely when his patient pleads, 'Can *You*.... feel for an operation that, to *You* must seem so trivial? – Trivial? he repeated – taking up a bit of paper, which he tore, unconsciously, into a million of pieces, *oui – c'est peu de chose – mais –* ' [it is a trivial matter – but –] he stammered, & could not go on' (611). In the end, sensibility triumphs over the horrors of Burney's physical experience, counterbalances the pain and the fear, by becoming intimately bound up in that experience.

Whether in Fielding's account of his final months in *The Journal of a Voyage to Lisbon*, or in the correspondence between George Cheyne and RIchardson, or in Burney's description of her mastectomy, we are offered a glimpse of the actuality of illness for eighteenth-century authors who were influenced by different fashions of medical speculation and rhetoric during the course of the century. Such influence on the expression of illness by these authors in their novels is unmistakable. The examination of medicine-by-post contemporaneous with these authors defines most precisely the meaning of illness for these authors as represented in their fiction.

Although we expect that moral and social issues will colour the description of illness in the eighteenth-century novel, it is also clear that changing medical speculation, and its associated rhetoric, in different decades of the Enlightenment modulated the meanings of illness in the public consciousness. The different significance of illness in *Tom Jones*, *Clarissa*, *Cecilia*, or *The Expedition of Humphry Clinker*, are all clearly derived from a medical Zeitgeist that resonated with real patients and shaped their rhetoric. Doctors, meanwhile, preserved their practices by announcing themselves as representatives of the social ideals of a given cultural moment. Illness, in the eighteenth century, was a collaborative effort between doctor, patient, and society, in which rhetoric played a vital role in the absence of meaningful therapy. In fact, rhetoric was the mainstay of eighteenth-century therapeutics – what gave form and meaning to illness, to the doctor–patient relationship, and what, in short, provided ultimate relief in times of physical distress.

Notes

1. S. Richardson, *Clarissa, or The History of a Young Lady* (1747–8), A. Ross (ed.), (New York: Viking, 1985). The first quotation is from Letter No. 436, 1265; the second from Letter No. 458, 1318.
2. G.J. Barker-Benfield, *The Culture of Sensibility: Sex and Society in Eighteenth-Century Britain.* (Chicago: University of Chicago Press, 1992), 6. The popularisation of medical rhetoric in popular magazines is discussed previously in Chapter 1.
3. A. Douglass, *Uneasy Sensations: Smollett and the Body* (Chicago: The University of Chicago Press, 1995), 22.
4. H. Fielding, from *The Champion*, 17 May 1740, in *The Complete Works of Henry Fielding, Esq.*, 16 volumes, W.E. Henley (ed.), (New York: Croscup and Sterling, 1902), Vol. 15, 314–15.
5. The great variety of alternative medicine available to the eighteenth-century patient is discussed more fully in Chapter 1; see also D. Porter and R. Porter, *Patient's Progress: Doctors and Doctoring in Eighteenth-century England* (Stanford, CA: Stanford U. Press, 1989),111–14.
6. H. Fielding, *The Journal of a Voyage to Lisbon* (1752), T. Keymer (ed.), (New York: Penguin, 1996), 16.
7. *Ibid.*, 20.
8. *Ibid.*, 16.
9. Joshua ('Spot') Ward (1685–1761), the proprietor of one of the most popular eighteenth-century quack nostrums, Ward's Pill and Drop, had a place of honour in Hogarth's engraving 'The Company of Undertakers,' which depicts prominent quacks in the company of established physicians.
10. Fielding, *op. cit.* (note 6), 17.
11. T. Keymer, 'Introduction' to Fielding, *op. cit.* (note 6), ix–x.
12. Fielding, *op. cit.* (note 6), 23.
13. Shallett Turner to James Jurin, 29 May 1726, Cambridge; Wellcome MS. 6139. See Chapter 2.
14. Keymer, *op. cit.* (note 11), x.
15. H. Fielding, *The History of Tom Jones, A Foundling* (1749), F. Bowers and M.C. Battestin (eds), (Connecticut: Wesleyan University Press, 1975), 111. Subsequent page references in text in parentheses.
16. H. Fielding, *Amelia*, M. C. Battestin (ed.), (Connecticut: Wesleyan University Press, 1983), 104.
17. A more critical picture of medicine is presented in the first edition of *Amelia*

(Bk. V, ch. ii), intended by the author 'to serve to inform Posterity concerning the present State of Physic' (542), but this chapter was deleted by Fielding in later versions of the novel. In this deleted episode, Booth and Amelia are anxious for their sick infant daughter. An apothecary, Mr Arsenic, and a doctor recommended by him, attend the child in a most perfunctory manner, prescribing excessive medications, and only heightening Amelia's concerns with their grim prognosis for the child. Booth consults an unorthodox physician (modelled on Dr Thomas Thompson), greatly offending the first doctor who demands: 'shall I meet a Man who pretends to know more than the whole College, and who would overturn the Whole Method of Practice, which is so well established, and from which no one Person hath pretended to deviate?' (541). The scene of professional contention strongly resembles a scene in Tobias Smollett's *The Adventures of Ferdinand Count Fathom* which pictures a nasty encounter between Fathom (in the role of doctor) and the arrogant Dr Looby (see Chapter 1).

18. A.J. Van Sant, *Eighteenth-Century Sensibility and the Novel: The Senses in Social Context* (New York: Cambridge University Press, 1993), 60–82. Though the subject of Van Sant's analysis is *Clarissa*, the same point can be made for Richardson's *Pamela*, though the character of Pamela lacks the rich complexity of Clarissa, and she is not a heroine of sensibility.
19. Richardson, *op. cit.* (note 1), Letter No. 366, Mr Belford to Robert Lovelace (Thursday, 27 July), 1129.
20. *Ibid.*, Letter No. 362; Clarissa to Mrs Norton (Monday night, 24 July), 1120–2.
21. *Ibid.*, Letter No. 424; Belford to Lovelace (entries of Wednesday, 3 o'clock and 9 o'clock), 1239–41.
22. *Ibid.*, Letter No. 419; Belford to Lovelace (Tuesday, 22 August), 1226.
23. *Ibid.*, Letter No. 424, 3 o'clock entry, 1120–2.
24. *Ibid.*, Letter No. 464; Belford to Lovelace (Tuesday, 5 September), 1336.
25. *Ibid.*, Letter No. 474; Belford to Lovelace (8 in the evening entry of Wednesday letter (473), 1352.
26. On the importance of touch in the culture of sensibility, see Van Sant, *op. cit.* (note 18). See, in particular, Chapter 5, 'The Centrality of Touch', 83–97.
27. S. Richardson, *Pamela, or Virtue Rewards* (1740), (New York: W.W. Norton, 1958); all quotations are from Pamela's letters dated: 'Thursday, Friday, Saturday, Sunday, the 28th, 29th, 30th, and 31st days of my distress', 177–88.
28. H. Fielding, *The History of the Adventures of Joseph Andrews and his Friend, Mr Abraham Abrams* (London, 1742). See Book III, Chapter 1: 'I declare here, once for all, I describe not men, but manners; not an individual, but a species.'

29. Frances Burney, *Cecilia, or Memoirs of an Heiress* (1782), P. Sabor and M.A Doody (eds), (New York: Oxford, 1988), 481. Subsequent page references are in text.

30. The condition of Cecilia's inheritance is that whomever she marries must relinquish his own family name and take on hers – unimaginable for the proud Delville family.

31. T. Smollett, *Travels Through France and Italy* (1766), F. Felsenstein (ed.), (New York: Oxford University Press, 1979).

32. L. Sterne, *The Journal to Eliza* (New York: Oxford University Press, 1984); entry 'London 24–25 April 1767,' 141–2. Additional page references are given parenthetically in text.

33. Tobias Smollett, *The Expedition of Humphry Clinker*, T.R. Preston and O.M. Brack, Jr (eds), (Athens, GA: University of Georgia Press, 1990). The letter, in the novel, is dated 18 April, from Hot-well, Bristol, 18. Subsequent references, including letter dates, are included in text in parentheses.

34. Douglass, *op. cit.* (note 3), 162–84. Douglass includes in her study of Smollett a chapter entitled 'The Body in Eighteenth-Century Narrative', 1–26, which traces the rise of sensibility (in medicine and literature) as a strategy to reclaim the body, deconstructed by Locke and Descartes, as a social, moral, and religious construct. Her analysis reinforces two important claims made in this study of medicine-by-post: first, that medical speculation was fully integrated into popular culture; second, that although the concept of sensibility was developing from the earliest part of the century, it was not till the 1740s that philosophers 'could rely on the impeccable support offered by experimental science' as iatromechanism was clearly supplanted by vitalism. In this respect, the work of Dr Robert Whytt, professor of medicine at the University of Edinburgh, was critical to allow philosophers in the second half of the century to claim 'that society, like the body, was united by a subtle, invisible force' (Whytt's 'sentient principle'), and that there was an analogy between the 'sympathetic' unity of the body and that of society (16–17).

35. The first page of the letter is dated 22 March 1812, but the letter was not completed till June. *The Journals and Letters of Fanny Burney (Madame D'Arblay)*, J. Hemlow (ed.), (Oxford: Clarendon Press, 1975), Vol. 6 (France 1803–12), Letter No. 595, 613. Subsequent page references are included in text in parentheses.

Bibliography

Baker, Robert, Porter, Dorothy and Porter, Roy (eds), *The Codification of Medical Morality: Historical and Philosophical Studies of the Formalization of Western Medical Morality in the Eighteenth and Nineteenth Centuries, Volume 1, Medical Ethics and Etiquette in the Eighteenth Century* (Boston: Kluwer Academic Publishers, 1993).

Barfoot, Michael, 'Dr William Cullen and Mr Adam Smith: A Case of Hypochondriasis?', *Procedings of the Royal College of Edinburgh*, 21 (1991), 204–14.

Barker-Benfield, G.J., *The Culture of Sensibility: Sex and Society in Eighteenth-Century Britain.* (Chicago: University of Chicago Press, 1992).

Barry, Jonathan, 'Piety and the Patient: Medicine and Religion in Eighteenth-Century Bristol', in Porter, R. (ed.), *Patients and Practitioners: Lay Perceptions of Medicine in Pre-Industrial Society* (New York: Cambridge University Press, 1985), 145–76.

Bate, W. Jackson, *Samuel Johnson* (New York: Harcourt Brace Jovanovich, 1975).

Battestin, Martin C., with Battestin, Ruth R., *Henry Fielding: A Life* (New York: Routledge, 1989).

Bazerman, Charles, *Shaping Written Knowledge: The Genre and Activity of the Experimental Article in Science* (Wisconsin: University of Wisconsin Press, 1988).

Behn, Aphra, *Sir Patient Fancy* (1678), in Todd, J. (ed.) *The Works of Aphra Behn*, 7 vols (Columbus: Ohio State University Press, 1996).

Boswell, James, *Boswell's Life of Johnson*, 6 vols, Hill, G.B. (ed.), (New York: Bigelow, Brown & Co., 1921).

Bibliography

Boswell, James, *London Journal, 1762–1765,* Pottle, F.A. (ed.), (New York: McGraw-Hill, 1950).

Brockliss, L.W.B., *Calvet's Web: Enlightenment and the Republic of Letters in Eighteenth-Century France* (New York: Oxford University Press, 2002).

Brown, Theodore M., 'Medicine in the Shadow of the *Principia,*' in *Journal of the History of Ideas,* 48, no. 1 (1987), 629–48.

Burney, Frances, *Cecilia, or Memoirs of an Heiress* (1782), Sabor, P. and Doody, M.A. (eds), (New York: Oxford University Press, 1988).

_____, *The Journals and Letters of Fanny Burney (Madame D'Arblay),* Hemlow, J. (ed.), (Oxford: Clarendon Press, 1975).

Burton, Robert, *The Anatomy of Melancholy,* 2 vols, Kiessling, N.K., Faulkner, T.C., and Blair, R.L. (eds), (Oxford: Clarendon Press, 1990).

Bynum, W.F. and Porter, R. (eds), *William Hunter and the Eighteenth-Century Medical World* (New York: Cambridge University Press, 1985).

Bynum, W.F. and Porter, R. (eds), *Medical Fringe and Medical Orthodoxy, 1750–1850* (Wolfeboro, NH: Croom Helm, 1987).

Cheyne, George, *The Letters of Dr. George Cheyne to the Countess of Huntington,* Mullet, Charles E. (ed.), (San Marino, CA: Huntington Library, 1940).

_____, *The Letters of Doctor George Cheyne to Samuel Richardson (1733–1743),* Mullett, Charles E. (ed.), The University of Missouri Studies, Vol. XVIII, No.1 (Columbia, MI: University of Missouri, 1943).

_____, *The English Malady (1733),* Porter, R. (ed.), (New York: Routledge, 1991).

Child, Paul William, 'Discourse and Practice in Eighteenth-Century Medical Literature: The Case of George Cheyne' (PhD thesis, Notre Dame, 1992).

Cody, Lisa Forman, 'The Politics of Reproduction from Midwives' Alternative Public Sphere to the Public Spectacle of Man-Midwifery', in *Eighteenth-Century Studies,* 32, no.4 (Summer 1999), 477–95.

Cook, Harold J., *Trials of an Ordinary Doctor: Joannes Groenevelt in Seventeenth-Century London* (Baltimore: Johns Hopkins University Press, 1994).

_____, 'Bernard Mandeville and the Therapy of 'The Clever Politician', *Journal of the History of Ideas* 60, no. 1 (1999), 102–24.

_____, 'Boerhaave and the Flight from Reason in Medicine', *Bulletin of the History of Medicine* 74 , no. 3 (Fall 2000), 221–40.

Corfield, Penelope J., *Power and the Professions in Britain 1700–1850* (New York: Routledge, 1995).

Defoe, Daniel, *A Journal of the Plague Year* (1722), Shakespeare Head edition (Oxford: Blackwell, 1928, reprinted 1974).

Doig, A., Ferguson, J.P.S., Milne, I.A. and Passmore, R. (eds), *William Cullen and the Eighteenth Century Medical World: A Bicentenary Exhibition and Symposium Arranged by the Royal College of Physicians of Edinburgh in 1990* (Edinburgh: Edinburgh University Press, 1993).

Doody, Margaret Anne, *The Daring Muse: Augustan Poetry Reconsidered* (Cambridge: Cambridge University Press, 1985).

Douglass, Aileen, *Uneasy Sensations: Smollett and the Body* (Chicago: The University of Chicago Press, 1995).

Estes, J. Worth, *Dictionary of Protopharmacology: Therapeutic Practices, 1700–1850* (Canton, MA: Science History Publications, 1990).

Fielding, Henry, *The Charge to the Jury; or, the Sum of the Evidence on The Trial of A.B.C.D. and E.F. All MD For the Death of one Robert at Orfud, at a Special Commission of Oyer and Terminer held at Justice-Colledge, in W___ck-Lane, before Sir Asculapius Dosem, Dr Timberhead, and Others, their Fellows, Justices, etc.* (London: Printed for M. Cooper, at the Globe in Pater-noster-Row,1745). This text located at the Wellcome Library for the History and Understanding of Medicine: no. 4 in a collection, bound as *Medical Tracts*, Old Series, Vol. 1, no. 52.

Bibliography

Fielding, Henry, *Remarks on Dr Cheyne's Essay on Health and Long Life, wherein Some of the Doctor's Notorious Contradictions, and False Reasonings are Laid Open: Together With Several Observations on the same Subject: Rectifying many of the Errors and Mistakes of that Performance. By a Fellow of the Royal Society* (London: for Aaron Ward, Sold by T. Cox). Found in same collection at Wellcome as above.

_____, *The History of Tom Jones, A Foundling* (1749), Bowers, F., and M.C. Battestin (eds), (Connecticut: Wesleyan University Press, 1975).

_____, *Amelia* ((1751), Battestin, M.C. (ed.), (Connecticut: Wesleyan University Press, 1983).

_____, *The Journal of a Voyage to Lisbon* (1752), Keymer T., (ed.), (New York: Penguin, 1996).

Fissell, Mary E., *Patients, Power, and the Poor in Eighteenth-Century Bristol.* Cambridge History of Medicine Series, Webster, C. and Rosenberg, C. (eds), (New York: Cambridge University Press, 1991).

Flynn, Carol Houlihan. 'Running Out of Matter: The Body Exercised in Eighteenth-Century Fiction', in Rosseau, G.S. (ed.), *The Languages of Psyche*, (Berkeley: University of California Press, 1990), 147–85.

Foucault, Michel, 'The Politics of Health in the Eighteenth Century' (1976), in Gordon, C. (ed.), *Power/Knowledge: Selected Interviews and Other Writings 1972–1977* (New York: Pantheon, 1980), 166–82.

_____, *The Birth of the Clinic* (New York: Vintage Books, 1975).

Fox, Christopher, *Locke and the Scriblerians: Identity and Consciousness in Early Eighteenth-Century Britain* (Berkeley: University of California Press, 1988).

Frank Jr., Robert G., 'Thomas Willis and His Circle: Brain and Mind in Seventeenth-Century Medicine', in Rousseau, G.S. (ed.), *The Languages of Psyche: Mind and Body in Enlightenment Thought*, Clark Library Lectures 1985–1986, (Berkeley: University of California Press, 1990), 107–46.

Gregory, John, *Lectures on the Duties and Qualifications of a Physician* (London s.n., 1772).

Bibliography

Guerrini, Anita, 'Case History as Spiritual Autobiography: George Cheyne's "Case of the Author",' *Eighteenth-Century Life*, 19, No. 2 (1995),18–27.

_____, 'Isaac Newton, George Cheyne and the Principia Medicinae', in French, R. and Wear, A. (eds), *The Medical Revolution of the Seventeenth Century*. (Cambridge: Cambridge University Press, 1989), 222–45.

_____, 'James Keill, George Cheyne, and Newtonian Physiology, 1690–1740', *Journal of the History of Biology* 18, no. 2 (Summer 1985), 247–66.

_____, "A club of Little Villains': Rhetoric, Professional Identity and Medical Pamphlet Wars', in Roberts, M. Mulvey and Porter, R. (eds), *Literature and Medicine During the Eighteenth Century* (New York: Routledge, 1993), 226–44.

_____, 'The Hungry Soul: George Cheyne and the Construction of Femininity', *Eighteenth-Century Studies* 32, no. 3 (1999), 279–91.

_____, *Obesity and Depression in the Enlightenment: The Life and Times of George Cheyne* (Oklahoma: University of Oklahoma Press, Norman, 2000).

Haakonssen, Lisbeth, *Medicine and Morals in the Enlightenment: John Gregory, Thomas Percival, and Benjamin Rush* (Amsterdam: Rodopi, 1997).

Habermas, Jürgen, *The Structural Transformation of the Public Sphere: An Inquiry into a Category of Bourgeois Society*, Burger, T. (trans), (Cambridge, MA: MIT Press, 1989).

Hippocrates, *Hippocratic Writings*, Lloyd, G.E.R. (ed.), Chadwick, J., and Mann, W.N. (trans), (New York: Penguin Classics, 1978).

Holmes, Geoffrey, *Augustan England: Professions, State and Society, 1680–1730*. (Boston: George Allen & Unwin, 1982).

Ingram, Alan, *The Madhouse of Language: Writing and Reading Madness in the Eighteenth Century* (New York: Routledge, 1991).

_____, (ed.) *Patterns of Madness in the Eighteenth Century: A Reader* (Liverpool: Liverpool University Press, 1998).

Jewson, N. D., 'Medical Knowledge and the Patronage System in 18th Century England', *Sociology*, 1974 (8), 369–85.

Bibliography

Johnson, Samuel, 'On the Death of Dr Robert Levet', in Green, D. (ed.), *Samuel Johnson* (New York: Oxford University Press, 1984).

_____, *The Letters of Samuel Johnson*, 6 vols., Redford, B. (ed.), (Princeton: Princeton University Press, 1992).

Jurin, James, *The Correspondence of James Jurin, 1684–1750: Physician and Secretary to the Royal Society*, Rusnock, Andrea (ed.), (Clio Medica series, Amsterdam-Atlanta, GA: Rodopi, 1996).

_____, 'An Expostulatory Address to John Ranby Esq; Principal SerjeantSurgeon to His Majesty, and FRS, Occasioned by his Treatise of Gunshot-Wounds, and his Narrative of the Earl of Orford's Last Illness. By a Physician' (London: Printed for M. Cooper at the Globe in Pater-Noster-Row. 1745).

Klein, Lawrence E., 'Gender and the Public/Private Distinction in the Eighteenth Century: Some Questions about Evidence and Analytic Procedure', *Eighteenth-Century Studies* 29, no. 1 (1995), 97–109.

Langford, Paul, *A Polite and Commercial People: England 1727–1783* (New York: Oxford University Press, 1989).

Lawrence, Christopher, 'Ornate Physicians and Learned Artisans: Edinburgh Medical Men, 1726-, in Bynum, W.F. and Porter, R. (eds), *William Hunter and the Eighteenth-Century Medical World* (New York: Cambridge University Press, 1985), 153–75.

_____, 'The Nervous System and Society in the Scottish Enlightenment', in Barnes, B. and Shapin, S. (eds), *Natural Order: Historical Studies of Scientific Culture* (Beverly Hills: Sage Publications, 1979), 19–40.

Lewis, Judith Schneid, *In the Family Way: Childbearing in the British Aristocracy, 1760–1860* (New Jersey: Rutgers, 1986).

Loudon, Irvine, *Medical Care and the General Practioner 1750–1850* (Oxford: Clarendon Press, 1986).

Mandeville, Bernard, *A Treatise of the Hypochondriack and Hysterick Diseases* (1730), in Vol. 2 of *Collected Works of Bernard Mandeville* (Facsimile editions), (New York: Verlag, 1981).

McIntosh, Carey, *Common and Courtly Language: The Stylistics of Social Class in 18th-Century English Literature* (Philadelphia: University of Pennsylvania, 1986).

_____, *The Evolution of English Prose 1700–1800: Style, Politeness, and Print Culture* (New York: Cambridge Press, 1998).

McKeon, Michael, 'Historicizing Patriarchy: The Emergence of Gender Difference in England, 1660–1760', *Eighteenth-Century Studies* 28, no. 3 (1995), 295–322.

Mullan, John, *Sentiment and Sociability: The Language of Feeling in the Eighteenth Century* (Oxford: Clarendon Press, 1988).

Ober, William B., *Boswell's Clap and Other Essays: Medical Analysis of Literary Men's Afflictions* (Edwardsville: Southern Illinois University Press, 1979).

Percival, Thomas, *Medical Ethics: Or a Code of Institutes and Precepts, Adapted to the Professional Conduct of Physicians and Surgeons* (Manchester: Printed by S. Russel, for J. Johnston, St. Paul's Church Yard, and R. Bickerstaff, Strand, London, 1803).

Pilloud, Séverine, Hächler, S., and Barras, V., 'Consulter par Lettre au XVIIIe Siècle' [Medical Consultation by Letter in the 18th Century], *Gesnerus : Swiss Journal of the History of Medicine and Sciences*, 61 (2004), 232–53.

Pope, Alexander, *The Poems of Alexander Pope*, Butt, J. (ed.), (New Haven: Yale University Press, 1963).

_____, *The Correspondence of Alexander Pope*, Sherburn, G. (ed.), (Oxford: Clarendon Press 1956).

Porter, Dorothy, and Porter, Roy, *Patient's Progress: Doctors and Doctoring in Eighteenth-Century England* (Stanford, CA: Stanford U. Press, 1989).

Porter, Roy, 'Civilization and Disease: Medical Ideology in the Enlightenment', in Black, J., and Gregory, J. (eds), *Culture, Politics and Society: Britain 1660–1800* (New York: Manchester University Press, 1991), 154–83.

_____, *The Greatest Benefit to Mankind: A Medical History of Humanity* (New York: W.W. Norton & Co., 1997).

Bibliography

Porter, Roy, 'Consumption: Disease of the Consumer Society?', in Brewer, J., and Porter, R., *Consumption and the World of Goods* (New York: Routledge, 1993), 58–81.

_____, *Disease, Medicine and Society in England, 1550–1860* (London: The MacMillan Press, 1993, 2nd edn).

_____, (ed.), *The Medical History of Waters and Spas*. In *Medical History*, Supplement no. 10 (London: Wellcome Institute for the History of Medicine, 1990).

_____, '"Expressing Yourself Ill": The Language of Sickness in Georgian England', in Burke, P., and Porter, R. (eds), *Language, Self and Society* (Cambridge: Polity Press, 1991), 276–99.

_____, *Health for Sale: Quackery in England 1660–1850* (New York: Manchester University Press, 1989).

_____, 'Laymen, Doctors and Medical Knowledge in the Eighteenth Century: The Evidence of the *Gentleman's Magazine*', in Porter, R. (ed.), *Patients and Practitioners: Lay Perceptions of Medicine in Pre-Industrial Society* (New York: Cambridge University Press, 1985), 283–313.

_____, 'Plutus or Hygeia? Thomas Beddoes and the Crisis of Medical Ethics in Britain at the Turn of the Nineteenth Century', in Baker, R., Porter, D. and Porter, R. (eds), *The Codification of Medical Morality* (Boston: Kluwer Academic Publishers, 1993), 73–91.

_____, 'The Patient's View: Doing Medical History from Below', *Theory and Society*, 14, no. 2 (1985), 175–98.

_____, 'Thomas Gisborne: Physicians, Christians and Gentlemen', in Wear, A., Geyer-Kordesch, J., and French, R. (eds), *Doctors and Ethics: The Earlier Historical Setting of Professional Ethics* (Clio Medica series no. 24), (Amsterdam-Atlanta, GA: Rodopi, 1993), 252–73.

_____, 'Barely Touching: A Social Perspective on Mind and Body', in Rousseau, G.S. (ed.), *The Languages of Psyche: Mind and Body in Enlightenment Thought* (Clark Library Lectures 1985–1986), (Berkeley: University of California Press, 1990), 45–80.

Bibliography

_____, *The Creation of the Modern World: The Untold Story of the British Enlightenment* (New York: W.W. Norton & Co., 2000).

Quincy, John, MD, *Lexicon Physico-Medicum: Or, A New Medicinal Dictionary, explaining The Difficult Terms used in the Several Branches of the Profession, and in Such Parts of Natural Philosophy as are Introductory thereto: With an Account of the Things Signified by Such Terms. Collected from the Most Eminent Authors; and Particularly these who have Wrote upon Mechanical Principles. The Third Edition, with New Improvements from the Latest Chymical and Mechanical Authors* (London s.n., 1726).

Redford, Bruce, *The Converse of the Pen: Acts of Intimacy in the Eighteenth Century Familiar Letter* (Chicago: University of Chicago Press, 1986).

Richardson, Samuel, *Clarissa, or The History of a Young Lady* (1747–8), Ross, Angus (ed.), (New York: Viking, 1985).

_____, *Pamela, or Virtue Rewarded,* (1740), (New York: W.W. Norton & Co., Inc., 1958)

Rousseau, G.S., (ed.), *The Languages of Psyche: Mind and Body in Enlightenment Thought* (Berkeley: University of California Press, 1990).

_____, 'Science', in Rogers, P. (ed.), *The Context of English Literature: The Eighteenth Century* (London: Methuen, 1978), 153–207.

_____, 'Nerves, Spirits, and Fibres: Towards Defining the Origins of Sensibility', *The Blue Guitar*, 2 (December 1976), 125–53.

Shapin, Steven, 'Trusting George Cheyne: Scientific Expertise, Common Sense, and Moral Authority in Early Eighteenth-Century Dietetic Medicine', *Bulletin of the History of Medicine*, Vol. 77 (Summer 2003), 263–97.

Shorter, Edward, 'The History of the Doctor–Patient Relationship', in Bynum, W.F., and Porter, R. (eds), *Companion Encyclopedia of the History of Medicine*, 2 vols (New York: Routledge, 1993).

Shuttleton, David E., 'Methodism and Dr George Cheyne's "More Enlightening Principles"', in R. Porter (ed.), *Medicine in the Enlightenment* (Amsterdam-Atlanta: Rodopi, 1995), 316–35.

Bibliography

Shuttleton, David E., "'Pamela's Library': Samuel Richardson and Dr. Cheyne's "Universal Cure"", *Eighteenth-Century Life* 23, no. 1 (February 1999), 59–79.

Sill, Geoffrey, 'Neurology and the Novel: Alexander Monro *Primus* and *Secundus*, *Robinson Crusoe*, and the Problem of Sensibility', *Literature and Medicine*, 16, no. 2 (Fall 1997), 250–65.

Smith, Frederick N., 'Scientific Discourse: *Gulliver's Travels* and *The Philosophical Transactions*', in Smith, F.N. (ed.), *The Genres of Gulliver's Travels*. (Newark: University of Delaware Press, 1990), 139–62.

Smollett, Tobias, *The Expedition of Humphry Clinker*, Preston, T.R. and Brack, O.M. (eds), (Athens, Georgia: University of Georgia Press, 1990).

_____, *Travels Through France and Italy*, Felsenstein, F. (ed.), (New York: Oxford University Press, 1979).

_____, *The Adventures of Ferdinand Count Fathom*, Beasley, J.C. (ed.), (Athens, GA: University of Georgia Press, 1988).

_____, *The Letters of Tobias Smollett*, Knapp, L.M. (ed.), (Oxford: Clarendon Press, 1970).

Sprat, Thomas, *The History of the Royal Society of London* (1667), Cope, J.I. and Jones, H.W. (eds), (St. Louis, MI: Washington University Studies, 1958).

Staves, Susan, 'Narratives of the Secret Disease: Representations of Venereal Disease in Eighteenth-Century England' (Paper delivered at Princeton University, October, 1985).

_____, 'Married Life: Venereal Disease, and Therapeutic Optimism' (Paper delivered at the American Society for Eighteenth-Century Studies, Pittsburgh, Pennsylvania, April 1991).

Steinke, Hubert, 'Why, What and How? Editing Early Modern Scientific Letters in the 21st Century', *Gesnerus: Swiss Journal of the History of Medicine and Sciences*, 61 (2004), 282–95.

_____, and Stuber, Martin, 'Medical Correspondence in Early Modern Europe: An Introduction', *Gesnerus: Swiss Journal of the History of Medicine and Sciences*, 61 (2004), 139–60.

Sterne, Lawrence, *A Sentimental Journey* with *The Journal to Eliza* and *A Political Romance* (1768), Jack, I. (ed.), (New York: Oxford University Press, 1968).

Straus, Ralph. *The Unspeakable Curll* (London: Chapman and Hall, 1928).

Swift, Jonathan, *The Prose Works of Jonathan Swift*, Davis, H. (ed.), (Oxford: Basil Blackwell, 1939–68).

_____, *The Correspondence of Jonathan Swift*, Williams, H. (ed.), (Oxford: Clarendon, 1963).

Temkin, Owsei, 'The Scientific Approach to Disease: Specific Entity and Individual Sickness', in Crombie, A.C. (ed.), *Scientific Change* (New York: Basic Books Inc., 1961), 629–58.

Thomson, John, MD, *An Account of the Life, Lectures, and Writings of William Cullen, MD* (1832), 2 vols (Edinburgh s.n., 1859).

Trotter, Thomas, *An Essay, Medical, Philosophical, and Chemical on Drunkeness and its Effects on the Human Body*, Porter, R. (ed.), (New York: Routledge, 1988).

Van Sant, Ann Jessie, *Eighteenth-Century Sensibility and the Novel: The Senses in Social Context* (New York: Cambridge University Press, 1993).

Vickers, Brian, 'The Royal Society and English Prose Style: A Reassessment', in *Rhetoric and the Pursuit of Truth: Language: Language Change in the Seventeenth and Eighteenth Centuries* (Clark Library Seminars, 8 March 1980), (Los Angeles: University of California Press, 1985), 2–76.

Vila, Anne C., *Enlightenment and Pathology: Sensibility in the Literature and Medicine of Eighteenth-Century France* (London: The Johns Hopkins University Press, 1998).

Ward, Jean E., and Yell, Joan (eds and trans.), *The Medical Casebook of William Brownrigg, MD, FRS (1712–1800) of the Town of Whitehaven in Cumberland. Medical History*, Supplement no. 13 (London: Wellcome Institute for the History of Medicine, 1993).

Wear, Andrew, 'Medical Ethics in Early Modern England', in Wear, A., Geyer-Kordesch, J., French, R. (eds), *Doctors and Ethics: The Earlier Historical Setting of Professional Ethics* (Amsterdam-Atlanta, GA: Rodopi, 1993), 98–130.

Bibliography

Wiltshire, John, *Samuel Johnson in the Medical World: The Doctor and the Patient* (New York: Cambridge University Press, 1991).

Winn, James Anderson, *A Window in the Bosom: The Letters of Alexander Pope* (Hamden, CT: Archon Books, 1977).

Index

A

abdominal fluids 245
Aberdeen 119, 120
accoucheur 258–9
alcoholic cirrhosis 97, 109(n68), 244–5
Alexander, Henry 106(n29)
alterative medicines 30
alternative medicine options 19–20,
    230(n12)
analogy use 154–5
anaphora 154
anatomical dissections 135, 185
Anglican church 75, 146
    see also Christian medical ethics
antimony treatments 97, 109(n66)
apothecaries 37–8, 41–2, 87–8
appetite 248
apprenticeship 58(n85)
Arblay, M. 259
Armitstead, Dr 223–4
arrogance 40
art of medicine 40, 190
ascites 245, 254
autopsy 76

B

Barry, John 36–8
Bath 130, 132, 156, 200
bedside medical training 188, 235(n57)
bladder stones 75–7, 80, 95
Blagden, Dr Charles 192
bleedings 18, 28, 33, 97, 205–6
blisters 94, 108(n61), 204
blood letting *see* bleedings

body–society connection 262(n34)
    see also mind–body connection
Boerhaave, Dr Hermann 62, 82, 99,
    163(n23), 189
book trade 130–1
Boothby, Hill 29
Boswell, James 22–4, 30–1
bowels 29, 97, 203–4, 221
    see also gastrointestinal symptoms
breasts
    cancer 27
    lump 258
    pain 81–94, 203, 204
    see also mastectomy
Bristol society 37–8
Brown, Thomas 68–70
bubonic plague 34–5, 36
Burney, Frances
    Cecilia 251–3
    mastectomy 12, 216, 256–9
Burton, Dr John 152–3
Buxton spa 217, 222–3

C

Cambridge University 61–2, 82,
    102(n2), 140
Cary, Bishop Mordecai 62, 81–94
Cary, Mrs, breast pain 81–94
celebrity status 134–5, 141
chalybeate waters 85, 107(n47)
character of physicians
    good 9, 24, 140, 247
    judge of 21
    moral 11, 13, 41, 43, 47, 194

Index

charges 17
see also fees; remuneration
charity hospitals 214–15, 234(n45),
240(n129)
charlatans 21, 22, 124
chemistry lectures 181
Cheyne, Dr George 113–73
celebrity status 134–5, 141
Cranstoun correspondence 159–60
Cullen contrast 204–5
dietary regimen 8, 117, 121,
135–6, 141–2, 145–6, 185,
209
The English Malady 121, 125–6,
141, 149–50
Fielding criticism 244
Huntingdon correspondence 141,
142–4, 150–7, 164(n33)
invented rhetoric 147–61
public private endeavour 121–32
publications 125–6, 130–2, 134–5,
148–9
Richardson correspondence 138–9,
148, 153, 155–6, 158–9,
161(n1)
self-fashioning 147
sensibility 10, 12, 14
society patients 21, 114
training and career 118–21
Christian medical ethics 49–50, 135,
143, 144
Church of England 75, 146
cirrhosis of the liver 97, 109(n68),
244–5
class *see* middle-class patients; social
class; upper-class patients
classical medical training 49–50,
53(n26), 135, 144
clinical details 64, 68, 257
Clutterbuck, Miss Mary 205–6
code of conduct 9, 21, 47–8, 125
colds 252

common prose 148–50, 227
compassion 43–4, 194
compliments 150–1, 153
confidentiality 124–5, 127, 165(n44),
214–16, 258
see also privacy
consciousness 134
constitutional weaknesses 198–201,
209
consumerism 23, 178
consumption 20
contra-naturals 104(n19)
conversational tone 31–2
copying machine 182, 231(n20)
corpulence 226
correspondence
extended 81–94
preciseness 80–1, 82–3, 89
publication 123–7, 129–32
see also individual writers; rhetoric
Cowmeadow, Mr 221–2, 232(n32-3)
Cranstoun, Dr 124, 126, 132, 159–60
credibility 9
Croft, Richard 169(n88)
Cullen, Dr William 12, 14, 15,
180–242
Armitstead correspondence 223–4
career and practice 180–1
Cheyne contrast 204–5
Cowmeadow correspondence
221–2, 232(n32-3)
dogmatist 191, 235(n60)
Fontescue correspondence 201–3,
237(n89)
Fraser correspondence 203–4
Hamilton correspondence 200–1
Hutchinson correspondence 192–3
individual attention 187
letters collection 181–4,
231(n18-19)
nosology 187, 197, 230(n11),
238(n100)

276

physical exercise 211
professor of medicine 191–2
Ross correspondence 198–200
Sandilands correspondence 210–11
Stapleton correspondence 219–21
sympathy expression 186–7, 196
teaching 191–4
Webster correspondence 226–7
Wedderburn correspondence
    217–18, 222–3
women patients 237(n86)
Wood correspondence 73–4, 224
Culpepper, Nicholas 75
cures
    customised 184–7
    folk 26
    vernacular 26–7, 29, 38, 85–8
    see also nostrums; regimen;
        treatments
Curll, Edmund 131
customised cures 184–7

D

Dallas, Mr James 217
deafness 227·
deathbed 249, 250
decorum 40–1
Defoe, Daniel
    A Journal of the Plague Year (1722)
        34–6, 245
    character traits 247
delicate constitution 198–201, 209
deliriums 71, 72
democratisation 226
diagnosis 207–9
dialogue *see* rhetoric
Diedier, Antoine 99, 100, 110(n73)
diet
    Lisbon Diet Drink 26
    milk 201–3
    milk and vegetables 123, 126–8,
        136, 139, 141, 155

regimen 8, 117, 121, 135–6,
    141–2, 145–6, 158, 185, 209
diplopia 68–70
discretion
    diagnosis 207–9
    medical condition 32
    see also confidentiality; privacy
distemper 28
diversion 159
doctors
    as friends 43
    ideal 38–41
    moral character 11, 13, 41, 43, 47
    see also physicians
doctor–patient relationship 7–13, 42–5,
    227–8
double vision 68–70
Douglas, Dr Andrew 22–3
drama
    effects 139, 154
    rhetoric 139, 154, 160–1, 179,
        197, 254–5, 256–9
    self-expression 199, 216–24
duality 197
Dubois, M. 258–9
Dyer, William 37–8
dyspepsia 192, 220–2

E

eclecticism
    Dr Cheyne 131–2
    medical marketplace 20, 34–8
    patients 26–34, 86
Edinburgh University
    Dr Cullen 180–1
    medical education 103(n5),
        188–94, 235(n57)
educated patients 9, 80–2, 93
    see also social class
education *see* medical education
electrical therapy 30, 37, 38
elegant style 150, 153–4

Elliot, Reverend 221
emmenagogues 87, 108(n54)
emotions
    frenzied behaviour 252–3
    prose style 256–9
    see also drama
empathy 127–8, 155
empirical nostrums 26–7, 29, 86
energy in rhetoric 157, 158–9
'English malady' 14, 117, 121, 135,
    137, 138, 139
    see also Cheyne, Dr George;
    hypochondria
English universities 188
Enlightenment 61
environment 96, 104(n19), 180, 182,
    191–2, 255–6
    see also non-naturals
epistolary accounts 73, 95–101, 132
    see also prose style; rhetoric
established physicians 53(n26), 140,
    141
ethics *see* medical ethics; practical ethics
evacuations 97, 98
exercise 132–47, 185, 211
    see also horse riding
expansiveness 157
expense 23
experience of illness 7, 8, 14, 114, 259

F
familiar style 151, 226
Farquhar, Sir Walter 105(n29)
fashion influence 48, 59(n103)
fecundity of expression 157
feelings *see* drama; emotions; sensibility
fees
    medical school 189
    physicians 74, 162(n13), 183–4
    see also remuneration
female bodies 11–12, 15
    see also women patients

Ferrers, Lady Mary 98–101,
    111(n74-6)
Ferrers, second Earl 98–100
Fielding, Henry
    Amelia 244, 247, 260(n17)
    criticism of Dr Cheyne 244
    iatromechanical medicine 243,
    244–5
    own illness 244–6
    praise of doctors 21–2
    satirical pamphlet 76
    The Journal of a Voyage to Lisbon
    244–8
    Tom Jones 246–8
Fizes, Dr 20, 219, 253
flattery 151, 156
Flynn, Carol Houlihan 157–8
folk cures 26
Fontescue, Mrs Frances 201–3,
    237(n89)
fractured arm 246
Fraser, Miss 203–4
friends 21–6, 43

G
Galen 67, 104(n19)
gastrointestinal symptoms 120,
    164(n29), 198–9
    see also stomach complaints
genteel prose 148–51, 152
gentlemen
    code of conduct 9, 47–8, 125
    physicians 193–4
Gillespie, Dr 30
Gisborne, Thomas 49, 50
Glasgow University 181
gonorrhoea 23, 26
good character 9, 24, 140, 247
gossip 123, 124
grammar *see* prose style
gratitude 42
Greek quotations 82

Gregory, Dr James 188, 213, 230(n14)
Gregory, Professor John 43–4, 48–9,
 185–6, 191, 193–4, 214
Guerrini, Anita 78–9, 145

H

Haakonssen, Lisbeth 21, 44, 47, 49
haemorrhoids 122–3, 164(n33)
Hamilton, Mrs 200–1
Handley, James 64–6
Harrogate 223
harsh treatments 91–3, 144
head injury 246
hepatic encephalopathy 109(n68)
home remedies 26–7, 29, 38, 85–8
horse riding 139, 204, 211
Horsley, John, minister 68–9
hospitals 214–15, 240(n129)
humanity 43–5
 see also sensibility
Hume, David 181, 212
humility 24–5, 34
Hunter, John 223–4
Hunter, William 219
Huntingdon, Countess of 12
 Burton correspondence 152–3
 Cheyne correspondence 122–3,
  132, 150–7
 medical condition 142–4
 milk and vegetable diet 126–7,
  128, 141, 155, 156
Hutchinson, Dr Francis 192–3
Hutton, Catherine 105(n29)
Huxham, John, physician 95–8
hydraulic medicine *see* iatromechanism
hyperbole use 77
hypochondria 117, 120–1, 137,
  163(n29), 209–13
 see also 'English malady'
hysteria 12, 191–2, 195, 196, 205, 209

I

iatromechanism
 Dr Cheyne 119, 135–7
 Henry Fielding 243, 244–5
 hydraulic concept 19, 34, 61–2, 67
 see also Newtonian principles
ideal doctor 38–41, 253
identity 133–4
illness
 clinical details 64, 68, 257
 experience of 7, 8, 14, 114, 259
 expression in novels 259–60
 mental 209–13, 251–2
 metaphor 7
 public nature 123–4, 257–8
 social significance 247, 251, 255–6
 terminal 248–50
 see also 'English malady'
impatience 220
imposter 38–41
improvement 181, 188, 191
individuals *see* patients
infirmary patients 234(n45), 240(n129)
Ingham, Dr William 205–6
integrity 41, 48, 49
intellect
 diversion 159
 effort 137
irresponsibility 136
irritability 191–2

J

Jeckyll, Sir Joseph 130
Johnson, Jacob 70–3
Johnson, Samuel
 phlebotomy 18, 55(n46)
 physician's character 24–6
 prose style 171(n128)
 rhetoric 21, 26–34
judgement 205

Jurin, Dr James 14, 61–111
  education and career 61–4
  letter to Paul Dudley 61, 80
  letter to James Handley 64–6
  letter to John Horsley 70
  letter to John Huxham 98
  pamphlet debate with John Ranby
    75–8

K
Klein, Lawrence 123

L
Lainberg, Richard 205
language 128, 148–9
  see also Latin text; prose style
Larrey, M., surgeon 258
Latin text 20, 33, 52(n11), 74–5
laudanum 222–3
Lawrence, Dr Thomas 18, 22, 24–5,
  29, 32–3
leg ulcers 32
leprosy 71–2, 74
Levet, Dr Robert 24–5, 26, 30, 31, 34,
  41, 54(n30)
Leyden University 62, 82, 102(n5), 189
lifestyle 146–7
  see also 'English malady'; regimen
Lisbon Diet Drink 26
literary applications 243–62
  see also under authors
literary style *see* prose style
lixivium lithontripticum 64, 76, 95, 96
Locke, John 133–4, 185
lovage root 30
lues *see* syphilis

M
magazines 243
male patients 12, 145, 197
Malvern waters 27

man-midwives 124, 165(n41),
  169(n88)
manners 44, 48, 59(n100)
masculinity 49, 176
mastectomy 12, 256–9
material luxuries 162(n15)
mathematics *see* Newtonian principles
Meadowbrook, Lord 213
medical education
  Edinburgh University 188–94,
    235(n57)
  theory and practice 190–1,
    235(n57)
  ward teaching 188, 234(n45),
    235(n57)
medical ethics 9–10, 21, 44–5, 132–47,
  214
  Christian 49–50, 135, 143, 144
  development 47–50
  see also practical ethics
medical regimen 132–47
medical rhetoric
  Dr Cheyne 131–2, 147–61
  language 148–9
  patients 80–94
  Samuel Johnson 26–34
medical students 215
medicine
  alterative 30
  alternative options 19–20,
    230(n12)
  art of 40, 190
  orthodox 38, 53(n26)
  social class 116
  status 79–80
  see also cures; nostrums;
    prescriptions; treatments
medico–religious language 128
melancholia 195, 196, 197, 211, 213
men *see* male patients
menses 83, 85, 92

mental illness 209–13, 251–2
   see also hypochondria; hysteria;
      melancholia
Mercer, Mrs 224
mercury treatments 27, 87, 91, 100,
   208, 254
metaphor use 7, 77, 154
middle-class patients
   Dr Cullen 182
   lifestyle 146–7
   medical histories 124
   prose style 148–9
   Puritanism 35–6
   rhetoric 225–6
   social mobility 116
midwives, male 124, 165(n41),
   169(n88)
milk diet 201–3
milk and vegetable diet 123, 126–7,
   128, 136, 139, 141, 155, 156
millipedes 85, 108(n49)
mind–body connection 45–6, 212,
   248–9, 251
model patient 42
modest rhetoric 225–8
Monro, Alexander, father and son
   190–1
mood 46
Moore, Dr John 45, 218
Moore, William 127–8, 132
moral issues
   character 11, 13, 41, 43, 47, 48,
      194
   example 250–1
   integrity 30–1, 48
   responsibility 25–6, 134
   strength 138
   see also sensibility

N

narratives *see* rhetoric
natural philosophy 79

naturals 104(n19)
negotiation 9
nervous system
   disorders 12, 14, 134
   final sensations 250

   functions 10, 116, 133, 137,
      228(n2)
   see also sensibility
new science
   empirical method 64, 66, 67–8
   rhetoric 10, 61–111
Newtonian principles 61–2, 64, 67,
   119, 163(n28), 189–90
   see also iatromechanism
non-naturals 67, 96, 104(n19), 136,
   142
nosology 187, 197, 230(n11),
   238(n100)
nostrums 26–7, 29, 34, 57(n73), 86
   see also cures; treatments
novels 243

O

obesity 113, 120
objectivity 32, 61, 97
ontology 191, 235(n58)
open air 211
optic nerve 68–70
orthodox medicine 38, 53(n26)
overindulgence 117
   see also 'English malady'
overseas advice 18, 51(n6)
Oxford graduates 61–2, 102(n2), 140

P

pain 249, 257
pain-killing drugs 222–3
pamphlet debates 75–80
parallelism 156–7
parasites 91–2
passions 136, 212

paternal attention 44
pathological processes 190–1
patients
    clinical details 64, 68, 257
    confidentiality 124–5, 127,
        165(n44), 214–16, 258
    epistolary accounts 95–101, 205
    expectations 10, 20
    individual therapy 206–7
    judgement 205
    medical rhetoric 80–94
    privacy 213–16
    responsibilities 42, 45, 47, 142
    self-determination 35–6, 42, 46,
        205
patriarchal society 98–100
patronage 19, 62, 114
Percival, Thomas 44, 214–15, 226
personal identity 133–4
personalised cures 184–7
pessimism 246
pharmacopoeia 181, 192
*Philosophical Transactions of the Royal
    Society* 66, 69, 104(n22)
philosophy
    France 233(n41)
    natural 79
    Scottish Enlightenment 189–90,
        192
phlebotomy 28, 55(n46)
    see also bleedings
physical appearance 113, 118
physical examinations 51(n3)
physicians
    established reputation 53(n26),
        140, 141
    public servant role 193
    see also character of physicians;
    doctors
Physick 87, 92–3, 108(n48)
physics *see* Newtonian principles
physiology 10

Pitcairne, Archibald 119–20
Pitodry, Mrs Likely 184, 227
polypharmacy 221
poorer patients 215, 231(n21)
    see also social class
Pope, Alexander 131
Porter, Roy 135, 167(n71-2)
postal service 182–3
practical ethics 25–6, 42, 47–50
    see also medical ethics
prescriptions 8, 86–7, 93
    see also nostrums
pride 23–4, 38
Pringle, Sir John 192
privacy 214–16
    see also confidentiality; discretion
private nostrums 34, 57(n73)
private patients 213–16
professional conduct 140
professional knowledge 10, 78–9, 179
prolixity 157
prose style 148–61, 171(n128)
    common 148–50, 227
    elegant 150, 153–4
    emotional 256–9
    familiar 151, 226
    figures of speech 74–5
    genteel 148–51, 152
    middle-class patients 148–9
    relaxed 82, 89
    upper-class patients 148–50
    see also rhetoric
protocol of correspondence 182–3
Providence 142, 144
pseudo-medico 38–41
psychological conditions *see* mental
    illness
public conversation 32
public health 176, 214–15
public illness 123–4
public servant role 193

publication
    correspondence 123–4, 126–7,
        129–32
    illness 257–8
    medical histories 124
purification 155
Puritanism 35–6, 48

Q

quacks 34, 35, 76, 107(n36), 141, 142
quarantine 36

R

Ranby, John
    pamphlet debate 75–8
    surgeon 21–2, 245, 247
regimen (diet, exercise and spirituality)
    132–47
relaxed prose 82, 89
religion
    analogy 154–5
    Christian ethics 49–50, 135, 143,
        144
    imagery 142
    inclinations 151
    language 128
    see also medical ethics
remedies *see* cures; nostrums
remuneration 74, 105(n29)
    see also fees
reputation
    man-midwife 169(n88)
    physicians 53(n26), 140, 141
responsibilities
    moral 25–6, 134
    personal 42, 45, 47, 134
    see also irresponsibility
rhetoric
    doctor–patient 7–11, 13, 42–3,
        182–3
    Dr Cheyne 131–2, 147–61
    faults 76–9

hyperbole 216–24
late-eighteenth century 225–8
new science 10, 61–111
patients 80–94, 197, 225–6
Samuel Johnson 26–34
Scottish Enlightenment 175–242
verbal energy 157, 158–9
see also correspondence; drama;
    prose style
rheumatism 30
Richardson, Samuel 12, 21
    character development 247
    Cheyne correspondence 138–9,
        141–2, 153, 155–6, 158–9,
        161(n1)
    Cheyne friendship 115–16
    Clarissa 21, 41–3, 45, 46, 143,
        161, 195, 247–51
    Fielding comparison 244
    medical condition 122, 136, 137
    Pamela 250–1
robust constitution 206
roles 47
Ross, Mrs Major 198–200
Royal College of Physicians of
    Edinburgh 181, 231(n18)
Royal College of Physicians of London
    24, 61, 75, 101(n2)
Royal Society 61, 62, 66, 74–5

S

Sandilands, Alexander 210, 212–13
Sandilands, James 210–11
satire 19, 21–6, 76
science *see* new science ; Newtonian
    principles
scorbutical 121, 164(n30)
Scotland
    Act of Union 1707 189
    medical influence 50, 180, 182,
        188, 230(n15)
    vitalism 176

Scottish Enlightenment 175–242
    customised cures 184–7
    hypochondria 209–13
    medical education 187–94
    medical philosophy 189–90, 192
    professional authority 179, 185
    sensibility 176–8, 184–7, 194–209
    sociability 178
    social and cultural revival 229(n7)
    sympathy 194–209
    women patients 194–209
scurvy 219
sea bathing 223
second opinions 18, 19
secrecy 214–15
self-advertisement 122, 126
self-determination 35–6, 42, 45, 205
self-expression 10, 14
self-fashioning 147
self-help 143
Selkirk, Earl of 183
sensibility
    concept 133
    customised cures 184–7
    Dr Cheyne 127–9
    Dr Cullen 191–2
    dualism 197
    expansion of cult 14, 175–8
    French philosophy 233(n41)
    interpretation 185–7
    male manifestation 176, 194–5
    model physician 43, 48
    nervous system 50, 114–16, 138,
        145, 244
    paradigm shift 10–11, 19
    passions 212
    women patients 194–209
    see also humanity; sympathy
serenity 250
Seymour, Dr 96–8, 109(n68)
Shafto, Henry 70–3, 81, 85
simile use 154

skin condition 71–2, 92–3
Sloane, Dr Hans 98–101, 110(n70)
smallpox inoculation 64
Smith, Adam 181, 211–12
Smollett, Tobias
    *The Adventures of Ferdinand Count
        Fathom* (1753) 38–41, 49
    The Expedition of Humphrey Clinker
        18, 23, 46, 216–18, 254–5
    illness and society 255–6
    medical career 58(n85), 241(n135)
    medical condition 12–13, 218–19
    Moore correspondence 45–6
    Travels through France and Italy 20,
        219, 255
sociability 178
social class
    diagnosis 207
    effect of medicine 116
    lifestyle 146–7
    mobility 116
    self-determination 35–8
social conversation 101
social ideology 178
social participation 209–13, 251
society
    body–society connection 262(n34)
    Bristol 37–8
    illness 247, 251, 255–6
solids 136, 168(n74)
solitude 210
spa waters 37, 85, 94, 107(n47), 156,
        217–18
    see also Bath spa; Buxton spa
spasms 206, 220–1, 238(n100)
spastic bowel 221
spirit 249–50
spirituality 132–47
spleen 121, 185
Sprat, Thomas, *The History of the Royal-
        Society of London...* 66–7
Stapleton, Thomas 219–21

Sterne, Lawrence
  A Sentimental Journey 256
  illness and society 255–6
  The Journal to Eliza 253–5
stomach complaints 198–9, 200,
    217–18, 220–2
  see also gastrointestinal symptoms
subjectivity 14, 61, 95, 96, 160, 179
superficial appearance 38–41
surgery
  mastectomy 256–9
  training 190–1
Swift, Jonathan 103(n17)
sympathy
  Cecilia 252–3
  feeling 175–6, 193–4
  model quality 50, 193–4
  women patients 194–209
  see also sensibility
syphilis 207–8, 253–5

T

Taylor, Reverend John 28
terminal illness 248–50
therapy 18, 206–7
Thompson, William 202
Thrale, Hester 27, 28, 32
touching of hands 250
treatments
  antimony 97, 109(n66)
  harsh 91–3, 144
  mercury 27, 87, 91, 100, 208, 254
  see also cures; nostrums
trust 122–3
  see also confidentiality; privacy
Turner, Shallett 94

U

ulcers 32
underqualified physician 26

upper-class patients
  Dr Cullen 182
  mobility 116
  prose style 148–50
  rhetoric 225–6
urgency 157, 160, 199
urine specimens 17, 83, 84, 160
utilitarian attitude 179–80

V

Van Sant, Jessie Ann 11, 195, 229(n11)
vegetables *see* milk and vegetable diet
venereal disease 98–101, 186–7, 207–9,
    216, 253–5
venesection 206
Venice treacle 36, 57(n76)
verbal energy 157, 158–9
vernacular cures 38, 85–8
vinegar of squills 30, 31, 56(n60)
virtuosi 189, 190, 234(n50)
visual examinations 17
vitalism 176
vomiting 65, 158, 172(n163)

W

Walpole, Sir Robert 75–7, 95
ward teaching 188, 234(n45), 235(n57)
wasting 94
Watt, James 182
weak constitution 198–201, 209
Webster, Jane 184, 226–7
Wedderburn, Mr Charles 217–18,
    222–3
Wesley, John 30, 37
Whytt, Professor Robert 175, 228(n2)
Willis, Thomas 133, 185
women patients
  hysteria 145–6
  non-compliance 142
  rhetoric 225

women patients (*cont...*)
    sensibility and sympathy 11–12,
        194–209, 237(n86)
    see also female bodies
Wood, Dr James 73, 224
worms 91–2
Worsley, Thomas 95
writing style *see* prose style

Printed in the United States
By Bookmasters

Printed in the United States
By Bookmasters